Introducing Psychology for Nurses and Healthcare Professionals

Introducing Psychology for Nurses and Healthcare Professionals

Dominic Upton

Professor of Psychology, Institute of Health and Society
University of Worcester

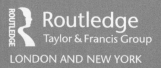

Routledge
Taylor & Francis Group

LONDON AND NEW YORK

First published 2010 by Pearson Education Limited
Second edition 2012

Published 2013 by Routledge
2 Park Square, Milton Park, Abingdon, Oxon OX14 4RN
711 Third Avenue, New York, NY 10017, USA

Routledge is an imprint of the Taylor & Francis Group, an informa business

Notices
Knowledge and best practice in this field are constantly changing. As new research and experience broaden our understanding, changes in research methods, professional practices, or medical treatment may become necessary.

Practitioners and researchers must always rely on their own experience and knowledge in evaluating and using any information, methods, compounds, or experiments described herein. In using such information or methods they should be mindful of their own safety and the safety of others, including parties for whom they have a professional responsibility.

To the fullest extent of the law, neither the Publisher nor the authors, contributors, or editors, assume any liability for any injury and/or damage to persons or property as a matter of products liability, negligence or otherwise, or from any use or operation of any methods, products, instructions, or ideas contained in the material herein.

ISBN 978-0-273-77007-7 (pbk)

British Library Cataloguing-in-Publication Data
A catalogue record for this book is available from the British Library

Library of Congress Cataloging-in-Publication Data
Upton, Dominic.
  Introducing psychology for nurses and healthcare professionals / Dominic Upton. – 2nd ed.
    p. cm.
  Includes bibliographical references and index.
  ISBN 978-0-273-77007-7
  1. Nursing – Psychological aspects.   2. Nurse and patient.   I. Title.
  RT86.U68 2012
  610.73–dc23

                                                                    2012002670

Typeset in 9.5/13 pt Interstate-Light by 73

Contents

Preface   xi
Acknowledgements   xvii

Chapter 1   Introduction: psychology in nursing care   1

	Learning Outcomes	1
	Your starting point	2
1.1	Introduction	3
1.2	A brief history of psychology	6
1.3	The language of psychology	10
1.4	What is a science?	10
1.5	Key qualities of a science	11
1.6	Researching psychology	12
1.7	Health and health psychology in a social world	17
1.8	The scope of psychology	21
1.9	Psychology in health and nursing care	22
1.10	Conclusion	24
1.11	Summary	24
	Your end point	24
	Further reading	25
	Weblinks	26

Chapter 2   Psychological approaches to understanding people   27

	Learning Outcomes	27
	Your starting point	28
2.1	How psychology helps us to understand why people do what they do	30
2.2	The psychodynamic approach	31
2.3	Psychoanalytic theory	32
2.4	Evaluation of the psychodynamic approach	38
2.5	Behaviourism	40
2.6	Classical conditioning	40
2.7	Operant conditioning	44
2.8	Reinforcement and the token economy system	45
2.9	Evaluation of the behaviourist approach	47
2.10	Social learning theory	48
2.11	Rotter's theory	48
2.12	Health locus of control	50

2.13	Bandura's theory	51
2.14	Self-efficacy	54
2.15	Evaluation of social learning theory	55
2.16	Cognitive psychology	56
2.17	Cognitive behavioural therapy	58
2.18	Humanistic psychology	61
2.19	Rogers' person-centred approach	63
2.20	Evaluation of the humanistic approach	65
2.21	Conclusion	66
2.22	Summary	68
	Your end point	69
	Further reading	70
	Weblinks	71

Chapter 3   Psychology across the lifespan   72

	Learning Outcomes	72
	Your starting point	73
3.1	Introduction	75
3.2	Piaget's theory of cognitive development	76
3.3	Attachment	82
3.4	Ecological systems theory	84
3.5	Vygotsky's socio-cultural theory of development	86
3.6	Erikson's theory of personality development	88
3.7	Adolescence – storm and stress	90
3.8	Putting theories into action	91
3.9	Working with older adults	92
3.10	Cognitive changes in adulthood	95
3.11	Social changes in late adulthood	96
3.12	Dementia	98
3.13	Death and dying	101
3.14	Children's understanding of loss	101
3.15	Models of grief	104
3.16	Conclusion	108
3.17	Summary	108
	Your end point	109
	Further reading	110
	Weblinks	111

Chapter 4   Social processes   112

	Learning Outcomes	112
	Your starting point	113
4.1	Introduction	115
4.2	Non-verbal communication (NVC)	115
4.3	Attitudes	122
4.4	Stereotyping	125
4.5	Persuasion, conformity and compliance	127

4.6	Power and status and its influence on obedience	137
4.7	Conclusion	140
4.8	Summary	141
	Your end point	141
	Further reading	142
	Weblinks	143

Chapter 5   Perception, memory and providing information   144

	Learning Outcomes	144
	Your starting point	145
5.1	Introduction	147
5.2	Perception	148
5.3	Memory	153
5.4	Attention	156
5.5	Information presentation	160
5.6	The role of cues	162
5.7	The role of perceived importance	163
5.8	Mnemonic aids	164
5.9	Compliance, adherence and concordance to treatment	164
5.10	Causes of non-adherence	167
5.11	Cognitive models of health behaviour	169
5.12	Social cognition models	173
5.13	Strategies for changing risk behaviour	175
5.14	Conclusion	181
5.15	Summary	181
	Your end point	182
	Further reading	183
	Weblinks	183

Chapter 6   Stress and stress management   185

	Learning Outcomes	185
	Your starting point	186
6.1	Introduction	188
6.2	What is stress?	189
6.3	Models of stress	190
6.4	Coping with stress – how to do it	195
6.5	The link between stress and health	198
6.6	How does stress affect health?	201
6.7	We need friends – social support	206
6.8	How to deal with stress	210
6.9	Does it work?	213
6.10	Stress and nursing practice	213
6.11	Conclusion	214
6.12	Summary	216
	Your end point	216
	Further reading	217
	Weblinks	218

Chapter 7   The psychology of pain   219

	Learning Outcomes	219
	Your starting point	220
7.1	Introduction	222
7.2	What is pain?	223
7.3	Concepts of pain	226
7.4	The gate control theory of pain	228
7.5	Psychological factors influencing pain	230
7.6	The assessment of pain	231
7.7	The management of pain	239
7.8	Behavioural approaches to pain and pain management	245
7.9	Cognitive approaches	246
7.10	Conclusion	249
7.11	Summary	250
	Your end point	251
	Further reading	252
	Weblinks	252

Chapter 8   Psychology of mental health   254

	Learning Outcomes	254
	Your starting point	255
8.1	Introduction	257
8.2	What is mental health?	257
8.3	Classification of mental health	258
8.4	Evaluation of the classification system	260
8.5	Schizophrenia	261
8.6	Anxiety disorders	265
8.7	Mood disorders	272
8.8	Personality disorders	275
8.9	Eating disorders	278
8.10	Substance misuse	282
8.11	The Mental Health Act	287
8.12	Conclusion	288
8.13	Summary	290
	Your end point	291
	Further reading	292
	Weblinks	292

Chapter 9   Developmental disorders: learning disability   294

	Learning Outcomes	294
	Your starting point	295
9.1	Introduction	296
9.2	Learning disabilities	297
9.3	Dyslexia	299
9.4	Attention-Deficit/Hyperactivity Disorder (ADHD)	302

9.5	Autism spectrum disorders	306
9.6	Communication	312
9.7	Quality of life	314
9.8	Emotional well-being	317
9.9	Psychological approaches	317
9.10	Conclusion	322
9.11	Summary	322
	Your end point	323
	Further reading	324
	Weblinks	324
	Glossary	326
	References	340
	Index	395

Preface

The role of psychology in nursing education and practice has become ever more significant in recent years and some would argue that it is *the* most important topic you will cover during your nursing or healthcare practitioner studies. Although psychology has always had a role in the nursing curriculum, in recent years this has come ever more to the fore. Even though psychology is a mandatory component of your programme, I hope that this text and the suggested additional reading will give you both an insight into, and a thirst for, psychology. More importantly, however, I hope that you will be able to use the material and the knowledge developed from this text within your practice for your clients' and patients' benefit.

The increase in interest and acknowledgement of the value of psychology has led to an increase in the number of texts, research and policy publications linking nursing, healthcare and psychology. This substantial body of literature has formed the backdrop of this book. Some of these publications are based on the classic texts of yesteryear, while others are more recent; there are also sources that have not even been published yet. When presenting this material, however, this text has taken an academically robust approach but attempted to do this in an appealing and readable manner. Hence, for example, even though the studies and reports have been read and reported here, the reference list has been kept to a minimum, although I hope the academic rigour that went into the preparation of this text comes through. There is a list of further reading for each of the topics and this will guide you into the deeper recesses of psychology (and I am sure you will want to go there . . .). In short, this is a textbook that is academic in tone and presentation and also useful and relevant for student nurses from all backgrounds with a range of professional aspirations. In this way this text is inclusive in nature and demonstrates the importance of psychology in both the nursing role and in healthcare in general. I am passionate about psychology and, importantly, communicating its relevance and effectiveness in nursing practice. I hope that this comes through.

The aim of the text was, therefore, to be inclusive, to demonstrate the value of psychology in nursing and healthcare from a British perspective. Although there are a number of American texts dealing with psychology there are few that have a British focus. There are, of course, other texts exploring health psychology or psychology in general but these do not explicitly link psychological aspects of health to the nursing role. Therefore, we have tried in this book to cover psychological aspects and concepts that have a direct role in health and nursing care. However, this text does not claim to be comprehensive – it does not cover every single aspect of psychology, for this would be impossible; it does not even cover every single aspect of psychology related to healthcare, as this too would be impossible. What has been achieved is a text that highlights the key areas in psychology related to nursing care. Every chapter has been honed to ensure that every single element is related to either your studies or your practice.

The choice, of course, is a subjective one and the decisions of what to include and what to exclude will (no doubt) be contentious – there are so many competing perspectives in psychology and its scope is so extensive (see Chapter 2 for further details). More could have been included on social groups and the nature of group-think and social loafing (which would have helped you when working in a team) or coping with chronic illness could have been further explored or why people go to their healthcare practitioner, or the role of nurses in promoting and extending health behaviours, and many more topics besides. However, something had to give – and these (amongst other things) were them.

This book has been produced with a number of aims in mind. First, for the student nurse to become familiar with how the role of psychology and health psychology can be applied to nursing and healthcare practice. Second, for the student nurse to be able to apply theories and ideas to both their own placement practice and student nurse portfolios. Third, to do this in a simplistic but robust manner with an interactive and supportive style. Finally, to ensure that there is a commitment to the role of psychology in nursing care.

Psychology has many perspectives which enable the student nurse to appreciate the individuality and diversity of patients. This is important in the construction and delivery of individualised care plans as stated throughout nursing courses and, of course, the Nursing and Midwifery Code of Conduct. Material presented in this text includes specific material dedicated to explaining how this can be successfully achieved in practice.

Creating a patient-led NHS – delivering the NHS Improvement Plan (DoH, 2005a) is a government health paper which highlights the importance of patient-centredness including patient choice and needs that should be addressed within any interaction with a patient. Hopefully, this book builds on the vision of such government statements and encourages the reader to appreciate the input psychology can have with such emerging visions of the future. There are, of course, many other policy developments that highlight the importance of a patient-centred NHS, ill-health prevention and promoting health and well-being (e.g. *Our Health, Our Care, Our Say: A New Direction for Community Services* (DoH, 2006); *Independence, Well-being and Choice: Our Vision for the Future of Social Care for Adults in England* (DoH, 2005b)) in which psychology has a key role to play.

Structure of this book

This book contains nine relatively short chapters that will engage you every step of the way. You will read, then stop and do some activities, discuss with colleagues (or friends, families, patients or the checkout operator at the local supermarket if you wish!), and then check your progress.

The book starts with **Chapter 1** (where better to start?), a basic introduction to psychology – from a historical perspective (don't yawn – it is brief and relevant), through to the role of psychology across the lifespan and its role in healthcare – from cradle to grave. That means that the roles of psychology in pregnancy, in childhood, in adulthood and in old age and death are all highlighted. Finally, the social context of psychology and healthcare is explored, demonstrating the interplay between psychology, the social world and other disciplines.

In **Chapter 2,** the various schools of thought are presented. Being a relatively young science psychology has a number of 'schools of thought' or perspectives on how and why people behave in a certain manner. This chapter presents these various perspectives and highlights how they can be applied to your practice. Some of these perspectives will be useful for those working with children, others will be useful for those working with people with a learning difficulty or mental health issue and there will be other perspectives applicable across all nursing practices. However, be warned – this is a weighty chapter but it does provide an important overview of the various approaches adopted in psychology to explain how and why people behave as they do.

Chapter 3 will explore psychology across the lifespan. It starts by exploring how psychologists have tried to explain the development of children from birth through to adolescence. It then explores how these developmental frameworks can be applied to nursing practice – whether this be at primary prevention level, dealing with mental heath issues or dealing with healthcare issues in the acute ward.

Chapter 4 looks at the social world – how we communicate with others through verbal and non-verbal means. It then looks at the power others have over us – conformity and obedience. Finally, we look at how these concepts and related issues can be put into practice when we introduce adherence to medical treatments.

The next chapter, **Chapter 5,** looks at cognitive psychology. It starts by exploring the concepts of perception and memory and how these can be related to nursing practice. The chapter then moves on from the 'pure' cognitive psychological areas and explores the social-cognition models of health behaviours and adherence (and the alternative forms of this term) to treatment. How these have been developed and how they can be used within practice to improve the care offered are explained.

Stress is the basis of **Chapter 6** – what it is, what causes it, what the consequences are. This is important from both a mental and physical health perspective as stress has the power to have negative consequences in a number of areas. The chapter finishes with some stress management techniques that are theory based – they are based on the models of stress presented earlier in the chapter.

The next chapter, **Chapter 7,** is the painful chapter. This chapter outlines the nature of pain, the models of pain and then how pain can be managed within a psychological framework. This is an application chapter (along with the stress chapter): you should be able to use your psychological knowledge and skills gathered from Chapters 6 and 7.

Chapter 8 explores mental health. Although this is a specific branch of nursing, it is a requirement for all nurses to understand issues related to mental health. This chapter presents an overview of these issues and highlights why this is important in healthcare. An overview of mental health issues is presented, along with reflections on the treatment considerations for those who have mental health problems.

The final chapter, **Chapter 9,** is also an area in which all nurses must have some exposure: learning disabilities. A broad, all-encompassing term is described and the various difficulties that are included within this description are outlined. The special considerations when nursing individuals with such disabilities are also outlined.

Is this book for you?

This book is geared towards nursing and healthcare students during their undergraduate studies, but it works equally well for those on postgraduate courses that require an additional psychological component. Nursing students from any nursing branch will find the text useful, as will those on midwifery programmes. We also hope that practising nurses and other healthcare professionals will find this text valuable and a useful reference source.

Features of this book

We have tried to use a variety of pedagogical devices throughout this book with the intent of interesting the reader, reiterating the relevance of key points, and acting as a revision device.

Here are the special features in each chapter, designed to make you a better student:

LEARNING OUTCOMES

Each chapter starts with the phrase 'At the end of this chapter you will be able to'. This is to guide you and orientate you to what the chapter contains and what you can expect to have achieved by the end of the chapter.

YOUR STARTING POINT

A series of five multiple choice/short answer questions to test where you are starting from – these will be returned to later in the chapter.

CASE STUDY

A brief case study that will help exemplify some of the issues contained within the chapter and highlight why the material presented is relevant to your clinical practice.

KEY MESSAGE

A one-sentence summary of the key message in a section.

QUICK CHECK

Asks you to recall or apply what you have just read. The answers can be found in the text and you should know the answer if you have read the text properly!

THINK ABOUT THIS

These ask the reader to consider a specific issue related to an individual topic under discussion. Obviously you can do this by yourself or with a colleague in order to increase your learning.

RESEARCH IN FOCUS

In this box we will present a recent research study that has been published that has direct relevance to the material presented in the chapter. This box demonstrates the importance of research in evidence-based nursing and healthcare.

SUMMARY

At the end of each chapter we present a summary of the chapter in a series of bullet points. We hope that these will match the Learning Outcomes presented at the start of the chapter.

YOUR END POINT

Another series of questions for you to answer – if you have read the text, followed the exercises and discussed the issues then you should get them all correct.

FURTHER READING

We have included a few items that will provide additional information – some of these are in journals and some are full texts. For each we have provided the rationale for suggesting the additional reading and we hope that these will direct you accordingly.

WEBLINKS

A list of useful websites ends each chapter. We hope you will access these for further information.

REFERENCES

All the references cited throughout the text are gathered here. If you want to explore an area further then use these, along with the Further Reading suggestions, to expand your knowledge.

GLOSSARY

Bold words in the text that may not be immediately familiar or are technical in nature are defined in the glossary.

WARNING

Finally, a warning for all readers. This text is written in a relaxed and informal style so that the key principles can be read, understood and appreciated easily. Hopefully, you will find the style appropriate so you will find the information and key principles relevant to your practice easy to digest. However, when writing your assignment, your research project, or even your journal article you should **NOT** copy the style of this text – you need to present your material in a formal academic style.

Acknowledgements

This project, like all such projects, has been a major undertaking and one that (on more than one occasion) has felt more distant than it should have been. The production involved the assessment of a range of sources – whether these be academic journal articles, internet sources or popular academic textbooks. This material then had to be digested into bite-sized, conversational pieces. I hope that I have done the researchers, clinicians and policy makers justice in the interpretation.

On a more personal level, several key colleagues have acted as researchers for us and have contributed their time, effort and opinions with vigour and a frankness that was as refreshing as it was useful. In particular I have to thank Danni Stephens and Felicity South who spent a summer working on updating material for this second edition and contributed to the glossary or found references for this book. I am extremely grateful for the time and effort they put into this work.

Many thanks also to the team at Pearson, in particular, David Harrison, for helping drive through this project. Obviously, for a text like this the design is of key importance so thanks to all of those involved in the production of this text – the designers and production editors for enhancing the text with some excellent features, which we hope have provided guidance, direction and added value for all readers.

I must offer thanks and acknowledgements to those who have supported me at both work and home. For colleagues at the University of Worcester many thanks for your help, advice, friendship and practical guidance over the gestation period of this text.

Finally, I would like to thank Penney for caring.

Publisher's acknowledgements

We are grateful to the following for permission to reproduce copyright material:

Figures
Figure 1.5 from Dahlgren, G., Whitehead M. 1991. *Policies and Strategies to Promote Social Equity in Health*. Stockholm, Sweden: Institute for Future Studies; Figure 5.12 from Wolfgang Stroebe, *Social Psychology and Health*, 2nd edn, 2000. Reproduced with the kind permission of Open University Press. All rights reserved; Figure 5.13 from Jane Ogden, *Health Psychology*, 3rd edn, 2004. Reproduced with the kind permission of Open University Press. All rights reserved; Figure 7.4 from Hockenberry MJ, Wilson D: *Wong's essentials of pediatric nursing*, ed. 8, St. Louis, 2009, Mosby. Used with permission. Copyright Mosby.

Tables
Table 3.2 adapted from http://www.cancer.gov/cancertopics/pdq/supportivecare/bereavement/Patient/allpages/

ACKNOWLEDGEMENTS

Photographs
(Key: b-bottom; c-centre; l-left; r-right; t-top)

Corbis: Laura Dwight 80; Getty Images: Christopher Furlong/Staff 94c, Getty Images/Handout 34, Dave Hogan/Stringer 94r, Image Source 147, Jupiterimages 148r, Juan Silva 148l, Miguel Villagran/Staff 94l; Science Photo Library Ltd: BSIP Laurent 235, Doug Goodman 77.

Cover images: *Front*: Getty Images

In some instances we have been unable to trace the owners of copyright material, and we would appreciate any information that would enable us to do so.

Chapter 1

Introduction: psychology in nursing care

Learning Outcomes

At the end of this chapter you will be able to:

- Understand the development of psychology as a science
- Appreciate some of the schools of thought in psychology
- Appreciate the research methods in psychology
- Understand the social context for health and health psychology
- Understand the role of psychology in many aspects of life
- Appreciate the role of psychology in all aspects of health and illness from the cradle to the grave.

Your starting point

Answer the following questions to assess your knowledge and understanding of the relationship between psychology and nursing and the key terms and principles underlying psychology.

1. By the 1920s a new definition of psychology had gained favour. Psychology was said to be the science of:

   (a) mind
   (b) consciousness
   (c) computers
   (d) behaviour
   (e) philosophy?

2. What is the independent variable, in experimental research:

   (a) a variable which nobody controls or changes
   (b) the variable which is manipulated in an experiment
   (c) the variable which is measured, to see results of an experiment
   (d) a variable which describes some durable characteristic of the subject
   (e) a variable which is held steady?

3. Cartesian dualism specifies that:

   (a) The body can interact with the mind via the pineal gland.
   (b) The mind can interact with the body via the pineal gland.
   (c) The mind and the body do not interact at all.
   (d) Both (a) and (b).
   (e) Neither (a) nor (b).

4. According to many, who was the founder of modern day psychology and first 'psychologist':

   (a) Wundt
   (b) Fechner
   (c) Weber
   (d) Helmholtz
   (e) none of the above?

5. Which of the following schools of thought would be most likely to reject the method of introspection to study human experience:

   (a) behaviourism
   (b) psychoanalysis
   (c) structuralism
   (d) functionalism
   (e) none of the above?

1.1 Introduction

Being a nurse is all about medicine and nursing practice, isn't it? It is all about biochemistry, physiology and anatomy? As a nurse you need to understand the patient's medical and nursing history, you need to understand their diagnosis and their treatment, you need to understand what is going on, inside the brain, the liver, the kidneys, the heart and so on. However, a human being is more than the sum of bodily parts (see Figure 1.1) and this has an important consequence for your nursing practice and the importance of psychology in healthcare.

It could be argued, of course, that your individual patient is not that concerned about their body parts – what they want is to get better in the shortest and most painless manner. They want to be treated with respect and dignity, they want to be involved in their care and they want the nurse to act in a thoroughly professional manner. All of these have a psychological element.

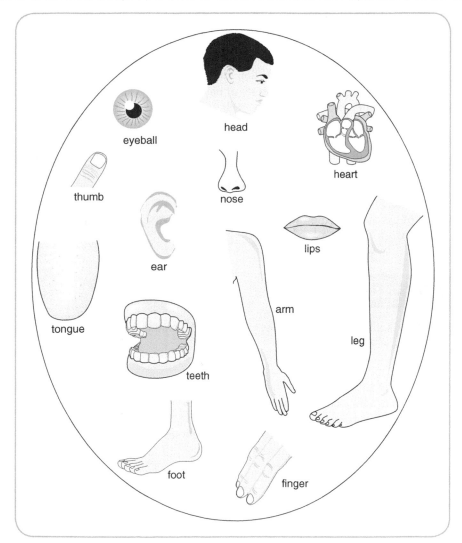

Figure 1.1 The human being is more than a sum of its parts

Key message

Humans are more than a collection of organs.

The patient also wants to know what caused their illness – is there something that can be done about it, and if so, what? How can they prevent it from occurring again and how can they be included in their care? Again, all of these have a psychological element.

Key message

Psychology is the most important subject you will study.

We must also appreciate the definition of health as provided by the World Health Organization (WHO, 1946): 'A complete state of physical, mental and social well-being and not merely the absence of disease or infirmity.' This suggests that health is not simply a problem with the biochemistry, physiology or anatomy of the individual patient but that there is a contribution, and an equal one at that, of social and psychological factors to the state of health.

And now for a bit of controversy: overall, psychology will be the most important subject you will study during your nursing degree.

If we look at Table 1.1, we see on the left-hand side all the benefits that a good knowledge of psychology brings, and on the right-hand side, all the things you can do without knowledge of psychology. The table has been limited to just half a page because of space considerations.

Key message

Psychology is the most important topic known to humankind.

As you can see from the table (which was completed in a totally unbiased fashion), psychology has many perspectives that enable the student nurse to appreciate the individuality and diversity of patients and clients. This is important in the construction and delivery of individualised care plans as stated throughout nursing courses and, of course, The Code (Nursing and Midwifery Council's Code of Conduct, 2008).

Quick check

What is the definition of health according to the WHO?

Table 1.1 The role of psychology in nursing practice

The role of psychology in nursing practice	Where psychology is not involved in nursing practice
✦ Understanding of mental health issues	
✦ Ability to communicate with peers	
✦ Ability to communicate with patients and clients	
✦ Ability to enhance adherence to treatment	
✦ Ability to change maladaptive behaviour	
✦ Ability to deal with the stresses and strains of practice	
✦ Stress management	
✦ Pain management	
✦ Design of systems and operations in theatre, ITU and on the wards	
✦ Ability to communicate with patients and clients irrespective of their needs, disability or health concern	
✦ Understanding of human behaviour from cradle to grave	

The word psychology means 'the study of the mind' (being made up of two Greek words – *psyche* – mind, soul or spirit and *logos* – knowledge, discourse or study). Many have subsequently defined psychology as the study of mind, behaviour, emotions and thought processes. It can assist us with understanding our patients and clients, and also ourselves.

The other definition that we should provide is 'health psychology'. This is, as the term suggests, how psychology can be applied to all aspects of health and the healthcare system – whether they be related to the aetiology of a particular condition, the treatment of a particular condition or the promotion of health in an individual's life. A longer, more formal definition is provided below.

Definition of health psychology

'Health psychology is the aggregate of the specific educational, scientific and professional contributions of the discipline of psychology to the promotion and maintenance of health, the prevention and treatment of illness, the identification of etiologic and diagnostic correlates of health, illness and related dysfunction, and the analysis and improvement of the health care system and health policy formation' (Matarazzo, 1982).

Think about this

What do you consider the most important topic you are studying on your nursing course? Why?

Quick check

What is the definition of psychology and health psychology?

1.2 A brief history of psychology

The schools of thought, or perspectives in psychology, that we will discuss in detail later in this book are indicated in Figure 1.2. However, the historical overview provides some information on those key figures who have been influential in psychology and how this relates to the current viewpoint and the perspectives that can be applied to healthcare.

The father of psychology is believed to be William Wundt, although he was originally a professor of physiology in Germany.

Wundt

Wundt wanted to apply the methodical, experimental methods of science to the study of human consciousness. To this end, he founded the first-ever psychology laboratory at the University of Leipzig in Germany in the 1880s. At his laboratory, Wundt spent hours exposing individuals to audio and visual stimuli and asking them to report what they perceived. In this way, he studied one component of consciousness, perception.

The school of thought that arose from the work of Wundt and his colleagues is called structuralism. The basic goal of structualists was to study consciousness by breaking it down into its components – mainly perception, sensation and affection. Their basic method was to

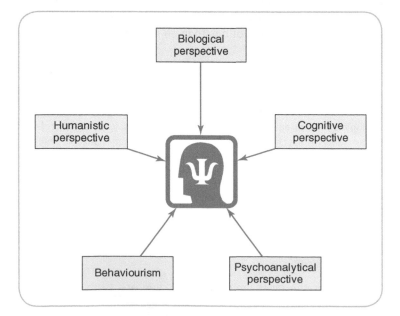

Figure 1.2 Schools of thought in psychology covered in this text

train their subjects in introspection, which was careful, systematic observation of one's own conscious experience.

> ### Key message 🔑
>
> Wundt believed in objective measurement – the initial scientific foundation of psychology.

Structuralism vs. functionalism

An opposing school of thought – functionalism – was led by William James and John Dewey. While structuralists essentially wanted to determine 'what is consciousness?', functionalists wanted to determine 'what is consciousness used for?' – in other words, they wanted to study the purpose, or function, of consciousness and basic mental processes.

The two camps debated passionately over which approach to psychology was best, each hoping to shape the direction of their fledging academic subject. Although neither won the war, the creative tensions led to the establishment of the first psychology lab in the USA (Johns Hopkins University).

Behaviourism

Around 1913, American psychologist John B. Watson founded a new movement that changed the focus of psychology. He believed that internal mental processes should not be studied, because they cannot be observed; instead, Watson advocated that psychology focus on the study of behaviour and thus his movement became known as behaviourism. As Watson saw it, behaviour was not the result of internal mental processes, but rather the result of automatic response to stimuli from the environment. Behaviourism became focused on how conditions of the environment affect behaviour and, specifically, how humans learn new behaviour from the environment. This movement took a strong hold in America and was the dominant school of thought for about 40 years. Watson's successor, as the leader of behaviourism, was B.F. Skinner, who developed an influential view that operant conditioning was the mechanism for learning.

> ### Key message 🔑
>
> Behaviourism has played a significant part in mental health and learning disability nursing.

> ### Think about this ❓
>
> In the past day, think about a time you have given a reward (i.e. reinforced a behaviour). What about receiving a reward (i.e. reinforcer)? Has it made the behaviour more likely?

> ## Key message
>
> Behaviourism confines itself to the effect of the environment on behaviour.

Gestalt theory

While behaviourism was becoming dominant in the USA, two other schools gained influence in Europe around the same time. Gestalt theorists' basic belief was that any psychological phenomenon, from perceptual processes to human personality, should be studied holistically; that is, they should not be broken down into components, but rather studied as a whole.

Psychoanalysis

The second major movement in Europe at this time was **psychoanalytic theory**. This theory, developed by Austrian psychologist Sigmund Freud, revolutionised psychology and other aspects of modern thought. Very much the opposite of behaviourism, it focused on humans' internal workings and proposed a whole new way of explaining them. The theory developed by Freud was quite extensive and intricate, but the main principle is that the unconscious is responsible for most thought and behaviour in all people and the disorders of the mentally ill. Freud's psychoanalytic theory gained a wide following and many of his ideas are commonly believed by the public today. However, there is limited evidence and most psychologists consider Freud to be of interest merely from a historical perspective.

> ## Key message
>
> Psychology owes a lot to Freud, but his theory is now considered to have a limited evidence base and hence receives limited support.

> ## Think about this
>
> Although Freud's theory is no longer considered valid, what value do his methods and theory still have in nursing practice?

Humanism

By the 1950s, a new movement began as an alternative to behaviourism and psychoanalytic theory. The followers of this movement considered behaviourism and psychoanalytic theory dehumanising and they took the name, humanism, for their movement. Instead of behaving as pawns of the environment or the powerful unconscious, humanists believed humans were inherently good and that their own mental processes played an active role in their behaviour. Free will, emotions and a subjective view of experience were important in the humanism movement.

Cognitive theory

The most recent major school of thought to arise has been the cognitive perspective, which began in the 1970s. This movement is much more objective and calculating than humanism, yet it is very different from behaviourism, as it focuses extensively on mental processes. The main idea of this movement is that humans take in information from their environment through their senses and then process the information mentally. The processing of information involves organising it, manipulating it, storing it in memory, and relating it to previously stored information. Cognitive theorists apply their ideas to language, memory, learning, dreams, perceptual systems and mental disorders.

Table 1.2 highlights how each of these areas is of central importance in psychology and in nursing practice and where they are covered in the following chapters of this text.

Quick check

Who is the founder of modern psychology?
Which school of thought grew in opposition to the introspection approach?

Table 1.2 Historical perspective on psychology's development

School of thought	Useful in nursing practice because . . .
Structuralism	Stressed the importance of scientific study of mental processes. An obvious link to mental health nursing and how psychological processes can impact on physical health (see Chapter 6).
Behaviourism	Emphasis was on the behaviour and how this could be influenced by the environment (see Chapter 2). Has a key role to play in working with children, people with learning disabilities, those with mental health issues and those in pain (i.e. many of the people nurses come across).
Gestalt	Importantly recognising that the human should be treated holistically and not as the sum of its individual parts (covered in Chapters 1 and 5).
Psychoanalysis	The importance of the unconscious was revealed and the link between psychological conflict and physical health was further highlighted (Chapter 2).
Humanism	The root of positive nursing practice.
Cognitive theory	The future (as some would see it) – a more scientific and information processing perspective that explores the way in which people make sense of their environment (see Chapter 2).

1.3 The language of psychology

All subjects have their own special language - you will have come across some terms in nursing that you probably have not come across before. Just as it is in nursing, so it is in psychology. Psychology has its own jargon and it is probably sensible that there is an introduction to this language before progressing any further. Psychology has its own terms including some words, phrases and approaches that may be familiar to you but mean different things to psychologists from normal (sic!) people.

For example, if a person says 'behaviour' then a psychologist would say 'define the behaviour'. If a person says 'personality' then a psychologist will ask 'which aspect of personality?'. Furthermore, psychologists from different traditions (see Table 1.2) would further refine the personality into an element that fits in with their understanding of the person. For example, a psychologist from the psychoanalytic tradition might suggest that a person has an 'anal personality' (stemming from the anal stage, a child who becomes fixated due to over-control). This phrase may be uncommon to you (and probably to many psychologists as well) but it is there simply to demonstrate the point that individual psychologists speak a different language from other professions, and often, from each other.

There are, of course, many other such examples and it would be impossible to go through all of these, but you get the point: psychologists have a language of their own, and this language may be further divided according to the psychologist's school of thought.

Having said that, however, there are a few terms that you should appreciate as being essential to the understanding of psychology. First, psychology is a scientific discipline based on models, theory, hypotheses and empirical study.

Think about this

List some terms you think of when thinking about psychology.

1.4 What is a science?

One common misconception about science is that it is all about statistics and hard maths. It is not - there are plenty of scientists who produced scientific theories without reaching for the calculator (think of Darwin or Piaget, for example). Nor is science about technology - there are plenty of examples of technology that have no scientific basis (e.g. 'lie detector') and plenty of science that has no technology (e.g. Newton). So, this is what science is not, but what are the central qualities of science and how does this relate to psychology?

Key message

Psychology is a science and uses scientific methods, language and approaches.

1.5 Key qualities of a science

All sciences share a common method of investigation: they are data driven and do not rely on personal biases or superstitions. This data is produced objectively and is subject to both replication by others and peer review. Hence, any study we conduct has to be clearly recorded and open to public scrutiny so it can be challenged and replicated. Furthermore, science examines solvable problems which are empirically derived and are not too all-encompassing (not looking for the meaning of life, for example). If we unpick this further, we see that for psychology to be defined as a science it has to have:

✦ **A defined subject matter:** we can clearly state the range of subject matter or phenomena that psychology studies.

✦ **Theory construction:** we can try to explain the observed phenomena in terms of theory (see Chapter 5 for how psychologists have attempted to do this).

✦ **Hypothesis testing:** we can make specific predictions based on our theory which we can test empirically.

✦ **Empirical testing:** used to collect data (or evidence) to support or refute the hypothesis.

In Figure 1.3 the scientific induction-deduction method is outlined and shows how science progresses. At the first stage there is the inductive process, where psychologists (or other scientists) observe instances of a natural phenomenon and derive a general law based on

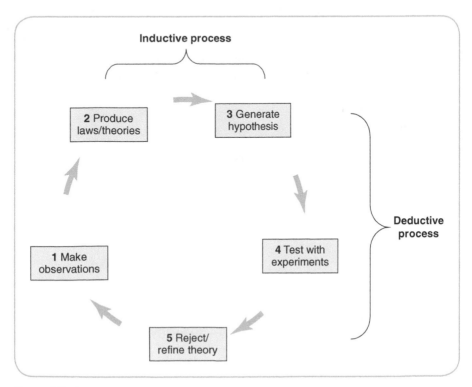

Figure 1.3 The scientific induction-deduction method

these observations. Hence, they are moving from the particular to the general. The next stage suggests that we move from the general to the particular – the theory has been derived and we now want to look for instances to confirm (or refute) our law or theories.

Quick check

List the central characteristics of a science.

Out of this perspective come a number of terms and methods that will crop up during this text:

+ **Hypothetical constructs**: These are not observable but can only be inferred from behaviour. For example, memory, intelligence and personality.
+ **Model**: A metaphor, involving a single fundamental idea or image.
+ **Theory**: Often the terms theory and model are used, incorrectly, interchangeably, but a model is a complex set of inter-related statements that attempt to explain certain observed phenomena.
+ **Hypothesis**: A testable statement about the relationship between two or more variables, based on a theory or model.
+ **Variable**: Anything that can vary and can be one of two kinds: an independent variable (IV), which the researcher manipulates to see if it affects the dependent variable (DV).

One argument against psychology is that major sciences have paradigms, which are general theories that encompass many smaller theories. However, psychology does not have any of these. Instead, it has levels of explanations that are used to explain phenomena. Thomas Kuhn (Kuhn *et al.*, 1990) said that because of this 'psychology is a pre-science'. He meant that psychology had not quite reached the stage of being a science, but may do so one day.

Think about this

How would you define and measure the following:

+ memory
+ personality
+ behaviour
+ thinking?

1.6 Researching psychology

Psychology, as you would imagine, generates a considerable number of research questions and consequently requires a range of methods for gathering evidence to answer them. This text will not consider the whole gamut of research methods available, but will just skim the surface so you understand some of the terms that may come up in this text. There are a number of textbooks related to research methods and these can be accessed for further information when you need it.

Between groups design

A between groups design allocates matched groups of people to different treatments. If the measures are taken at one time this is a cross-sectional design, whereas if they are tested over two or more time periods then this would be a longitudinal design. For example, if we want to see whether a certain psychological approach (e.g. behavioural) to pain management works we would have one group that has the intervention (the experimental group) and another group (the control group) that does not. If we followed these people over time to see whether the behavioural intervention worked then it would be a longitudinal design.

We also have to remember to use an appropriate control group – we could not give the group nothing as the mere fact that the experimental group was receiving the intervention might be enough to cause improvement. So, we have to include a **placebo** control as treatment. This might be a non-specific treatment that does not involve the behavioural intervention.

Within participants design

This type of design is used when the same people provide measures at more than one time and differences between the measures at the different times are recorded. An example would be a measure taken before an intervention and again after the intervention. For example, you introduce a psychological intervention to try to improve the mental health of a group of people with learning disabilities living in supported accommodation. You measure the levels of mental health before the treatment, and then again after you have undertaken the intervention. There are obvious problems with this – did we keep everything else constant? How can you be sure that it was down to the intervention specifically?

Quick check

List the advantages and disadvantages of a between participants and within participants design.

Cross-sectional studies

These studies obtain the responses from a group of participants on one occasion only. With appropriate randomised sampling methods, the sample can be assumed to be a representative cross-section of the population under study. So, for example, we can explore how many people are under stress at any one point in time. If we collect enough participants then we can probably also compare specific sub-groups: is stress greater in men than women, is it greater in nurses or doctors (or psychologists)? These studies are quite common, but we must make sure the sample is representative and we cannot infer any cause and effect.

Observations

A simple kind of study involves observing behaviour in a relevant setting. Hence, we can explore interactions within a consultation setting: how do patients react to bad news? How do nurses react to giving good news?

Structured interviews

An interview schedule is prepared with a standard set of questions that are asked of each person, by telephone or by face-to-face interview. A semi-structured interview is more open ended and allows the interviewee to address issues that they feel are relevant to the interview.

Longitudinal design

These designs involve measuring responses of a single sample on more than one occasion over a period of time. These can either be prospective (where the recordings are taken and then planned for the future) or retrospective (where the recordings are obtained from already collected records). These types of designs are among the most powerful designs available for the evaluation of treatment and of theories about human behaviour.

Meta-analysis

This is a statistical analysis of the results from a number of studies already completed. A useful definition was given by Huque (1988): 'A statistical analysis that combines or integrates the results of several independent clinical trials considered by the analyst to be "combinable".'

Questionnaires

This is a popular and frequently employed method of study in psychology. Questionnaires consist of a standard set of items with accompanying instructions. Ideally a questionnaire will be both reliable (i.e. measure the same thing on more than one occasion) and valid (i.e. measure the thing that they say they are measuring). Questionnaires can be designed specifically for the study under discussion or they can be picked 'off the shelf' since many have already been designed (see Bowling (1995) for further details).

Surveys

This is a systematic method for determining how a sample of participants respond to a set of questions (or questionnaires) at one or more times. For example, we may want to know what people with alcohol problems think of the service they are receiving and how this compares to the views of the service providers. In this case we would do two surveys – one with the service users, and one with the service providers.

Randomised controlled trials

Randomised controlled trials (RCTs) involve the systematic comparison of interventions using a fully controlled application of one or more 'treatments' with a random allocation of participants to the different treatment groups. This design is the 'gold standard' to which much research in psychology and healthcare aspires. People are allocated at random (by chance alone) to receive one of several interventions. One of these interventions is the standard of comparison or control. The control may be a standard practice, a placebo or no intervention at all. RCTs seek to measure and compare the outcomes after the participants receive the interventions.

Think about this

What design would you use to investigate whether:

+ a behavioural approach to pain management works in older people
+ painting the walls blue increases the quality of life in a children's ward
+ people with a learning disability in supported housing have better language skills than when living within their families
+ stress causes mental health problems
+ 'hard' drug users have a different personality to non-drug users?

What methodological and ethical considerations should you take into account?

Qualitative techniques

The methods discussed so far are quantitative techniques favoured by many in psychology and healthcare. However, there are also a number of qualitative techniques that may be of use. For example, there are diary studies which can help the researcher collect information about the temporal changes in health status (e.g. dealing with a life-limiting condition). There are also narrative approaches in which the desire is to seek insight and meaning about health and illness through the acquisition of data in the form of stories concerning personal experiences (e.g. dealing with substance abuse). Cases studies provide a 'thick description' of a phenomenon that would not be obtained by the usual quantitative or qualitative approach. Focus groups are a common approach which involves a group of participants discussing a focused question or topic which can lead to the generation of interactive data.

Key message

Qualitative and quantitative techniques are both useful and valid techniques. You must use the most appropriate method for your research question.

Action research

Action research is increasingly being used within health, nursing and psychology and has been recommended by the Department of Health as a valuable approach for public health research (DoH, 2001). At its heart is the idea of using research to directly change practice. While other quantitative and qualitative research approaches may go through a long process of data collection, analysis and eventually producing a final report which researchers hope

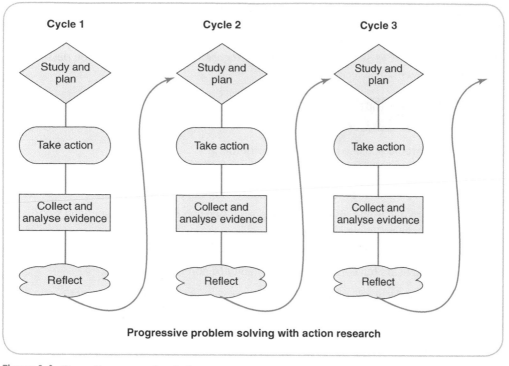

Figure 1.4 The action research spiral

that practitioners will use to inform their work, action research works directly with practitioners or community members so that findings are used immediately and continually to develop practice. Hence, a core idea within action research is that it is done *with* participants rather than *on* them. Lewin, who is considered the founder of action research, suggests that it 'proceeds in a spiral of steps each of which is composed of a circle of planning, action and fact-finding about the result of the action' (Lewin, 1946: 15).

This basic principle of a spiral of steps lives on in the design of many action research studies. A simple diagram of the action research spiral is shown in Figure 1.4.

Many action research studies now aim to empower the disempowered and to challenge the social structures that create such power imbalances. These developments have led to what has become known as 'participatory action research'. Participatory action research is built on the concept of a group of co-researchers working together as equal participants trying out various actions, evaluating and reflecting on their effectiveness as a group and then developing and, hopefully, improving their actions. Through this process the co-researchers begin not only to analyse the situation they are in, but also to build a sense of empowerment as they are able to take action to respond to their analysis.

Key message

Action research is a useful technique for involving users in research in order to improve services.

1.7 Health and health psychology in a social world

The definitions of health and illness can be the subject of a book themselves – indeed many texts have been written on this subject. However, for the purposes of this book we will use the definition of health provided by the World Health Organization (1946): 'Health is a state of complete physical, mental and social well-being and not merely the absence of disease or infirmity.'

We will use this definition not necessarily because it is the best one, but because it is the one that all of us know and that many people cite. Despite its flaws (e.g. it is too idealistic) it does provide a good basis for future study and aspirational care. What this does suggest is that health is not merely about bugs, germs, accidents or biochemistry – it is about social and psychological variables as well.

Think about this

How else can you define health?

Hence the current focus is on the **biopsychosocial** model of health and illness. This model considers illness to be a result of a number of factors and hence the individual is not seen as passive: the person can contribute to their health and to their ill-health. The person takes an active role in their treatment – they are responsible for taking their medication, for example, and more importantly changing their beliefs and behaviours. In contrast, the original biomedical model suggested that the causes of illness were outside the control of the individual – all physical disorders could be explained by disturbances in physiological processes, which result from injury, biochemical imbalance, bacterial or viral infections and so on. Psychology had very little role in either health or illness and no relationship was postulated between the mind and physical illness (the so-called **Cartesian dualism**). Luckily most people have come to their senses and recognise that psychology has a role to play in health and illness!

If we explore what causes illness from a biopsychosocial perspective then it is not simply a case of looking for a biological causative agent or physiological or genetic marker; we have to look additionally at both social and psychological factors.

Bio	Psycho	Social
Viruses	Behaviour	Class
Bacteria	Beliefs	Gender
Genetics	Stress	Ethnicity

Biological factors are, perhaps, more apparent and include such factors as the genetic make-up of the individual along with anatomy, physiology and chemical balance. Illness is caused by involuntary physical changes caused by such factors as chemical imbalance, bacteria, viruses and genetic predisposition.

Psychological factors include such variables as lifestyle (e.g. smoking, drinking) along with personality. They also include such variables as cognition – thinking and interpreting, and beliefs. Emotional factors are also important in determining whether we seek out medical or some other form of healthcare assistance. Motivational factors are another factor under the psychological variable: if we are motivated when we start an exercise programme we are more likely to keep up with the programme.

Quick check

What is Cartesian dualism and how does it relate to healthcare?

Social factors are both broad and deep. All of us live in a social world – we all have relationships with others, whether these be our family, our friends or our work colleagues. Children may start smoking if their peer group encourages it because it may make them feel more grown up. These may be referred to as social norms of behaviour (whether it is OK to smoke or thought 'cool' to drink to excess) and relate to social values on health.

Think about this

Consider an individual who comes to you with one of the following diagnoses:

+ myocardial infarction/heart attack
+ schizophrenia
+ hepatitis
+ kidney stones
+ depression
+ alcohol abuse.

What biological, psychological and social factors could be implicated? Is any one of the factors alone sufficient?

Now consider how you would treat them. What intervention would you suggest? How would you employ psychological and social variables?

The role of social factors in health, illness and psychology is of paramount importance. In Figure 1.5, an example framework for considering the general determinants of health is presented. The framework is multi-layered like an onion with the fixed factors over which we have no control (e.g. age, sex and genetic factors) at the core but surrounded by four layers of influence that we can do something about, either through psychological or social change.

This is a useful framework for understanding health and illness and the role of psychology within it. As Marks (2005) points out, the framework has six positive characteristics:

+ It is concerned with all of the determinants of health, not simply with the course of events during the treatment of illness.
+ It places the individual at the core but acknowledges the primary determining influence of society through the community, living and working conditions, and the surrounding socio-economic, cultural and environmental conditions.
+ It places each layer in the context of its neighbours, reflecting the whole situation including possible structural constraints upon change.

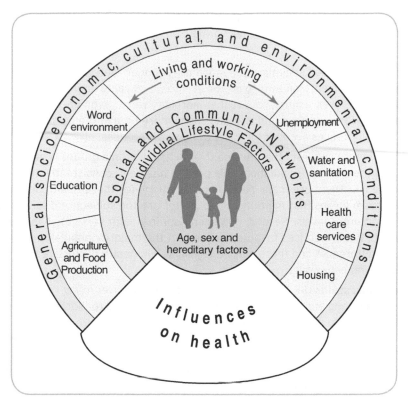

Figure 1.5 A framework for the determination of health

Source: Dahlgren, G. and Whitehead, M. (1991) *Policies and Strategies to Promote Social Equity in Health*, Stockholm, Sweden: Institute for Futures Studies.

✦ It has a true interdisciplinary flavour and is not purely a medical or quasi-medical model of health.

✦ It is even-handed and makes no claims for any one discipline as being more important than others.

✦ It acknowledges the complex nature of health determinants.

Think about this

In light of the framework of Dahlgren and Whitehead (1991), what factors would you consider to be involved in the following:

✦ myocardial infarction/heart attack

✦ schizophrenia

✦ hepatitis

✦ kidney stones

✦ depression

✦ alcohol abuse?

This means that we have to be aware of the socio-cultural variables and their potential impact on both psychology and health. We should be aware of the following broad factors:

✦ **Gender:** in industrialised societies today men die younger than women, yet women have poorer health than men. Men tend to die, on average, 6–8 years younger than their female counterparts. However, women have higher morbidity rates – women suffer more chronic and acute illnesses than men, and visit and spend more time in the hospital. Psychosocial and lifestyle differences account for many of these differences.

✦ **Ethnicity:** evidence suggests that the health of minority ethnic groups is generally poorer than that of the majority population. This pattern has been consistently observed in the USA and the UK. There are many possible explanations for these health differences. For example, racism means that minority ethnic groups are the subject of discrimination at a number of different levels. Second, ethnocentrism in health services, health promotion and access to health services favours the needs of the majority population. Finally, there are cultural differences and these may be highlighted in health protective behaviours and health damaging behaviours.

✦ **Socio-economic status (SES):** evidence from many studies over many years has indicated that there is a strong and consistent relationship between SES (or social class) and health. Specifically, the data suggests continuously increasing poor health as SES changes from high to low. The mediators of SES effects on health experience are likely to be behavioural and psychosocial. The behavioural factors include diet, exercise and smoking while the psychosocial factors include such processes as self-efficacy, self-esteem and perceived control (Siegrist and Marmot, 2004).

Think about this

When treating or interacting with a patient, what psychosocial variables must you take into account?

Key message

Psychology as applied to health cannot be taken in isolation – you have to take note of the cultural context.

Quick check

What are the layers on the Dahlgren and Whitehead (1991) model? Why is this model of value?

1.8 The scope of psychology

Psychology has strong links with a range of other disciplines. At one end of the spectrum we have sociology and social anthropology – exploring societies and communities. This can be linked to social psychology and, as we will see in this chapter, the link to health and health psychology is also strong. One example is stress and social support. We get considerable support from our social relationships and this can be of benefit both psychologically and physically. As we will see in Chapter 4, the benefits derived from social networks can be considerable and can reduce the impact of stress and thereby improve health and well-being.

At the other end of the psychological spectrum we have the biological basis of our actions and activities. For example, when we look at pain in Chapter 7 we note that pain is both a psychological and a biological construct: both of these factors are central to our understanding of pain and, consequently, to its management (see Figure 1.6 for an indication of the scope of psychology and its links across to other disciplines).

Think about this

What other disciplines can psychology and nursing link with? Expand the diagram.

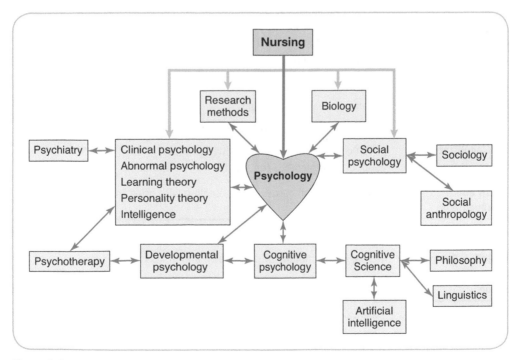

Figure 1.6 Scope of psychology and link to other disciplines

1.9 Psychology in health and nursing care

Given the nature of psychology and its links with a considerable number of other disciplines it will come as no surprise that psychology has a central role in health and illness. Consequently, when exploring psychological links to health, illness and healthcare, we find that at every step of the journey there is a role for psychology both through an untroubled life (see Table 1.3) and if there was an ill-health episode (see Table 1.4).

Table 1.3 Psychology's involvement across the lifespan

Event	Example of psychology's input
Conception ↓	Psychology can assist with family planning to ensure that either safe sex is practised (or isn't in the case of conception!) and that the psychological and physical states are maximised for the developing foetus (e.g. behaviour change to maximise health state).
Pregnancy ↓	Behaviour change to enhance health states (e.g. stop smoking sessions).
Labour and birth ↓	Social support reduces time in labour and pain associated with it.
Child growing up ↓	Appreciation of the cognitive stage of development and the impact this has on understanding of health and illness.
Adolescence ↓	Potential optimum time to develop positive health behaviours. Mental health difficulties may appear – interventions required.
Adulthood ↓	Enhancing health behaviours. Changing health behaviours. Support for any maladaptive psychological or physical ill-health.
Late adulthood ↓	Coping with physical and cognitive decline. Support and methods for dealing with potential social isolation.
Death and bereavement	Support through bereavement, dealing with grief and preparing for death.

Table 1.4 Examples of the role of psychology during health and illness

Stage	Example of psychology's input
Person is healthy ↓	Maintaining health. Promoting healthy behaviours. Reducing stress and promoting mental health. Reducing inappropriate health behaviours.

(Continued)

Table 1.4 Examples of the role of psychology during health and illness (*Continued*)

Stage	Example of psychology's input
Person feels ill ↓	How does a person become aware of symptoms?
	How does a person respond to sensations?
	How does a person perceive that they are unwell?
	How does a person interpret symptoms?
Plans to visit healthcare professional ↓	Why does a person make the choice to go to the healthcare professional at that time?
	What prompts (or who prompts) the person to go?
	How does the person respond to symptoms?
	What is the role of family and friends in deciding to visit the healthcare professional?
Visits healthcare professional ↓	What does the person tell the healthcare professional?
	How does the person communicate (both verbally and non-verbally) in the consultation?
	What are the factors that influence the consultation?
	How does the healthcare professional react?
	What cognitive processing does the healthcare professional go through to reach their conclusion?
Diagnosis and treatment ↓	How does the healthcare professional come to their diagnosis and choice of treatment?
	How does the patient react to the diagnosis?
	How does the patient react to the treatment plan?
	How does the person react to becoming a patient?
	Is the person satisfied with the consultation?
	Did they understand and remember the diagnosis and treatment?
Living with an illness ↓	How does living with an illness affect the self?
	How has the illness affected the individual's quality of life?
	What impact does the diagnosis have on family and friends?
	What is the role of family and friends in dealing with the diagnosis and illness?
	How does the illness affect the emotions of the person?
	How does the family and individual adjust to the diagnosis?
Dealing with pain ↓	What is pain?
	How can pain be affected by the illness and the reaction to the illness?
	What is the role of the family in managing pain?
	How does pain influence quality of life?
Coming to the end of life ↓	What stages does the person go through on diagnosis?
	How can the healthcare practitioner help the person come to terms with their impending death?
	How can the family and friends be supported?

Both of these are rather extreme examples, going from a perfectly fit person through to a dead person within a few steps. However, they are there to serve a point: psychology plays an important role in our lives, whether we be healthy or ill, whether we are young or old, or whether we are at the start of our life or at the end of it.

1.10 Conclusion

This book has been designed to provide you with the insight you need to demonstrate how important psychology is to your professional role. Whilst not all of the topics highlighted in Tables 1.3 and 1.4 are covered in this text, there is enough information here for you to find useful and informative, and to help move your professional career forward.

1.11 Summary

✦ Psychology has an important role to play in nursing.

✦ The WHO definition of health encompasses both biological and psychosocial elements.

✦ Psychology is the study of the mind and behaviour.

✦ Psychology has its origins in the systematic, experimental study of human consciousness.

✦ Psychology has its own language and terminology.

✦ Psychology is a science and employs a number of methods in order to complete research studies.

✦ Action research is a useful technique for involving users in research in order to improve services.

✦ The role of psychosocial factors should not be overlooked.

✦ Psychology has links with a number of other disciplines.

✦ Psychology has a role across the lifespan both in health and in illness.

Your end point

Answer the following questions to assess your knowledge and understanding of the relationship between psychology and nursing and the key terms and principles underlying psychology.

1. The cognitive revolution in psychology was a response to the limitations of which school of thought:

    (a) psychoanalysis
    (b) behaviourism
    (c) human information-processing
    (d) gestalt psychology
    (e) all of the above?

→

2. Psychologists employ a variety of tools and methods to study human behaviour. Which of the following methods do psychologists rely on to make systematic observations and draw conclusions about human behaviour:

    (a) speculation and common sense
    (b) generalisation and common sense
    (c) hindsight and experimentation
    (d) controlled measurement and experimentation
    (e) personal experience and collective wisdom?

3. The study of psychology is most concerned with which field of scientific inquiry:

    (a) the science of philosophy
    (b) the science of behaviour and mental processes
    (c) the science of developmental processes
    (d) the science of physical processes
    (e) the science of emotional and mental processes?

4. Which of the following might affect an individual's view about issues in psychology:

    (a) socio-cultural context
    (b) political beliefs
    (c) sources of funding
    (d) all of the above
    (e) none of the above?

5. What is the main focus of the nature/nurture debate in psychology:

    (a) child development
    (b) experimental studies
    (c) cognitive maps
    (d) mind reading
    (e) none of the above?

Further reading

Angoff, W.H. (1988) The nature–nurture debate, aptitudes and group differences. *American Psychologist* **43**, 713-720.

Eysenck, M.W. (2000) *Simply Psychology*. Hove, UK: Psychology Press.

Fischer, C.T. (2006) *Qualitative Research Methods in Psychology: Introduction through Empirical Studies*. Boston: Academic Press.

Fisher, S. and Greenberg, R.P. (1996) *Freud Scientifically Reappraised: Testing the Theories and Therapy*. Chichester, UK: Wiley.

Gravetter, F.J. and Forzano, L.A.B. (2002) *Research Methods for the Behavioural Sciences*. New York: Thompson/Wadworth.

Kimble, G.A., Wertheimer, M. and White, C.L. (1991) *Portraits of Pioneers in Psychology*. Washington, DC: American Psychological Association and Hillsdale, NJ: Lawrence Erlbaum Associates.

Whitehead, D. (2001) Health education, behavioural change and social psychology: Nursing's contribution to health promotion? *Journal of Advanced Nursing* **34**(6), 822-832.

Weblinks

http://www.behavenet.com
Behavioural Health Care Information. This site contains all the latest news and developments in behavioural healthcare. There are also links to the latest behavioural healthcare articles.

http://www.onlinepsychresearch.co.uk
Online Psychology Research. This site actually gives you the chance to take part in real psychology studies online. Make a contribution to psychological knowledge today.

http://www.behavior-analyst-online.org
Behaviour Analyst Online. This site contains links to behaviour analysis journals.

http://www.all-about-psychology.com
All About Psychology. This site, as the name suggests, is all about psychology. It contains definitions, history, topic areas, theory and practice.

http://www.dcity.org/braingames/stroop/index.htm
Stroop Test Demonstration. This site allows you to take part in a classic psychology test. The test demonstrates the difficulties we can all have in processing information. Have a go!

Check point

Your starting point		Your end point	
Q1	A	Q1	B
Q2	D	Q2	D
Q3	C	Q3	B
Q4	A	Q4	D
Q5	A	Q5	E

Chapter 2

Psychological approaches to understanding people

Learning Outcomes

At the end of this chapter you will be able to:

+ Name, define and explain psychological approaches to understanding the person
+ Understand the psychoanalytical approach to understanding the person
+ Appreciate the concepts, terminology and approach of the behavioural explanation
+ Develop the cognitive approach to the person and how this can be applied to nursing and healthcare
+ Explain how social learning theory has been applied to understanding the person
+ Understand the humanistic approach to the person
+ Express the ideas of major theorists within each approach
+ Evaluate each approach in terms of its strengths and weaknesses
+ Demonstrate the application of each approach to nursing and health practice.

Your starting point

Answer the following questions to assess your knowledge and understanding of the psychological approaches to understanding the person.

1. Which of the following approaches to understanding the person came first:

    (a) psychoanalytic theory
    (b) behaviourism
    (c) cognitive psychology
    (d) social learning theory
    (e) humanism?

2. According to psychoanalytic theory:

    (a) All behaviour is learned.
    (b) Behaviour is the result of maladaptive thinking.
    (c) Behaviour is the result of physiological processes.
    (d) Behaviour is the result of innate drives and early experiences.
    (e) Behaviour is the result of vicarious reinforcement.

3. Behaviourism is concerned with:

    (a) unobservable mental states
    (b) modelling
    (c) defence mechanisms
    (d) observable behaviour
    (e) none of the above.

4. According to the information processing approach:

    (a) The mind is analogous to a computer.
    (b) It doesn't matter what goes on inside the 'black box'.
    (c) Culture plays a major role in cognitive development.
    (d) Thinking is information processing.
    (e) (a) and (d).

5. Social learning theory is concerned with:

    (a) cognition
    (b) observation
    (c) modelling
    (d) vicarious reinforcement
    (e) all of the above.

Case Study

Gary is a 55-year-old office administrator, who spends a large amount of time at his work with little opportunity to relax at home with his family. This has led to an increase in his levels of stress recently and he has been drinking regularly after work with his work colleagues for a number of years. Gary also smokes heavily and has done so since he was a teenager. Given his current workload and his drinking patterns, Gary has also stopped going to the gym and his diet consists of take-aways. Gary does realise that his current behaviours are damaging his health.

Recently Gary has been in and out of the GP's due to a general feeling of being unwell. Specifically, he has been experiencing pain when breathing. Given the background and his current level of smoking, the GP decides to send Gary for tests at his local hospital. Gary and his wife Mabel wait in anticipation for Gary's results. When the results come through they are a tremendous shock for both Gary and Mabel: the consultant informs them that Gary has lung cancer and that it is essential for Gary to begin treatment as soon as possible. Gary becomes extremely upset and frightened as his father died of cancer when he was a child and he fears that he too will leave his children fatherless. However, after the consultation Gary's demeanor changes and he gets angry and storms off, leaving Mabel alone in the car park.

When Gary arrives home he busies himself with his work around the house and decides to have a cigarette. When Mabel tries to get him to stop, and to talk about the situation and how they should tell their 10-year-old son, Jack, she gets a very frosty response. Gary refuses to acknowledge the situation and tells Mabel to leave him to his work. Mabel becomes very confused and upset at her husband's behaviour leading to her becoming extremely anxious.

When Jack comes home from school, he goes in to help his father but sees him getting extremely angry with his mother in the middle of a big argument. Ultimately, he sees his father kicking the bin and then storming out of the room. Jack then decides to follow what his dad has done and kicks the furniture. When Mabel realises that Jack is home and is copying his father's behaviour she calls him over and gives him a cuddle to calm him down and then gives him some sweets thinking that it may help in telling him the bad news.

Why is this relevant to nursing practice?

Why has Gary acted in such a manner? Why has Jack copied his father? Why is Mabel acting in the way she does? Why does Gary smoke? All of these fundamental questions have been posed by psychologists - they want to try and explain how and why people behave in a certain manner. If we can unpick the core reasons then this will help us in all other areas - including clinical practice. Explaining the person will help us understand why people smoke, drink, eat and behave the way they do. It will help us reflect on why certain people follow advice and others do not. It will be of use throughout all areas of our lives - whether they be personal or professional.

2.1 How psychology helps us to understand why people do what they do

Why do people do what they do and behave in a particular way? Why is it that some people leave their assignment to the day before it is due in, while others do it in an organised and systematic manner? Why is it that certain individuals are aggressive and outspoken, and others patient and understanding? Why is it that certain people want to become nurses, while others want to become psychologists, physiotherapists or police officers? Why is it that certain nurses enjoy working with older people, whereas others enjoy working with children? These and various other sorts of questions have been addressed by psychologists in a range of different ways to help formulate approaches in which a person's behaviour can be explained.

An approach is a perspective (i.e. view) that involves certain beliefs about people and the way they function. Although there may be several different theories within each approach, they will all share some common underlying assumptions. Unfortunately (or fortunately depending on your perspective), there are several different approaches in psychology. There are many reasons for this; first, it is because all psychologists enjoy the experience of arguing and debating with one another. Second, there is no real agreed position, and there may be several factors that influence the way we behave – there is no conclusive evidence for any one of the approaches.

However, the final and most important reason for different approaches existing is that our behaviour is determined by several factors: for example our genetic endowment, physiological processes, personal characteristics such as intelligence, personality and **psychopathology**, the environment, specific stimuli and cognitive processes such as perception, thoughts, and memories.

Think about this

Why do people act in this way:

+ yawn
+ eat too much
+ drink alcohol
+ are short tempered
+ don't follow your advice
+ get depressed
+ have phobias about spiders, needles or uniforms?

The idea that there are various explanations for human behaviour can be illustrated by taking a concrete example. For example, most people now agree that substance abuse and substance dependence are determined by a range of factors: 'a multiply determined phenomenon' (Lowe, 1995; Sanson *et al.*, 2011).

Think about this

Think about all the factors associated with substance misuse. List them all. Is there any way you can group them into different themes? (As a clue, what about social, biological and so on?)

When we have listed all the factors associated with substance misuse we may come up with variables such as social factors (e.g. stressful living conditions or unemployment) or you may suggest some biological factors (such as the genes the individual inherited from their parents) (Anderson and Teicher, 2009). You may also come up with other suggestions – personality characteristics which make the individual prone to substance abuse or the reduction in tension and raised spirits that substance use may bring about (which could be broadly described as psychological factors) (Iigen *et al.*, 2011). Indeed all of the variables you listed may simultaneously contribute to substance abuse/dependency behaviours.

Of course, due to the complex nature of human behaviour it cannot be understood simply by one approach; we have to accept the inevitable – it is multi-faceted. Just as trying to explain a complex behaviour, like substance misuse, is confusing, so is trying to understand relatively simple behaviours such as arriving early or late for appointments or food preference.

Within this chapter we will discuss the key psychological approaches and how these could be applicable within clinical practice. We will begin by examining the basic ideas underlying the psychodynamic approach. After reviewing the shortcomings of these ideas we will consider the assumptions of behaviourism and how these aimed to overcome the issues evident within the psychodynamic approaches. We will then proceed in examining social learning theory, which attempts to extend behaviourist ideas, before considering the cognitive approach. Finally, we will consider the humanistic approaches.

Key message

Attempting to understand the person by just one psychological perspective is impossible.

2.2 The psychodynamic approach

The term 'psychodynamic' refers to a collection of theories that try to account for the dynamics of human behaviour; 'dynamics' are what drive us or motivate us to behave in particular ways. The **psychodynamic approach** explores how the mind (especially the unconscious mind) is responsible for everyday behaviour. In relation to this the most influential psychodynamic theorist is Sigmund Freud (1856-1939).

Freud was a medical doctor in Austria who became interested in how the 'mind' could influence physical symptoms of the body. He began to experiment with **hypnosis**, but soon found that its beneficial effects were short-lived, proving ineffective for a permanent cure. At this point he decided to adopt a method which had been suggested by his colleague and close friend Josef Breuer. This later came to be known as the **talking cure** (Parker, 2010). Breuer had discovered that when he encouraged his neurotic patients to talk openly about the earliest experiences of their symptoms, their symptoms gradually subsided.

In collaboration with Breuer, Freud developed the idea that many **neuroses** (e.g. phobias, paranoia, hysterical paralyses and pain) had their origins in traumatic events experienced in childhood but which were now forgotten. The belief that all behaviour originates from childhood experiences that reside within the unconscious is called **psychic determinism**.

Key message

Psychoanalysis highlights the importance of unconscious drives.

Basic assumptions behind the psychodynamic approach

+ Much of our behaviour is determined by unconscious thoughts and desires.
+ Maladaptive behaviour is the result of unresolved unconscious conflicts originating in childhood.
+ Resolution occurs through accessing and confronting unresolved conflicts.

2.3 Psychoanalytic theory

Freud's **psychoanalytic theory** seeks to explain behaviour in terms of an interaction between innate drives (i.e. those we were born with and which we all have) and early experiences in childhood. In order to fully understand Freud's theory and its application to your clinical practice, we first need to explain some important concepts, for instance:

+ Freud's topography and structure of the mind
+ defence mechanisms
+ the theory of infantile sexuality
+ the oedipus complex.

Freud's topography of the mind

According to Freud, the mind has three levels: the **conscious**, **pre-conscious** and **unconscious**. The conscious part of the mind deals with present situations, for instance the here and now. The pre-conscious part of the mind contains feelings, thoughts and experiences from the past that can easily be retrieved from memory and brought back into conscious awareness. The unconscious part of the mind contains information that the individual is not aware of; this information is very difficult and sometimes impossible to retrieve. Freud often used an iceberg analogy (see Figure 2.1) to illustrate the amount of importance given to the unconscious. Just as the major portion of an iceberg lies below the water's surface, a major portion of the human psyche lies below the level of awareness. Freud believed that causal factors responsible for human behaviour reside at this level of the mind. Therefore to understand human behaviour, the unconscious must be revealed.

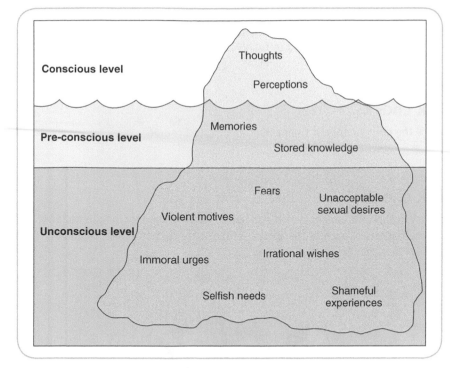

Figure 2.1 Freud's analogy for the human mind

Freud's topography of the mind forms the main premise of **psychoanalysis**. Psychoanalysis is a form of therapy which explores a patient's unconscious thoughts and emotions in order to allow them to gain a deeper insight and understanding of their behaviour. Although nurses cannot practise psychoanalysis without full and correct training, the principles of this approach may be useful in situations where the cause of a patient's complaint is not apparent and may warrant further exploration (Hoffmann, 2009; Gross, 2010).

Freud's structural model of the mind

Freud also assumed that the mind could be divided into three basic sections; the **id**, **ego** and **superego**. This constitutes Freud's structural model of the mind and is said to represent impulsivity, rationality and morality respectively.

✦ The id is the part of the mind which contains innate sexual (libido) and aggressive instincts and is located in the unconscious, which Freud considered the basic motivating force of human behaviour. The id is based on the 'pleasure principle' which drives the desire for immediate satisfaction.

✦ The second component is the superego, which contains the morals and rules of society. The superego develops as a result of the Oedipus complex (which will be discussed later on in this chapter) and usually emerges between the ages of three and six years. The main purpose of the superego is to prevent gratification of the id's desires by observing the rules and regulations that operate within society.

✦ Finally, the third component is the ego. The ego is based on the 'reality principle' and mediates between the id's innate desires and the moral standards of the superego.

An important part of Freud's theory was the notion that there are frequent conflicts among the id, ego and superego, which cause the individual to experience anxiety. Consequently the ego spends much of its time trying to resolve these conflicts. This is usually accomplished through the use of ego defence mechanisms.

Quick check

What are the components of the mind according to Freud?

Quick check

We can try to apply the concepts of id, ego, superego by looking for manifestations or representations of each of these concepts in some text or aspect of life. For example, in *Sex and the City* we may get:

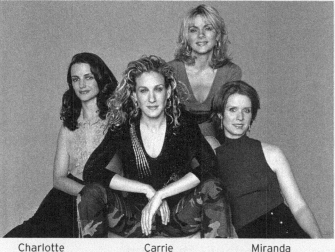

| Charlotte | Carrie | Miranda |
| (Superego) | (Id) | (Ego) |

Source: Getty Images/Handout

Now you try to find characters that fit into each of these concepts:

Topic	Id (emotion)	Ego (pure rationality)	Superego (command)
Books			
Films			
Heroes/heroines			
Songs			
TV programmes			
Your work colleagues			
Your student peers			
YOUR PATIENTS			

Ego defence mechanisms

The ego protects itself by employing a number of **defence mechanisms**. According to Hough (2002), defence mechanisms are strategies designed to protect the individual against painful anxiety and ensure that the ego is not overwhelmed (for a recent discussion on defence mechanisms see Kramer, 2010). Over a dozen defence mechanisms have been proposed by Freud and his followers. Among those commonly described are displacement, sublimation, projection, reaction formation, rationalisation, repression, regression and denial. Some of these defence mechanisms are outlined in Table 2.1.

Defence mechanisms are indicative of high levels of anxiety. A nurse who is familiar with defence mechanisms can help the patient move forward psychologically by tailoring communication to encourage and facilitate catharsis (Fillingham, 2010).

Table 2.1 Some of the defence mechanisms described by Freud

Defence mechanism	Definition	Example
Repression	The purposeful forgetting of anxiety-laden thoughts, memories or desires. Extreme reactions as well as high levels of anxiety can be indicative of repressed thoughts and feelings.	An adult unable to recall being abused as a child. In order to resolve these issues, the patient or client should be invited to talk about their anxieties and encouraged to discharge negative emotions, thoughts, memories and so on. This is referred to as **catharsis** (although please note that specialist education is required to practise psychoanalysis properly).
Displacement	Involves the expression of an unconscious impulse, but against a substitute person, animal or object.	'Kicking the cat' instead of whoever caused the anger or upset. In recent years there have been several highly publicised cases in which carers have neglected or mistreated elderly patients. For example, research suggests that the stress of caring is often identified as a trigger for elder abuse (Wieland, 2000), although this has not always been found (e.g. Action on Elder Abuse, 2004).
Sublimation	Socially unacceptable impulses or idealisations are consciously transformed into socially acceptable actions or behaviours.	An individual with strong aggressive impulses trains to be a boxer. Or an individual with a strong sexual energy transfers this into a different emotion in order to avoid confrontation with the sexual urge.

(Continued)

Table 2.1 Some of the defence mechanisms described by Freud (*Continued*)

Defence mechanism	Definition	Example
Projection	This involves getting rid of one's own undesirable characteristics by attributing them to others. The person who is projecting may accuse others of hating them or wishing them harm, when actually they are the one guilty of these thoughts and emotions.	A patient who dislikes a nurse could project by openly accusing the nurse of being unfriendly or hostile. Nurses therefore need to be aware of projection and, if such a situation arises, not take the feelings of the patient personally.
Reaction formation	An anxiety-laden impulse, thought or feeling is replaced in consciousness by its opposite.	For example, a patient with a loss of control, self-esteem and/or self-worth can result in the patient concealing such feelings and instead portraying a blasé, overconfident or even aggressive façade. In fact Ferns (2007) found that factors such as pain, fear and anxiety were closely linked to aggression in acute care settings.
Denial	In denial the ego is incapable of dealing with threatening facts and therefore fails to acknowledge the reality of this information. Aligned with health practice, denial can manifest itself as a mechanism for denying the presence of illness and medical diagnoses (Kreitler, 1999). Denial itself can be healthy to a certain extent and is part of the normal coping process featured within many of the grief framework models (Rana and Upton, 2009). However, denial can become problematic when it interferes with compliance with medical advice or ongoing treatment.	For example a patient who cannot accept that she has terminal cancer. Research suggests that nurses should work with rather than confront patient denial. According to Houldin (2000), direct confrontation of patient denial will only result in the increased use of this defence mechanism, therefore it is better to support the patient and discuss issues of concern which they will be able to think about at their own pace.
Regression	In regression, during times of stress, individuals will retreat to behaviours that are comforting and characteristic of an earlier stage of development. Regression is another type of defence mechanism which is closely linked to **fixation** and the theory of infantile sexuality.	For example, an individual who is diagnosed with cancer may seek comfort and thus retreat to a childhood state by rocking backwards and forwards. Displaying regression should indicate to the nurse that the patient is anxious and coping by comforting themselves. Nurses should aim to reduce patient anxiety by offering appropriate information and coping strategies which encourage relaxation.

Quick check

List the ego defence mechanisms.

Think about this

Looking back at the case study, what ego defence mechanisms can you identify?

Consider these ego defence mechanisms – how can they be applied to your practice?

How do you think they will manifest themselves in long-term conditions?

Freud's theory of infantile sexuality and the Oedipus complex

Freud's **theory of infantile sexuality** has its origins in Breuer's earlier discovery that traumatic childhood events have devastating negative effects upon the adult. According to Freud, the newborn infant is essentially an id, driven by the desire for sexual pleasure and demanding total immediate satisfaction (Zamanian, 2011).

In the early years of life the sexual instinct is satisfied through oral contact, i.e. through the act of sucking and biting the nipple and other objects. Freud termed this the **oral stage** of development, which occurs between the ages of 18 to 24 months where children only have the id. Accordingly, the stage is characterised by an inability to delay gratification, and displays of selfish demanding behaviour. Following the oral phase the locus of sexual gratification shifts to the anus, particularly in the act of defecation; appropriately Freud termed this the **anal stage**. This stage is continuous until the age of between 42 and 48 months. Freud argued that the process of toilet training is the first time children become aware of the effect of their actions on other people, and begin to modify their behaviour to gain gratification from them. Realistic expectations of these outcomes are evidence of the beginning of the ego development.

The penis or the clitoris becomes the focus of the libido during the **phallic stage**, which continues until the age of 5 or 6. In this stage the superego begins to develop. According to Freud all children experience the **Oedipus complex**. The Oedipus complex is named after the mythical Greek character Oedipus who unknowingly kills his father and then commits incest with his mother. According to the theory, the complex occurs when the young boy lusts after his mother, driven by the urges of the id and therefore views his father as a sexual rival. The young boy has the ability to judge the realistic consequences of these actions and is able to recognise that they would meet with his father's disapproval. Additionally, the young boy also acknowledges that he will not be able to defeat his father. Through observation, the young boy establishes that girls do not have a penis, resulting in the conclusion that it has been cut off by a jealous father (this is termed **castration anxiety**), and that he too will castrate him to prevent him from becoming a future rival for his mother. Anxious to avoid this, boys repress their lustful feelings towards their mother and *identify* with their father by adopting many of their father's attitudes and developing a superego.

While Freud regarded boys' and girls' relationships to the phallus as central to their psychosexual development, the Oedipus complex tends only to refer to the experience of male

Table 2.2 Mental health problems associated with a failure to move through Freud's stages of development

Stage	Associated problem
Oral	Depression, dependency, narcissism
Anal	Obsessive-compulsive disorder, obstinacy
Phallic	Paedophilia, homosexuality, antisocial personality
Latent	Inadequate or excessive self-control
Genital	Identity diffusion

children. Thus Freud posited a theoretical counterpart to the Oedipus complex known as the **feminine Oedipus attitude**. (In 1913 Carl Jung proposed the name the **Electra complex** for Freud's concept, deriving from the Greek myth of Electra, who wanted her brother to avenge the death of her father by killing her mother.) The feminine Oedipus attitude or Electra complex operates in much the same way as the Oedipus complex but in reverse, i.e. girls desire to possess the father and displace the mother. Freud attributes the nature of this psychosexual stage in girls to the notion of **penis envy**. According to the theory, penis envy leads to resentment of the mother, who is believed to have caused the girl's 'castration'. The father figure now becomes the girl's love object and she substitutes her penis envy with the wish to have a child; this ultimately leads to identification with the mother. Following these traumas both sexes enter a **latency period** in which sexual motivations become much less pronounced. This lasts until puberty or what is known as the **genital phase** in which the locus of pleasure or energy release refocuses around the genital area.

Freud postulated that the developmental process is essentially a movement through a series of conflicts, the resolution of which is detrimental to adult mental health (Table 2.2). Freud believed that many mental illnesses can be traced back to unresolved conflicts which otherwise disrupt the normal pattern of child development. For example, neuroses, paedophilia or homosexuality could be seen as resulting from a failure to resolve the Oedipus/Electra complex, whereas obsessive compulsive disorders concerning cleanliness or hand washing could be seen as failure to resolve conflicts at the anal stage.

Think about this

Consider how these concepts can be applied to everyday behaviour. Now consider how the Freudian concepts could be applied to mental illness. What does this mean for your practice?

2.4 Evaluation of the psychodynamic approach

Freud is considered as one of the most influential and authoritative thinkers of the twentieth century although more recently many of his ideas have fallen out of favour or have been adapted to incorporate more social rather than sexual influences. A criticism repeatedly made of Freudian and other psychodynamic theories is that they do not easily translate into measurable observations and are therefore untestable. A related problem is that Freud's (and other psychodynamic) theories are unfalsifiable and therefore lack scientific credibility. Around the middle of the twentieth century concerns grew about the nature of Freud's data and the validity of the interpretations that he drew from data (Hoffman, 2010). For instance, Freud's method of investigation was to focus on the individual (known as an **idiographic approach**), examining particular cases in great detail. Although this has the advantage of providing rich, detailed information, it is hardly justifiable to use such unique observations to formulate general theories about human behaviour. Besides, the case histories that Freud based his theories on were mainly of white middle-class women suffering from neurotic disorders; the fact that he relied on such cases to construct a theory of normal development is questionable in itself. Finally, Freud's theories are highly **deterministic** and **reductionist**. They are deterministic to the extent that infant behaviour is determined by innate drives and that adult behaviour is determined by childhood experiences, and overly reductionist because they reduce human behaviour to a basic set of abstract concepts (i.e. the id, ego and superego). Thus too much emphasis is placed on innate biological drives.

Despite much criticism, the psychodynamic approach brings forth several areas that are valuable for the nurse to consider. For instance:

✦ It acknowledges that unconscious desires influence behaviour.

✦ It recognises that childhood is a critical period of development and that experiences encountered during this time shape future behaviour (Zamanian, 2011).

✦ It offers an approach for understanding reactions to health problems.

An appreciation of psychodynamic concepts, and in particular ego defence mechanisms, will enable nurses to offer appropriate care and communication (Fillingham, 2010). Tailoring communication and care as well as recognising the diverse components which contribute to patient well-being will encourage and facilitate the patient to move forward both physically and psychologically.

Strengths and weaknesses of the psychodynamic approach

Strengths

✦ Freud's ideas have had a significant impact on psychology.
✦ Acknowledges that unconscious desires influence behaviour.
✦ Recognises that childhood is a critical period of development.
✦ Recognises that childhood experiences are fundamental determinants of adult behaviour.

Weaknesses

✦ Many psychodynamic concepts cannot be observed or measured (e.g. the Oedipus complex).
✦ Many psychodynamic concepts are unfalsifiable and lack scientific credibility.
✦ Theories are post hoc, i.e. based on historical reconstruction.
✦ Freud's theories were based on a very small, unique sample of people and so may lack generalisability.
✦ Freud's theories are highly reductionist and deterministic.
✦ Too much emphasis on innate biological drives.

2.5 Behaviourism

Behaviourism was proposed in 1913 by the US psychologist J.B. Watson and monopolised psychology, particularly in the USA, until the early 1960s (Hoffman, 2010). Watson, who was influenced by the Nobel Prize-winning work of Russian physiologist Ivan Pavlov (1849-1936) on conditioned reflexes, became increasingly critical of the **introspective approach** which previously dominated psychology. He postulated that introspective reports were unreliable and difficult to verify and he made a radical break from traditional introspective psychology. According to Watson: 'psychology as the behaviourist views it is a purely objective experimental branch of natural science. Its theoretical goal is the prediction and control of behaviour' (Watson, 1913: 158).

Behaviourism rejects claims that unconscious conflicts drive human behaviour. Instead it has the propensity to focus on the influences of reinforcement and punishment in producing particular acts of behaviour. According to behaviourists, we all learn our behaviour from our environment (to the near exclusion of innate or inherited factors; this is in keeping with the **tabula rasa view of mind**). It can be reduced to simple stimulus response associations and, regardless of its complexity, can be described and explained without reference to internal states (motivation, emotion, etc.) or mental events (i.e. perception, attention, memory, thinking and so on). Thus learning and experience are fundamental to the behaviourist approach.

Key message

According to behaviourism all behaviour is learnt from the environment.

Assumptions of the behaviourist approach

+ Psychology is the science of behaviour. Psychology is not the science of the mind.
+ Only observable behaviour should be studied.
+ Behaviour is determined by the environment.
+ All behaviour can be reduced to simple stimulus response associations.
+ Behaviour can and should be described without making reference to unobservable mental states or internal psychological processes.

2.6 Classical conditioning

Early behaviourist theories suggest that learning and behaviour are the result of conditioning. Conditioning was first reported in the early 1900s by the Russian physiologist Ivan Pavlov. During his experiments Pavlov observed that dogs would often start salivating before their food was presented to them, for example when they saw their food bowl or when they heard the footsteps of the laboratory assistant who was coming to feed them. These observations

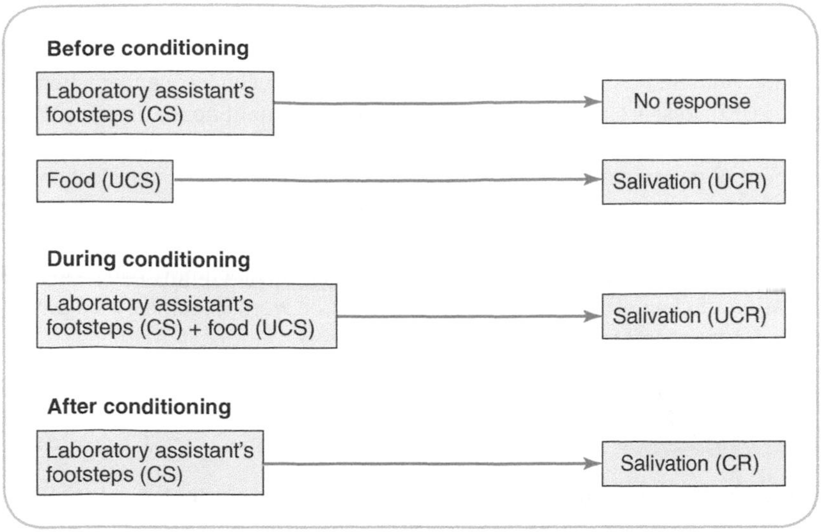

Figure 2.2 Classical conditioning

caused Pavlov to abandon his research on digestion and led to the study of what is now called **classical conditioning**.

Classical conditioning (see Figure 2.2) is a process of learning whereby an initially neutral stimulus comes to elicit a particular response, as the result of being paired repeatedly with an unconditioned stimulus. So let us break this down:

✦ The food (in the demonstration above) is an **unconditioned stimulus** (UCS) because it naturally evokes an unlearned **reflexive response** (salivation) which is known as the **unconditioned response** (UCR).

✦ The sound of the laboratory assistant's footsteps is a neutral stimulus that comes to be linked with the food when the two events repeatedly occur close together in time. Once the two events become associated with one another the footsteps become a **conditioned stimulus**.

✦ After satisfactory repetition this conditioned stimulus will produce a salivation response. When the salivation response is produced by the conditioned stimulus as opposed to the unconditioned stimulus, salivation becomes a **conditioned response** (CR).

Quick check

What are CS and UCS?

One of the most famous early examples of the classical conditioning response is 'Little Albert'. Within this experiment a young infant was repeatedly presented with a furry animal at the same moment as a loud noise. This led to an association between the furry animal and the frightening noise, resulting in little Albert becoming afraid of the animal. However, early studies such as this were rendered unethical due to the potentially severe implications of the conditionings implemented (Powell, 2011).

Nonetheless, there have been a large number of successful applications derived from classical conditioning theory. An example that has been extensively researched is anticipatory nausea and vomiting (ANV) experienced by patients receiving cancer chemotherapy (Roscoe *et al.*, 2010). Research has shown that prior to treatment approximately 29 per cent of patients experience anticipatory nausea, while anticipatory vomiting occurs in approximately 11 per cent of patients (Morrow *et al.*, 1998). In the 'language' of classical conditioning the first few chemotherapy infusions are the learning trials. The chemotherapy drugs are the UCS that, in some patients, induce post-chemotherapy nausea and vomiting (UCR). During repeated treatments, the hospital or ward, a previously neutral stimulus, is associated with the administration of chemotherapy. Thus the hospital or ward becomes a CS which elicits ANV as a CR in future chemotherapy cycles.

Key message

Classical conditioning can explain physiological reactions to psychological stimuli.

A number of studies provide empirical support for the role of classical conditioning in the aetiology of ANV. For example, Morrow and Rosenthal (1996) report that ANV prior to chemotherapy is uncommon and few patients experience ANV without prior post-chemotherapy nausea. Additionally, Roscoe *et al.* (2010) reported that in most published work in this area nausea is reported by approximately 20 per cent of patients at any one chemotherapy cycle to occur before chemotherapy was administered and by 25 to 30 per cent of patients by their fourth chemotherapy. Although other mechanisms have been posited, classical conditioning provides the best explanation for the aetiology of ANV in cancer chemotherapy patients (Roscoe *et al.*, 2010; Stockhorst *et al.*, 1998).

Think about this

How would classical conditioning explain the following:

✦ a child crying when approached by a nurse

✦ an adult with an anxiety reaction to needles

✦ anxiety feelings after taking an emetic

✦ the use of biofeedback to relax?

An interesting phenomenon in classical conditioning is **stimulus generalisation**. Stimulus generalisation is the tendency of a CR to occur in a weaker form in response to stimuli similar to, but different from, the original CS (see Schechtman *et al.*, 2010; Derenne and Breitstein, 2010). For example, it is not uncommon for patients to report ANV when they see the oncology nurse who administers their drugs or when they attend the same hospital for another matter. In one experimental study Bovbjerg *et al.* (1992) found that a new form of drink could induce nausea when paired with several chemotherapy infusions.

Think about this

How would generalisation be employed within your nursing practice? Consider how this may affect an individual's behaviour in one of the key settings of your practice, whether it be in mental health, physical health or child health, whether in secondary or primary care.

Anti-emetic drugs do not seem to control ANV once it has developed (Morrow *et al.*, 1998); so what can nurses do to prevent adverse associations, or if they are inevitable, lessen their effects? According to behaviourists, what can be learned can be unlearned (Feeney, 2010). For example, Pavlov found that when a CS was repeatedly presented in the absence of food, the CR of salivation became weaker and eventually stopped; this is called **extinction**.

Think about this

How can extinction be used to resolve post-chemotherapy vomiting?

Although prevention is the best strategy (i.e. avoiding post-chemotherapy nausea and vomiting during the initial stages of treatment), a variety of behavioural interventions have been shown to mediate the effects of ANV. For example, **systematic desensitisation** (also called counter-conditioning) appears to have an anti-emetic effect (see Foa, 2010). In this step-by-step approach, patients are taught to replace an anxiety-laden maladaptive response (such as ANV) with a more appropriate and healthy response (such as muscle relaxation). First, patients are taught progressive muscle relaxation techniques. Next, the patient and the therapist construct what is known as an 'anxiety hierarchy', a list of feared situations relating to the chemotherapy treatment (e.g. driving to the hospital or seeing the oncology nurse). This hierarchy of anxiety-provoking situations is ordered from the least to the most unpleasant. As the patient reaches a state of deep relaxation they are asked to imagine or are confronted by the least threatening situation in the hierarchy. The patient repeatedly imagines or is confronted by this situation until it fails to elicit anxiety, indicating that the counter-conditioning has been successful. This process is repeated while working through all of the situations in the hierarchy.

Several studies and reviews have demonstrated the beneficial effects of systematic desensitisation in the treatment of ANV (Figueroa-Moseley *et al.*, 2007; Gude, 2011; Roscoe *et al.*, 2010). In one particular study, 60 patients who developed ANV while undergoing cancer-related chemotherapy were randomly assigned to receive systematic desensitisation, counselling or no intervention. It was discovered that the frequency and severity of ANV decreased significantly in the group of desensitised patients compared to patients assigned to the other two conditions (Morrow and Morrell, 1982).

Think about this

How could you use systematic desensitisation in those with a phobia?

Another method based on the principles of classical conditioning (as well as operant conditioning and reinforcement) that has been found to reduce ANV in cancer-related chemotherapy patients is **biofeedback**. In biofeedback training, patients learn to control a specific physiological response (e.g. blood pressure) by receiving information about moment-to-moment changes in that response (Inman, 2010). Burish *et al.* (1981) found that when combined with **progressive muscle relaxation training** (PMRT) biofeedback proved fruitful in reducing anticipatory nausea.

Key message

Classical conditioning can explain some physiological reactions to physical stimuli.

Quick check

Explain the following terms:

✦ extinction

✦ systematic desensitisation

✦ stimulus generalisation.

2.7 Operant conditioning

Operant conditioning (sometimes called instrumental learning) was first studied by American psychologist Edward Thorndike in the late 1800s. Thorndike's experimental procedure typically involved confining a hungry cat to a puzzle box from which it could escape and obtain food only by performing a specific behaviour, i.e. operating a latch on the puzzle box door. Each time the cat escaped and ate the food, it was returned to the box and the whole process was repeated. At first the cat struggled to get out, behaving aimlessly until by accident it tripped the latch and managed to escape. However, after repeated trials the cat took less and less time to operate the latch until eventually he had learned what he had to do to release himself. This led Thorndike to state his 'law of effect'. The **law of effect** states that behaviours (opening the latch) that lead to reward (food) tend to increase in strength, whereas those that lead to punishment tend to decrease in strength. This concept has continuously been altered and developed and continues to be examined within present research (Navakatikyan and Davison, 2010).

During the 1930s and 1940s, Thorndike's ideas were developed further by the American psychologist B.F. Skinner. Skinner's basic premise, much like Thorndike's, was that when behaviour was rewarded it would increase the frequency with which it would be displayed; subsequently behaviour which is unrewarded will decrease in frequency. Skinner also constructed a form of puzzle box known as the Skinner box; however, it was modified so that the food could be delivered automatically. This would allow for measurement of the rate of responding without the need to repeatedly handle the animal. For example, a rat was placed in a Perspex cage containing a lever or bar. If the lever was pressed a pellet of food was dispensed. At first the rat pressed the lever by accident, but soon learnt that there was a link between pressing the lever and obtaining the food. In these procedures, the response being conditioned (i.e. pressing the lever) is called the operant, because it operates on the environment. In turn the food reward is termed a **reinforcer** as it reinforces the likelihood of the behaviour occurring again. Although these studies focus predominantly on the conditioning of animals such as rats and cats, recent research has posited the link between previous animal studies and the potential positive outcomes on human conditioning (Castro and Wasserman, 2010).

Think about this

How can you use operant conditioning within your practice?

Quick check

What is a reinforcer?

2.8 Reinforcement and the token economy system

One of the key concepts derived from Skinner's exploration of operant conditioning was that of **reinforcement**. Wade and Tavris (2003: 241) define reinforcement as 'the process by which a stimulus or event strengthens or increases the probability of the response that it follows'. There are two types of reinforcement: positive reinforcement and negative reinforcement.

Differentiating between positive and negative reinforcement can be difficult and the necessity of the distinction is often debated. Positive reinforcement occurs when a particular behaviour results in the experience of something pleasurable, thus increasing the likelihood of the behaviour occurring again. For example, if every time you behaved in the way I wanted you to, I gave you a doughnut then you would repeat that behaviour (assuming you liked doughnuts). However, there are certain aspects you have to consider when attempting to use these forms of rewards (see Table 2.3).

Contrastingly, negative reinforcement occurs when, as the result of a particular behaviour, something unpleasant stops; this also increases the likelihood of the behaviour occurring again. For example, an individual who has depression or an anxiety-related disorder may strive to avoid situations that evoke anxiety or unpleasant feelings. The avoidance of anxiety or unpleasant feelings will therefore tend to reinforce the avoidance behaviour.

Operant conditioning describes how behaviour patterns develop through the consequences of a behaviour. An understanding of operant conditioning and the principles of reinforcement will enable the nurse to appreciate what is required in order to enhance or reduce particular patient behaviours. One of the first applications of operant conditioning in the clinical context involved the development of the token economy system. The token economy system is a form of behaviour modification that was often used in psychiatric hospitals to

Table 2.3 Use of rewards

Aspect	Comment
Timing	The sooner the reward is given after the behaviour the better.
Nature	The reward can be physical (e.g. doughnut, money) or emotional (e.g. smile, praise).
Appropriateness	Ensure that rewards are appropriate – giving an overweight person a doughnut if they had lost 2 kilos would not be sensible.
Schedules of reinforcement	Continuous reinforcement (i.e. every time you do something you get the reward) leads to quicker learning. Partial reinforcement (i.e. rewards for completing the behaviour are given only part of the time) is learned more slowly but lasts longer.

manage the behaviour of individuals who might be aggressive or unpredictable (Scanlan, 2009). The system was based on selective positive reinforcement, whereby patients are rewarded with tokens for behaving in an appropriate way; inappropriate behaviour is not rewarded. These tokens can later be exchanged for various privileges (e.g. time watching television or cigarettes). Initially tokens are awarded often and in higher amounts, but as individuals learn the appropriate behaviour, opportunities to earn tokens decrease. The amount and frequency of token dispensing is termed a **reinforcement schedule**. Paul and Lentz (1977) carried out a classic study using token economies with long-term hospitalised patients with **schizophrenia**. Researchers found that as a result of the intervention patients developed various social and work-related skills, they were able to take better care of themselves and their symptoms reduced. Remarkably this also coincided with a substantial reduction in the number of drugs being administered to patients. As a result the token economy system has been recommended within mental health psychiatric units (Lin *et al.*, 2006).

Think about this

How would you use reinforcers with the following individuals:

+ a person with learning disability being taught cooking skills
+ a person with substance misuse
+ a person with diabetes
+ a person with poor adherence to treatment
+ a colleague who is always late for their shift?

Quick check

What are the key principles with the use of rewards?

2.9 Evaluation of the behaviourist approach

A large number of successful applications relevant to nursing practice have derived from the behaviourist approach, i.e. behavioural therapy (see Tai and Turkington, 2009; Hoffman *et al.*, 2010) and behaviour modification (see Soderlund, 2009; Joubert *et al.*, 2009). In contrast to other psychological approaches, the focus is very much on the patient's behavioural symptoms rather than on the underlying causes of the behaviour itself. This is one of the central criticisms of the behaviourist approach.

Generally speaking the behaviourist approach is grossly oversimplified and mechanistic (machine-like). It de-emphasises the influence of knowledge, motivation, subjective experience and emotion, denies the role of innate factors (i.e. the *tabula rasa* view of mind) and excludes the role of cognition (Gross, 2010). It is a reductionist approach in that it reduces complex human behaviour to stimulus response associations and is deterministic to the extent that behaviour is seen as being determined by the environment.

There are ethical problems associated with some forms of treatment based on the behavioural model. For example, most forms of treatment focus solely on behaviour modification and it could be argued that it is dehumanising to neglect patients' internal experiences and feelings. It is also important to reflect on the fact that behaviourist principles are used to control others; this can be seen with the use of token economy systems in psychiatric institutions. Thus therapies derived from the behavioural model can be seen as manipulative.

In spite of the criticisms levelled at the behaviourist approach, an understanding of behaviourist theories and associated behaviour modification techniques can help the nurse to understand and discourage maladaptive behaviours (Stayt, 2011).

Key message

Behavioural approaches to some treatment conditions can be viewed as being manipulative – for example, eating disorders.

Strengths and weaknesses of the behaviourist approach

Strengths

+ Scientific.
+ Emphasises objective measurement.
+ Large number of successful applications (e.g. therapy).

Weaknesses

+ Mechanistic.
+ Reduces complex human behaviour to stimulus response associations.
+ Environmental determinism.
+ De-emphasises the influence of knowledge, motivation, subjective experience and emotions; denies the role of innate factors and excludes the role of cognition.
+ Oversimplified.
+ Therapies derived from the behaviourist approach can be seen as manipulative and unethical.

Think about this

How do the behaviourist and psychodynamic approaches differ?

2.10 Social learning theory

So to recap on the two approaches we have had so far – one has been based on the iceberg of the unconscious and the other on the environment to the exclusion of the 'mind', with the latter being a response to the former (perhaps an over-response?). It is now generally accepted that the behaviourist approach is grossly oversimplified and that it is unlikely that behaviour is solely determined by situational factors. A major alternative to the 'orthodox' learning theories proposed by behaviourism comes from **social learning theory** (SLT).

SLT originated in the USA in the 1940s and 1950s. It is a neo-behaviourist (new behaviourist) approach because it still largely emphasises the role of learning as a way of explaining behaviour. However, a central difference between orthodox learning theories and SLT is the introduction of mental states. Although social learning theorists agree that we should only study what is observable, they also believe that there are important cognitive variables which mediate between stimulus and response, without which we cannot adequately explain behaviour. These cognitive variables cannot be directly observed but can only be inferred from the observation of behaviour. Hence, it is a development of behaviourism rather than an over-reaction to it.

While social learning theorists do not deny the importance of classical and operant conditioning, they do think that these processes provide an inadequate account for the development of novel behaviours.

Assumptions of social learning theory

✦ All behaviour is learned.
✦ Classical and operant conditioning cannot adequately account for all human behaviour.
✦ Cognitive variables mediate between stimulus and response.
✦ Cognitive variables or mental states cannot be directly observed, only inferred from observing actual behaviour.

Quick check

What are the key principles of social learning theory?

2.11 Rotter's theory

The first major theory of social learning was put forward by Julian Rotter (1954) who suggested that when we are reinforced for a particular behaviour, this increases our *expectancy* (or belief) that the behaviour will achieve the same outcome again in the future; for example, when we are rewarded for a particular behaviour this increases our expectancy that the behaviour will be rewarded in the future. Thus expectancies are formed on the basis of past experience. It is important to note, however, that expectancy is subjective. There may be no relationship between the individual's assessment of how likely a reinforcement will be and the actual objective probability of it occurring. People can either over- or underestimate this likelihood, and both distortions can be problematic (Mearns, 2008).

Key message

Expectancies play a key part in reinforcing our behaviour.

If people have low expectancies, they do not believe their behaviours will be reinforced – so if a person believes their increase in physical activity will not be reinforced by their colleagues then this will impact on the subsequent likelihood of undertaking that behaviour. Consequently they put little effort into their behaviours and are therefore more likely to fail. When they do, it confirms their low expectancies, creating a vicious cycle. When patients have low expectancies, the nurse should endeavour to increase the patient's confidence by helping them to gain insight into the irrationality of their expectancies and/or attempt behaviours they have been avoiding out of fear of failure (Mearns, 2008; Francis *et al.*, 2010).

Think about this

How can you, the nurse, increase an individual's expectancies about:

+ quitting smoking
+ improving their diet
+ being able to take their medication successfully?

Another important concept is the notion of **reinforcement value** - the extent to which we prefer one reinforcer over another when the probability of obtaining each reinforcer is equal. For instance, desirable reinforcers, things we want to happen, or we are attracted to, have a high reinforcement value, whereas undesirable reinforcers, things we wish to avoid, have a low reinforcement value. According to Rotter (1954), an individual may devote a great deal of time and effort to achieving a particular goal because they attach considerable reinforcement value to it. As with expectancy, reinforcement value is subjective, meaning that the same reinforcer can differ vastly in desirability, depending on the individual's life experience (Mearns, 2008). If people set unrealistic or unobtainable goals for themselves, they are likely to experience frequent failure, triggering the development of the vicious cycle described above. In this situation the nurse would help the patient to set realistic, achievable goals – 'it is better to strive step by step, to achieve a series of goals than it is to set one distant, lofty goal for oneself' (Mearns, 2008: 4).

Key message

Realistic goals identified as achievable are extremely useful in reaching larger goals.

> ## Think about this
>
> Using the concept of a series of goals rather than a 'distant, lofty goal' how would you now approach helping a patient:
>
> + quit smoking
> + improve their diet
> + take their medication successfully?

In the mid-1960s Rotter extended his approach, arguing that some people believe that they have an enormous amount of personal control over the rewards and punishments they receive, while others believe that they have little or no control over what happens to them. Rotter (1966) devised a **locus of control** (LoC) scale to measure these differences. According to Rotter, those who believe that what happens to them depends on their own actions have an **internal LoC**, whereas those who feel that they have little control or that things simply occur by chance or by the actions of powerful agents have an **external LoC**.

2.12 Health locus of control

The concept of LoC was further developed by Wallston and Wallston (1982) who specifically applied it to the area of health; the notion being that those individuals with an internal **health LoC** (HLoC) would be more likely to behave in a health protective manner than those with an external HLoC. Why? Those with an internal HLoC believe that what happens to them depends on their own behaviour and are therefore more likely to take action (e.g. starting an exercise programme or engaging in self-screening behaviours). In contrast, those with an external HLoC believe that what happens to them is beyond their control, down to genetics, fate or God's will and are therefore not convinced that their behaviour will affect their later physical health.

Wallston and Wallston (1982) developed a measure of HLoC. This measure categorised people into one of three types:

+ **Internal,** if an individual regards their health as controllable by them (e.g. 'I am directly responsible for my health').
+ **External,** if an individual believes their health is not controllable by them and is in the hands of fate (e.g. 'whether I am well or not is a matter of luck').
+ **Powerful others**, if an individual regards their heath as under the control of powerful others (e.g. 'I can only do what my doctor tells me to do').

If individuals do not value their health, it is thought that they are unlikely to engage in health protective behaviour (even if they feel they have control over their health), because their health is not a high priority.

It should be obvious that people with different types of locus of control will act in a different manner. For example, it could reasonably be expected that those individuals with an internal HLoC, or a powerful other HLoC, are more likely to behave in a health protective manner compared to those with an external HLoC. Combes and Feral (2010) examined the

HLoC with drug compliance with schizophrenics; finding that the more patients believed their schizophrenia could be controlled by themselves and/or doctors, the more they followed their prescriptions than those who had an external HLoC. However, of course, what action this takes may differ – those with a high internal LoC would be more likely to take their own action, for example starting an exercise programme at the gym. In contrast, somebody with a powerful other HLoC would be more likely to go to a local health clinic and get some diet advice. This type of person would be more likely to seek advice, direction and 'cures' from medical and healthcare practitioners. Those with an external LoC would suggest it was not under their control or was due to other factors such as fate, genetics or God's will (Johnson et al., 2009).

Key message

Health locus of control can influence a person's reaction to health messages.

Norman and Bennett (1995) argue that HLoC is better at predicting health-related behaviour if studied in conjunction with **health value** (i.e. the value people attach to their health). Indeed, Weiss and Larsen (1990) found an increased relationship between internal HLoC and health when the health value was taken into account.

To conclude, Rotter showed that orthodox learning theories could be extended and improved by adding various cognitive processes (e.g. expectancies and reinforcement value).

Think about this

Looking back at the case study, what HLoC does Gary have?

How would a person with internal, external or powerful others HLoC react to the following:

+ a health promotion message to go for breast screening
+ a nursing command to stop smoking
+ some advice to 'lose some weight'
+ an article read in the newspaper?

2.13 Bandura's theory

Rotter's general approach was taken much further by Albert Bandura who tried to reinterpret Freud's concept of identification in terms of conditioning processes. More specifically, he endeavoured to make the concept more 'scientific' by studying it in the laboratory in the form of imitation.

According to this approach, learning can take place both directly through traditional conditioning processes (i.e. classical and operant conditioning) and indirectly through observation. **Observational learning** was first demonstrated by Bandura *et al*. (1961) in the famous Bobo doll experiment. During the experiment children sat and watched a film in which an adult model punched and kicked a large inflated Bobo doll which bounced back every time it was hit. After 10 minutes the children were moved to another room, where there were some toys, together with a Bobo doll. Once in the room they were left to play, during which time they were observed through a one-way mirror. Children who had watched the adult model were violent in their play and imitated some of the behaviours they had observed in the film (see Figure 2.3). In comparison, children who had watched no model or had watched an adult model behave in a non-aggressive manner were non-aggressive in their play activities.

Key message

We learn by observing others.

What Bandura's experiment shows is that observational learning can take place without any reinforcement; mere exposure is sufficient for learning to take place. However, whether this learning actually translates into behaviour depends largely upon the consequences of that behaviour. This was demonstrated by Bandura (1965) in his investigation of **vicarious reinforcement**.

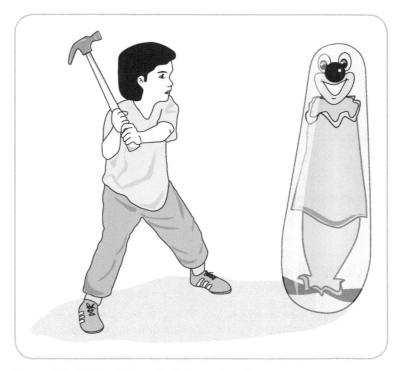

Figure 2.3 Child and the Bobo doll experiment

Vicarious reinforcement occurs when another person is observed to be rewarded for a particular action, thus increasing the likelihood that the observer will imitate that action. Bandura (1965) carried out another study in which young children watched a short film of an adult model behaving aggressively toward a Bobo doll. Group 1 saw a film in which the model kicked and punched a Bobo doll; group 2 saw the same film, but this time the model was rewarded for his behaviour; and group 3 watched the same film, but the model was punished and warned not to be aggressive in the future. The children were then allowed to play with the Bobo doll. Those children who had seen the model rewarded exhibited the most aggression, whereas those children who had seen the model punished exhibited the least aggression. Bandura wondered whether these group differences in overt behaviour were matched by differences in learning. Accordingly, he rewarded all the children for imitating as much of the model's aggressive behaviour as they could remember. All three groups demonstrated comparable levels of observational learning; however, those who had seen the model rewarded were most likely to apply this learning to their own behaviour. Recent research exploring the effects of vicarious reinforcement is supportive of the effects discovered by Bandura (Fox and Bailenson, 2009).

Think about this

How would vicarious learning occur within the healthcare setting? Try to think of both physical and mental health examples.

Bandura's SLT explores how individuals learn from observing and imitating others around them; it also provides a cognitive explanation of why phobias run in families. For example, Ost and Hugdahl (1985) report that 12 per cent of adults with a dental phobia can trace their fear back to a vicarious experience in their past (a figure confirmed by Coelho and Purkis, 2009). Further research has demonstrated the effects of social learning in the acquisition of dental anxiety in children. Townsend *et al.* (2000) found that mothers of anxious children were significantly more anxious than mothers of non-anxious children, suggesting that children are vicariously developing dental anxiety through observing the behaviour of their parents.

Many interventions have drawn upon the principles of observational learning, especially for those patients who may have a particular fear that becomes a barrier to the care that they are receiving. Melamed *et al.* (1975) provide an example in which children were instructed to sit through a 13-minute film of a four-year-old coping with a typical dental visit. The children who had watched the film of the young boy coping with the visit received lower ratings of anxiety by independent raters and dentists in comparison with children who were shown an unrelated film; they were also more cooperative with the dentist and showed fewer disruptive behaviours. The principles of observational learning and imitation are equally applicable to student nurses. According to Pearcy and Elliot (2004), students' learning is directly affected by their observations of practitioners and it is only via observing that students are able to develop specific skills. In fact there is evidence to suggest that role modelling in the clinical workplace can be one of the most important parts of early nurse education, although it is often underused (Murray and Main, 2005). Furthermore, recent research has explored the positive impact of internet-based observational learning for health professionals (Cook *et al.*, 2010).

Think about this

Looking back at the case study, can Bandura's theory relate to Jack's behaviours?

How can the nurse use modelling in their practice? Think about it in terms of:

+ preparing a patient for surgery
+ working with an adult with learning disabilities to go shopping
+ dealing with an aggressive patient
+ working with children with diabetes requiring daily injections.

Key message

We can model good health behaviour that will result in positive change.

2.14 Self-efficacy

An overarching concept in SLT is **self-efficacy** – an individual's expectation about their capacity to succeed in a particular task. For example, an overweight man who feels that he should do more exercise but has very little confidence that he will be able to do so would be said to have low self-efficacy. In contrast, a woman who is motivated to attend for cervical screening and feels confident that she can do so would be said to have high self-efficacy. Self-efficacy judgements are not concerned with the skills one has, but with the judgements of what one can do with the skills one possesses (Bandura, 1977a). Thus the main aim of SLT is to build on self-efficacy, i.e. to enhance the individual's perception of their capacity to succeed.

According to Bandura (1977b), expectations of personal efficacy in any given situation are based on four major sources of information: performance accomplishments, vicarious experience, verbal persuasion and emotional arousal. The impact of this information on efficacy expectations will depend on how it is cognitively appraised.

+ **Performance accomplishments:** are based on previous experiences of success and/or failure in a given situation. Success raises efficacy expectations, while repeated failures lower them. Once established, enhanced self-efficacy tends to generalise to other situations, although generalisation effects most often occur when activities are similar to those in which self-efficacy was established.

+ **Vicarious experience:** many expectations of personal efficacy are derived from vicarious experience. Observing others cope successfully or unsuccessfully in a given situation can generate expectations in observers that they too will succeed or fail if they persist in their efforts.

+ **Verbal (social) persuasion:** self-efficacy may increase if an individual is led to believe, through suggestion, that they have the skills required to succeed in a particular situation.

✦ **Emotional arousal:** high levels of arousal are often associated with stressful and taxing situations, and depending on the circumstances may have informative value concerning personal competency. Because high arousal usually hampers performance, individuals are more likely to expect failure if they are tense and emotionally agitated.

Understanding the concept of self-efficacy is important for the nurse as it can determine (among other things) the initiation of health behaviours (Bandura, 2000). It can also enable the nurse to understand a patient's motivation to follow through with goals that become challenging (Gatchel *et al.*, 2007), adherence to medical advice and/or treatment and the successful (or unsuccessful) management of chronic pain (Oliver and Ryan, 2004). Self-efficacy is not just an important determinant of health behaviour but has been shown to be amenable to change; for this reason self-efficacy as a construct has a vital role to play in behaviour modification programmes and patient management (see Luszczynska *et al.*, 2009; Gwaltney *et al.*, 2009).

Key message

Self-efficacy is an important determinant of health behaviour.

Quick check

What are the four major sources of information that change personal efficacy?

2.15 Evaluation of social learning theory

Although relatively overlooked by other theorists, Bandura's research on observational learning and modelling has been very influential. There is no doubt that observation is important in the acquisition of behaviour; however, Bandura has exaggerated this somewhat. It could also be argued that Bandura's experiments lack ecological validity; there is also the problem of **demand characteristics** as Bandura's experiment almost 'invited' participants to behave in predictable ways. Durkin (1995: 406) pointed out: 'Where else in life does a five-year-old find a powerful adult actually showing you how to knock the hell out of a dummy and then giving you the opportunity to try it out yourself?'

On a more general note, SLT has had a considerable impact on nursing and health practice, with major applications in nurse education, patient empowerment, self-management and expert patient programmes (Perry, 2009; Livsey, 2009). Unlike the other approaches presented in this chapter, SLT clearly illustrates how behavioural, cognitive and environmental factors interact. However, the biological reality underlying cognition and behaviour has been largely ignored, not to mention factors such as emotion and personality. Nonetheless, SLT can account for cultural and individual variation in behaviour; it can also explain why we behave in a particular manner in one situation but not in others, namely **context-dependent learning**. Finally, SLT can be considered a bridge or transition between behaviourist and cognitive theories. Within the next section we will discuss the apparent cognitive explanations of human behaviour.

Strengths and weaknesses of social learning theory

Strengths

✦ Considerable impact on nursing and health practice.

✦ Numerous applications.

✦ Illustrates how behavioural, cognitive and environmental factors interact.

✦ Can account for cultural and individual variations in behaviour as well as context-dependent learning.

✦ Can be considered a bridge or transition between behaviourist and cognitive approaches.

Weaknesses

✦ Ignores biological factors underlying cognition and behaviour.

✦ Does not consider the role of emotion or personality.

✦ Observers do not always show strong tendencies to imitate the behaviour of a model.

✦ Bandura's experiments have low ecological validity and high demand characteristics.

Think about this

Self-efficacy is of key importance in health behaviour and behaviour change. How can you, as a nurse, increase self-efficacy?

2.16 Cognitive psychology

Cognitive psychology first emerged in the late 1950s, a period often referred to as the '**cognitive revolution**', and grew in part out of increasing dissatisfaction with behaviourist explanations. Cognitive psychology is concerned with human thought processes and the ways in which these processes interact with behaviour (Eysenck and Keane, 2010). There are many facets of cognitive psychology but some of the major areas include memory, learning, intelligence, thinking and language. Like behaviourism it too rejects introspection as a valid method of investigation and maintains that the only true source of knowledge is that which is obtained through observation and experiment (Eysenck and Keane, 2010). Yet somewhat incongruous to this is the fact that it explicitly acknowledges the existence of unobservable mental processes. Although there have been many contributors to cognitive psychology, no specific person can be identified as central to its development. What is more, unlike other approaches cognitive psychology does not yet have a unifying theory.

Assumptions of the cognitive approach

✦ Acknowledges the existence of unobservable mental processes and emphasises their importance in determining and predicting behaviour.

✦ Accepts empiricist ideas and use of the scientific method.

✦ Is based mainly on laboratory experiments.

✦ Views the mind as an information processor, i.e. it computes answers to problems in a manner analogous to a computer.

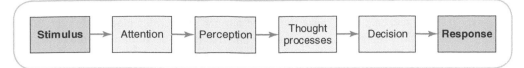

Figure 2.4 Information processing model

Information processing

Psychologists have often tried to understand human **cognition** by comparing it with something less abstract and better understood. Hence the advent of the modern digital computer provided psychologists with an ideal metaphor for conceptualising how the mind worked and inspired what is now the main **paradigm** within cognitive psychology: the **information processing approach** (e.g. Forgas and Jennifer, 2001). According to this approach, the mind is analogous to an information processing system: inputting, storing and retrieving data. This system is used in flexible ways to handle all kinds of cognitive tasks, from reading the newspaper to playing a game of chess. An early version of the information processing approach is shown in Figure 2.4. According to the model, external stimuli are attended to, perceived and then various thought processes are applied to them. Finally a decision is made as to what to do with the stimuli and an appropriate response is produced.

The greatest value of the information processing approach is that it identifies the structures and processes involved in cognition. However, the approach is limited in several ways. First, evidence for the information processing approach is largely based on experiments under controlled, scientific conditions; yet most laboratory experiments are artificial and could be said to lack **ecological validity**. Second, although the information processing approach identifies the structures and processes involved in human cognition, it rarely specifies how individuals acquire those processes. You will find the information processing approach discussed further in Chapter 5.

Schemas

The concept of **schema** is perhaps one of the most important contributions made by cognitive psychology. A schema is a cognitive structure that contains knowledge about a thing, its attributes and the relations among its attributes (Fiske and Taylor, 1991). It guides individuals and influences how they perceive and interpret events around them, providing the basic building block of our cognitive processes.

When we receive information we locate it within a schema (Launder *et al.*, 2005). This saves time and energy through the use of an already established knowledge base. There are many different kinds of schema; for example, schemas about events are called **scripts** and thus guide us when we are performing commonplace activities such as shopping or going to the cinema. **Role schemas** tell us about different roles and how particular groups of people are likely to behave; this would include a schema for a nurse or midwife, or simply a male or female (e.g. Bornstein, 2010). Role schemas also include our expectations about social groups and can result in **stereotyping** (see Chapter 4); **self-schemas** embody our self-concept.

Quick check

What are schemas and scripts?

Schemas are socially determined and derived from our past experiences. They allow us to form expectations and help us to make the world a more predictable place. However, schemas do not necessarily represent reality; thus we can use the concept of a schema to explain negative thought patterns or irrational beliefs which are maladaptive to a patient's health and well-being. According to the renowned counsellor and psychotherapist Aaron Beck, some individuals develop self-defeating attitudes as children. Such attitudes often result from past experiences, family relationships or the judgements of others around them. These maladaptive attitudes ultimately develop into schemas against which the child evaluates every experience. The negative schemas of these persons may lie dormant for years. But later in life, upsetting situations such as prolonged stress, illness or hospitalisation can trigger an extended round of negative thinking. Any situation where the patient has negative thoughts or holds beliefs or schemata that are irrational and maladaptive to their health requires the nurse to challenge such beliefs.

Key message

Some people have irrational or illogical beliefs – CBT can help change these.

2.17 Cognitive behavioural therapy

Cognitive behavioural therapy (CBT) combines both cognitive and behavioural principles. The cognitive aspect concentrates on modifying or replacing irrational beliefs or thought processes associated with self-destructive patterns of behaviour, while the behavioural aspect concentrates on modifying or replacing maladaptive behaviours. CBT is a short-term structured approach which can be implemented individually, within a group (Salehzadeh et al., 2011), or on a computer-based programme (Khanna and Kendall, 2010), all of which have been shown to be effective. CBT has been shown to help with many different types of disorders, including: anxiety, depression, stress, bipolar disorder, bulimia, obsessive compulsive disorder, post-traumatic stress disorder and psychosis. However, CBT is most often recommended with disorders and illnesses that encompass anxiety and depression (Anderson et al., 2008; Curran et al., 2006; Stallard et al., 2011). Most cognitive behavioural experts recommend that CBT is only used by those who have undergone an accredited diploma in CBT (Oldham, 2007); however, nurses will often find that they need to identify triggering factors for particular behaviours and for this purpose the CBT framework is particularly effective.

Key message

CBT is a key treatment modality in mental health practice.

The ABC model

The **ABC model** (Ellis, 1962) (also see Chapter 9) is from the **rational emotive** [therapy] component of **cognitive behavioural therapy** and provides a framework that nurses can work within when challenging a patient's negative schemata. Within this framework the nurse will endeavour to change the mental script of the patient so that new ways of thinking will result in behaviour change. The ABC model will encourage the patient to explore the causative factors of their current thinking and to consider the implications of their behaviour. As a result, alternative perspectives that do not result in negative consequences for the patient's health will be sought. Each letter in the ABC model represents a stage, the application of which is as follows (Gates, 2007):

A. **Activating event** – this could be some action or attitude of an individual or an actual physical event. The patient, with the help of the nurse, could explore triggering factors in this initial stage, which impact upon current behaviour.

B. **Beliefs about the event** – this involves the exploration of irrational beliefs.

C. **Consequence** – this involves exploring the emotional or behavioural consequences of unhealthy negative beliefs or schemata.

D. **Disputing** – the nurse will dispute the cognitive, emotional and behavioural aspects of the patient's current belief system.

Patients can receive many benefits when the ABC model is applied.

1. It acts as a catalyst for the patient to reflect on their thinking and to relate their emotional experiences to behavioural reactions.

2. It allows the patient to go through a process of self-analysis and self-discovery.

3. It helps the patient understand that people are not disturbed by things or events but by the views they take of them.

4. It helps the patient understand that there are different ways of seeing the same event and thus helps develop alternative ways of thinking.

5. Once patients have been educated about the ABC concept, they often report feeling a sense of hope and control (Lam and Gale, 2000). Finally, patients can apply the principles of the ABC model to challenge negative or irrational beliefs outside professional healthcare.

Although the ABC model is most often applied within mental health settings, it may also be helpful to those individuals who:

+ hold irrational beliefs
+ distort reality
+ have faulty cognition
+ engage in black and white or all or nothing thinking
+ over-generalise
+ feel they have no control over their lives
+ engage in emotional reasoning
+ feel a sense of hopelessness or **learned helplessness**.

Think about this ?

Where could you use the cognitive behavioural approach? How could you use it within your own practice?

Would you advise Mabel to have cognitive behavioural therapy, and if so, why?

Evaluation of the cognitive approach

The cognitive approach has broad appeal and has become very influential in recent years. It focuses on the way that mental or cognitive processes work and the ways in which these processes interact with behaviour. Any explanation that incorporates mental concepts is essentially using a cognitive perspective. What is more, it combines easily with other approaches to produce, for example, social learning theory.

The cognitive approach grew out of discontent with the behaviourist model and its focus on environmental factors; the irony is that cognitive psychology today is rather similar to behaviourism in that it excludes certain other internal factors such as motivation and emotion (Eysenck and Flanagan, 2007; Eysenck and Keane, 2010). For this reason the cognitive approach has been described as overly reductionist and deterministic. It has also been described as mechanistic because cognitive explanations themselves are based on the 'behaviour' of machines.

Much of the research in cognitive psychology is experimental and conducted in laboratories. Some would argue that laboratory experiments create an artificial environment and that subsequent results have low ecological validity. Nevertheless, there are many successful 'real world' applications of cognitive psychology relevant to nursing and health practice, ranging from suggestions about how to improve communication and information giving, to how theories of perception promote holistic care (see Chapter 5).

Strengths and weaknesses of the cognitive approach

Strengths

✦ Scientific.

✦ Large number of successful applications.

✦ Focuses on processes unique to human beings (i.e. thought).

✦ Combines easily with approaches, e.g. cognitive behavioural therapy.

✦ Many empirical studies to support theories.

Weaknesses

✦ Mechanistic.

✦ Lacks human element, i.e. ignores social factors and the role of emotion.

✦ Research on which cognitive explanations are based is rather artificial.

✦ Ignores biology (e.g. hormones).

2.18 Humanistic psychology

Humanistic psychology emerged in the 1950s as a reaction to the dominant paradigms in psychology – namely the behaviourist and psychodynamic approaches. Thus it was said to be the 'third force' in psychology by one of its founding members, Abraham Maslow (1970). Humanist psychologists considered psychoanalysis to be too pessimistic due to its emphasis on pathological, irrational and unconscious fragmentation aspects of personality. Additionally, behaviourism was rejected due to its mechanistic underpinnings and approach to understanding the human condition.

The humanistic approach strives to provide a more holistic vision of both psychology and the person. It has roots in **existentialist** thought which holds that human beings have free will and freedom of choice (**personal agency** is the humanistic term for exercising free will). It is further assumed that people are basically good in nature and have an innate need to grow, develop and achieve their full potential; this has been captured by the term **self-actualisation** which will be discussed later. Thus the subjective, conscious experience of the individual is of primary interest; humans are not simply objects of study but must be described and understood in terms of their own subjective views of the world, their perceptions of self and their feelings of self-worth.

Key message

Humanistic psychology is the third force in psychology.

Consequently, humanistic psychology focuses on issues that are uniquely human such as health, hope, love, creativity, individuality and meaning – in a nutshell, the personal nature of human experience. The major proponents of this approach are Abraham Maslow and Carl Rogers.

The five main principles that underpin humanistic psychology

✦ Human beings cannot be reduced to components.

✦ Human beings have in them a uniquely human context.

✦ Human consciousness includes an awareness of oneself in the context of other people.

✦ Human beings have choices and responsibilities.

✦ Human beings are intentional; they seek meaning, value and creativity.

(Bugental, 1965)

Maslow's hierarchy of needs and motivations

According to Maslow, the primary cause of psychopathology is the failure to gratify one's fundamental needs. Maslow (1954) outlined these needs within his model (see Figure 2.5), which are presented in order from the most basic needs (deficiency drives) to higher level needs (growth drives). Both drives are leading the person to self-actualisation. Maslow argued that

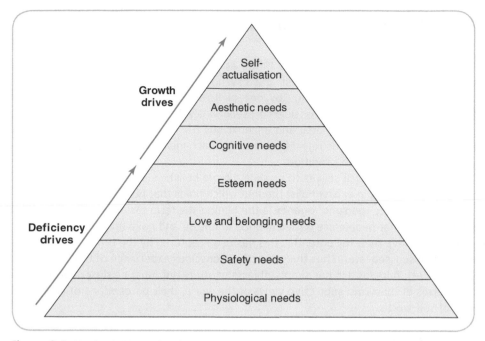

Figure 2.5 Maslow's hierarchy of needs

people have to work their way up from the bottom of the hierarchy to the top and that higher order needs cannot be met until lower order needs have been satisfied.

+ **Physiological needs:** is the first level of Maslow's hierarchy and encompasses the most basic physical needs of the human being (e.g. oxygen, water, protein, vitamins, minerals and so on).

+ **Safety needs:** when physiological needs have been satisfied, the need for safety and security comes into play. This level encompasses needs such as protection, stability and freedom from anxiety.

+ **Love and belonging needs:** when physiological and safety needs have been met, you begin to feel the need for friends, a partner, children, affectionate relationships in general and even a sense of community. In our day-to-day life these needs manifest themselves in our desire to marry, have a family or be part of a community, church or club. Failure to satisfy these needs can lead to feelings of loneliness and social anxiety.

+ **Esteem needs:** next we begin to look for self-esteem. Maslow distinguished between two levels of esteem needs. The lower level is the need for the respect of others, the need for status, recognition, appreciation and dignity. The higher level involves the need for self-respect and includes feelings of confidence, achievement, independence and freedom. Failure to satisfy these needs can result in low self-worth and inferiority complexes.

The levels discussed so far are deficiency drives. If you are lacking at any one level you feel deficient. According to Maslow, all these needs are survival needs; even love and esteem are needed for the maintenance of health. In terms of development, we move through these levels a bit like stages. For example, as newborns our focus is on physiological needs, i.e. feeding or having our nappy changed. Soon we begin to recognise that we need to be safe and secure, after which we crave love and affection; esteem needs soon follow. All of these deficiency drives are encountered within the first few years of life.

Under stressful conditions we can regress to a lower need level. For example, when we are ill we may seek food, liquids, sleep and attention. There is also the possibility of fixation at any of the four deficiency levels. For instance, if you face significant problems during your development, such as the loss of a family member through death or divorce or significant neglect or abuse, you may fixate on a particular set of needs for the rest of your life. This is how Maslow understands neurosis. When all of the deficiency drives have been satisfied, growth drives then come into play:

✦ **Cognitive needs:** these stem from the need for understanding and knowledge.

✦ **Aesthetic needs:** these include the need for order and beauty.

When cognitive and aesthetic needs have been satisfied the individual progresses to a higher state of psychological functioning. The highest need is referred to as the need for self-actualisation.

✦ **Self-actualisation:** a number of terms have been used to refer to this need level including growth motivation and being needs (or B-needs). These needs do not involve 'balance' but a continuous desire to fulfil potential; hence the term self-actualisation. Once these needs have been engaged they continue to be felt. This is in contrast to the lower order deficiency needs which surface when unmet. In order to self-actualise, lower order needs must be satisfied: when lower order needs are unmet, you cannot fully devote yourself to fulfilling your potential. It isn't surprising then that only a small percentage of the world's population is truly self-actualising.

Quick check

List the elements in Maslow's hierarchy.

It is important for the nurse to keep Maslow's hierarchy of needs in mind. This will act as a reminder that many basic needs have to be met before a patient can effectively manage their own state of health. This can also be applied to the nurse and their professional practice – in order for the nurse to work effectively, they should be aware of their own basic needs and ensure these are being met. If not, then the nurse should make this a workable target within their personal development. Many lifestyle behaviours such as smoking or excessive drinking are influenced by multiple internal and external factors. Simply stating that someone has to change will not motivate an individual to do so (Hunt and Pearson, 2001). Instead, motivation itself as outlined in Maslow's hierarchy may need to be addressed before initiating any proposed change.

2.19 Rogers' person-centred approach

By far the most significant practical contribution of any humanistic psychologist is Rogers' person-centred therapy (also known as non-directive therapy and client-centred therapy). At the heart of this approach is the basic trust in human beings and in the movement of every person towards constructive fulfilment of their possibilities. Rogers called this a person's 'actualising tendency'. Central to Rogers' theory is the notion of self-concept; the organised, consistent set of perceptions and beliefs about oneself (Rogers, 1959). It consists of the ideas and values that characterise the 'I' and the 'me' and includes perception and valuing of 'what I am' and 'what I can do'. Consequently, the self-concept influences both our perception of the world and perception of oneself. Rogers suggested that if a person's self-concept is close to their ideal self they will experience a high level of self-esteem. On the other hand, if there is very little match the person may experience psychological distress. When a client or patient's actual self and ideal self are distant, it is the role of the therapist or nurse to reverse this situation and help the client become a more fully functioning person.

Think about this

How can you use the person-centred approach in your practice? And would this be appropriate in Mabel's case?

Rogers believed very strongly that people are able to solve their own problems if they are given the opportunity and a supportive environment. He pointed to three core conditions which he described as 'necessary and sufficient' for therapeutic movement to occur. These core conditions are empathy, unconditional positive regard and congruence.

Key message

Empathy, unconditional positive regard and congruence are essential in humanistic psychology.

Empathy

Empathy is the ability to understand what the client is feeling. This refers to the therapist's or nurse's ability to understand sensitively and accurately (not sympathetically) the client's experience and feelings in the here and now (Webb, 2011).

Many studies have cited empathy as being crucial within any helping relationship. For example, Olsen (1997) examined the relationship between nurse-expressed empathy, patient-perceived empathy and patient distress. Seventy nurses and 70 patients from medical-surgical acute care units were involved in the study. Each nurse completed two measures of nurse-expressed empathy while each patient completed a measure of perceived empathy and distress. Researchers found negative relationships between nurse-expressed empathy and patient distress and between patient-perceived empathy and patient distress. A moderate positive relationship was found between nurse-expressed empathy and patient-perceived empathy, demonstrating that empathy is an important aspect of the nurse–patient relationship. Further support comes from Wilkin and Silvester (2007). Forty patients were interviewed and asked to recall a time when a nurse had shown empathy to them, how they did this and any outcomes. The same questions were asked for an occasion when a nurse had not shown empathy. As far as patients were concerned they regarded empathy as important to their recovery process, with one patient stating that engaging in personal conversations 'was the difference between feeing like you were going to die here or go home for Christmas'. Wilkin and Silvester concluded from their study that nurses lacking in empathy cause patients to suffer fear, confusion and depression, lower their confidence in the care provided and subsequently decrease their motivation to comply with treatment.

Sympathy and empathy – what is the difference?

Sympathy has been defined as 'a means to share another's emotions such as sorrow or anguish' (*Health and Age*, 2006). This differs from empathy, as when expressing sympathy the listener becomes emotionally involved. This can become a barrier to care as becoming emotionally involved may distort clear and measured thinking.

Unconditional positive regard

The next core condition is unconditional positive regard. Unconditional positive regard means that the counsellor (or nurse) must accept the client unconditionally and non-judgementally, irrespective of their illness, lifestyle or previous medical history (Webb, 2011). It is important that the client is free to explore all thoughts and feelings (good or bad) without danger of rejection or condemnation. Crucially, the client must be free to explore and express thoughts and feelings without having to meet any particular standards or 'earn' positive regard from the counsellor or nurse (Webb, 2011).

Unconditional positive regard should be expressed from the outset of the helping relationship, especially when the nurse may not agree with the patient's perspective. In order to display unconditional positive regard, the nurse should not express judgement or expectations towards the patient. In turn the patient will feel accepted and worthy and ready to initiate change (Webb, 2011).

Congruence

The final condition to initiate change is congruence: also called genuineness. According to Rogers, congruence is the most important attribute in counselling. Genuineness can be defined as 'the basic ability to be aware of inner experiences and to allow the quality of that inner experience to be apparent in relationships' (Rana and Upton, 2009). Thus the counsellor or nurse does not present a detached professional façade, but is present and transparent to the client. There is no air of authority and the client does not have to speculate what the counsellor or nurse is 'really' like.

In order for empathy and unconditional positive regard to be successful in initiating change, the patient has to perceive them as genuine feelings. If a patient does not perceive the nurse to be genuine, therapeutic change is less likely to occur. The nurse should be aware that congruence is expressed both verbally and non-verbally; thus self-awareness of one's own behaviour is paramount.

2.20 Evaluation of the humanistic approach

The three core conditions for therapeutic change described by Rogers are key to the understanding of patient-centred care. Likewise, the motivation model provided by Maslow is a useful framework that explores how patients can be motivated to initiate behavioural change.

According to Wilson *et al.* (1996), the humanistic approach isn't a comprehensive theory, but a collection of diverse theories that have similar underlying principles created by people optimistic about human potential. For this reason it has wide appeal to those who seek an alternative to the more mechanistic theories provided by the psychodynamic and behaviourist approaches. Related to this, humanistic psychology has been criticised because its theories are difficult to test empirically. Since humanistic psychology is descriptive rather than explanatory it is subject to what is known as the **nominal fallacy** (Carlson and Buskist, 1997) and so cannot really be called a theory. Humanistic psychology intuitively appeals as positive and optimistic (Henriques, 2011). However, Rogers and Maslow are criticised for having an overly optimistic and simplified view of human nature. Finally, a frequent criticism of the humanistic approach is that delivering the three core conditions proposed by Rogers is what all good counsellors and nurses do anyway. However, this criticism may reflect a misunderstanding of the real challenges of consistently providing the patient with empathy, unconditional positive regard and congruence.

In spite of its shortcomings, the humanistic approach has helped bring the 'person' back into psychology. It recognises that people determine their own behaviour and are not simply slaves to environmental contingencies or to their past (Gross and Kinnison, 2007). However, the greatest contribution of humanistic psychology may lie in its encouragement of humane and ethical treatment of persons, approaching psychology and healthcare as a human science rather than a natural science. Nonetheless, it is suggested that in order for us to understand human behaviour in a complete and multidimentional way it is imperative that researchers adopt a combination of psychological approaches (Henriques, 2011).

2.21 Conclusion

Contemporary psychology is a complex multidisciplinary subject characterised by a range of different approaches. Given their different assumptions the approaches are sometimes in conflict. Proponents of one approach often criticise the naïve interpretations and treatment efforts of others, yet no approach is complete in itself.

Each approach focuses mainly on one aspect of human functioning and none can explain all aspects of behaviour. Ultimately it is up to you, the nurse, to decide which approach makes best sense to you in the context of the situation you are faced with. According to Raudonis and Acton (1997: 138):

Theory provides nurses with a perspective with which to view client situations, a way to organise the hundreds of data bits encountered in the day-to-day care of clients, and a way to analyse and interpret the information. A theoretical perspective allows the nurse to plan and implement care purposefully and proactively. When nurses practise purposefully and systematically, they are more efficient, have better control over the outcomes of their care, and are better able to communicate with others.

Think about this again . . .

On the basis of the material presented here, why do people act in this way:

✦ yawn
✦ eat too much
✦ drink alcohol
✦ are short tempered
✦ don't follow your advice
✦ get depressed
✦ have phobias about spiders, needles or uniforms?

Research in Focus

Nilsson, T., Svensson, M., Sandell, R. and Clinton, D. (2007) Patients' experiences of change in cognitive behavioral therapy and psychodynamic therapy: a qualitative comparative study, *Psychotherapy Research* **17**(5), 553-566.

Background

Research suggests that different therapeutic approaches produce roughly the equivalent outcome despite their theoretical and technical differences. A number of hypotheses have been suggested as to why this may be. It may be that differences do exist in the effect of particular forms of treatment, but research methodology and effect measures have not been sufficiently sensitive to elucidate them. Another explanation, the common factors hypothesis, suggests that specific or unique ingredients matter less than the ingredients that are common or similar among the different forms. And finally another explanation, the interaction or matching hypothesis, suggests that different forms of psychotherapy vary in their degree of suitability for individual patients. It has been suggested that when researchers only test for main effects, ignoring the interaction between patient factors and types of psychotherapy, different treatments will appear to have equal mean effects. McLeod (2001) has consistently argued that qualitative research methods need to be used as a complement to conventional quantitative outcome studies. If this is not done, the full array of psychotherapy effects will not emerge, including the negative effects, side effects, and so on. Therefore this study was to qualitatively compare two theoretically distinct forms of psychotherapy: psychodynamic therapy (PDT) and cognitive behaviour therapy (CBT).

Methods

Participants: 31 patients who had terminated CBT or PDT were recruited.

Interviews: Semi-structured interviews about the patients' experiences of change during psychotherapy were conduced; these lasted around 60 minutes. The interviews covered six specific domains, with equal emphasis on the part of the interviewer: nature of change, course of change, therapist's methods, therapist and the therapeutic relationship, external influences on change, and patient's own contribution to change.

Results

Common experiences among satisfied patients: General experience was that therapy helped in the long term. Specifically in helping patients find new coping tools, feeling less anxious.

Satisfied PDT patients: The most distinctive change was that patients could understand themselves better than before.

Satisfied CBT patients: The most distinctive change was that the patients now regained a feeling of being a normal person and being able to cope with difficult situations.

Differences between the satisfied CBT and PDT patients: The treatment results were not as immediately obvious to the PDT patient as to the CBT patient. Nevertheless,

→

both CBT and PDT patients continue to improve after termination, albeit in clearly different ways. The CBT patient became gradually more capable of applying new coping methods and the PDT patient continued to use self-reflection in coping with new experiences.

Common experiences among dissatisfied patients: Therapy only had an insufficient change and the termination was too abrupt.

Dissatisfied PTD patients: Patients had a feeling of frustration and feeling lost, and felt that the change was not good enough.

Dissatisfied CBT patients: The CBT patients felt that there was really no change or that the therapy had only helped in the short term.

Differences between the dissatisfied CBT and PDT patients: Both patients experienced major problems in their relations to the therapists, but in different ways: CBT patients considered the therapist to be intrusive and oppressive; PDT patients felt the therapist was withdrawn, disengaged. The CBT patients were very disappointed and negative whereas the PDT patients were ambivalent.

Implications

Dissatisfied patients should be identified and asked about the reasons for their feeling and advised to try some other type of psychotherapy or another therapist who may better meet their needs and complaints.

2.22 Summary

+ Psychological approaches to the person attempt to explain why people behave in a certain manner.

+ Understanding the person requires an appreciation of a number of psychological perspectives.

+ The psychodynamic approach explores how the unconscious mind is responsible for behaviour.

+ Freud's psychoanalytic approach suggests behaviour is a result of an interaction between innate drives and early experiences in childhood.

+ According to Freud, the mind has three levels: the conscious, pre-conscious and unconscious.

+ Freud also assumed that the mind could be divided into three basic sections the id (innate), ego (reality) and superego (morals).

+ The ego protects itself by a number of defence mechanisms.

+ Freud's ideas have fallen out of favour or have been adapted to incorporate more social rather than sexual influences.

+ A criticism of Freudian and other psychodynamic theories is that they do not translate into measurable observations and are therefore untestable.

+ According to behaviourists, all behaviour is learnt from the environment (to the near exclusion of innate or inherited factors).

✦ Early behaviourist theories suggest that learning and behaviour are the result of conditioning (classical or operant).

✦ The focus of the behavioural approach is on the patient's behavioural symptoms rather than on the underlying causes of the behaviour itself.

✦ Social learning theorists suggest we should only study what is observable, but believe that there are important cognitive variables that mediate between stimulus and response.

✦ Expectancies and realistic goals are useful in setting and reaching large goals.

✦ Health locus of control impacts on an individual's behaviour and response to health messages.

✦ According to Bandura, we learn by observing others and through vicarious learning.

✦ Good health behaviour can be modelled by health professionals and will result in positive change.

✦ An important concept is self-efficacy: an individual's expectations about their capacity to succeed on a particular task.

✦ Cognitive psychology is concerned with human thought processes and the ways in which these processes interact with behaviour.

✦ The concepts of schema and scripts are some of the most important contributions made by cognitive psychology.

✦ Cognitive behavioural therapy is often recommended with disorders and illnesses that encompass anxiety and depression.

✦ The humanistic approach strives to provide a more holistic vision of both psychology and the person.

✦ Humanistic psychology focuses on issues that are uniquely human such as health, hope, love, creativity, individuality and meaning – in a nutshell, the personal nature of human experience.

✦ According to humanism, the primary cause of psychopathology is the failure to gratify one's fundamental needs.

✦ Rogers' person-centred therapy emphasises the basic trust in human beings and the movement of every person towards constructive fulfilment of their possibilities.

Your end point

Answer the following questions to assess your knowledge and understanding of the schools of thought in psychology.

1. According to Freud, the unconscious:
    (a) deals with the here and now
    (b) contains thoughts and feelings from the past that can easily be retrieved from memory
    (c) contains information that the individual is not consciously aware of
    (d) is all of the above
    (e) is none of the above?

→

2. The iceberg analogy illustrates:

   (a) the Oedipus complex
   (b) defence mechanisms
   (c) the amount of importance given to the unconscious
   (d) the theory of infantile sexuality
   (e) none of the above?

3. According to Freud's structural model of the mind, the id:

   (a) contains innate sexual instincts
   (b) contains innate aggressive instincts
   (c) is located in the unconscious
   (d) is all of the above
   (e) is none of the above?

4. Classical conditioning is concerned with:

   (a) learning through association
   (b) learning through reinforcement
   (c) vicarious learning
   (d) observational learning
   (e) none of the above?

5. The major proponent of operant conditioning is:

   (a) Watson
   (b) Skinner
   (c) Pavlov
   (d) Bandura
   (e) Upton?

Further reading

Psychological approaches are described and elaborated in most introductory psychology texts.

Armstrong, N. (2008) Role modelling in the clinical workplace. *British Journal of Midwifery* **16**(9), 596–603.

Bandura, A. (1977) Self-efficacy: Toward a unifying theory of behavioural change. *Psychological Review* **84**(2), 191–215.

Kreitler, S. (1999) Denial in cancer patients. *Cancer Investigation* **17**, 514–534.

McCormack, B. and McCance, T. (2010) *Person-Centred Nursing: Theory and Practice*. Oxford: Wiley-Blackwell.

Rana, D. and Upton, D. (2009) *Psychology for Nurses*. Harlow, Essex: Pearson Education.

Stockhorst, U., Klosterhalfen, S. and Steingruber, H.J. (1998) Conditioned nausea and further side-effects in cancer chemotherapy: A review. *Journal of Psychophysiology* **12** (suppl 1), 14–33.

Summers, R.F. and Barber, J.P. (2009) *Psychodynamic Therapy*. New York: Guildford Press.

Thornton, S.P. (2006) Sigmund Freud (1856–1939). *The Internet Encyclopaedia of Philosophy*. Available at http://www.iep.utm.edu/f/freud.htm

Watson, J.B. (1913). Psychology as the behaviourist views it. *Psychological Review* **20**. Available at http://psychclassics.yorku.ca/Watson/views.htm

Weblinks

http://www.psychexchange.co.uk/index.php
PsychExchange. A resource exchange for psychology teachers with useful video clips including: an interview with Albert Bandura and original footage from his Bobo doll experiments; an interview with B.F. Skinner, showing operant conditioning with pigeons; and an excerpt from a 1960s film about Freud.

http://psychclassics.yorku.ca/index.htm
Classics in the History of Psychology. This site provides a substantial collection of historically significant documents from the scholarly literature of psychology, including original articles written by J.B. Watson, B.F. Skinner, Albert Bandura and Edward Thorndike.

http://www.simplypsychology.pwp.blueyonder.co.uk/
Simply Psychology. This site provides information on the various psychological approaches, including video clips and weblinks.

http://des.emory.edu/mfp/self-efficacy.html
Information on Self-Efficacy. This site provides a substantial collection of links to self-efficacy and social learning theory.

Check point

Your starting point		Your end point	
Q1	A	Q1	C
Q2	D	Q2	C
Q3	D	Q3	A
Q4	A	Q4	B
Q5	E	Q5	B

Chapter 3

Psychology across the lifespan

Learning Outcomes

At the end of this chapter you will be able to:

✦ Understand children's development as characterised by Piaget, Vygotsky and Bronfenbrenner

✦ Appreciate Erikson's staged personality development and its application to nursing and healthcare

✦ Review how children define and perceive health and illness

✦ Understand how child development theories can be applied to health and illness

✦ Understand the definition and extent of 'old age' in the UK

✦ Appreciate that stereotypes of old people are inaccurate and unhelpful

✦ Understand the cognitive and social changes that occur in later life

✦ Explore the nature of death and dying

✦ Understand the process of grieving.

Your starting point

Answer the following questions to assess your knowledge and understanding of psychology across the lifespan.

1. Piaget proposed that cognitive development proceeded in four distinct stages. What is the correct order?

   (a) Pre-operational, concrete operational, formal operational, sensori-motor.
   (b) Pre-operational, concrete operational, sensori-motor, concrete operational.
   (c) Concrete operational, pre-operational, formal operational, sensori-motor.
   (d) Sensori-motor, pre-operational, concrete operational, formal operational.
   (e) None of the above.

2. In Piaget's 'conservation of mass' task, children younger than five or six years of age tended to respond by saying that the lengthened item had increased in mass. What did Piaget conclude from this?

   (a) The child lacks visual perception.
   (b) The child has the ability to process two aspects of an object at the same time.
   (c) The child does not understand the concept of conservation of mass.
   (d) The child cannot 'decentre'.
   (e) None of the above.

3. What is 'attachment'?

   (a) The behaviour shown when a mother and child watch, copy and respond to each other's behaviour.
   (b) An enduring emotional connection between people characterised by a desire for continual contact as well as feelings of distress during separation.
   (c) The ability of a parent to know what their child wants when they cry.
   (d) The emotional connection between mother and father.
   (e) None of the above.

4. Which of the following statements is false? In old age:

   (a) Some people find that the marital relationship becomes more rewarding.
   (b) The most long-lasting relationships are usually with siblings.
   (c) Family becomes more important.
   (d) Social networks are no longer important.
   (e) None of the above.

5. What is separation anxiety?

   (a) The child feels fearful when in the company of a parent for too long.
   (b) The child feels fearful when the parent tries to leave the child alone.
   (c) The child feels fearful when the parent tries to play when the child is tired.
   (d) The child feels fearful when strangers approach them.
   (e) None of the above.

Case Study

Mrs Dahlia Patel had to rush to hospital with her middle child – Roshi – who is five years of age. Roshi had fallen over and cut her head open on the concrete during a playground incident at her primary school. Mrs Patel has three children in total, with a daughter of 14 years of age being the eldest (Soha), and the youngest being an 11-month-old son, Gabe.

After falling while playing, Roshi was whisked to hospital by her mum with a deep cut to her forehead. Due to the position of the wound it was decided that it needed to be stitched in order to close it successfully. Both Roshi and Mrs Patel were extremely and visibly anxious and Mr Patel was rushing to the hospital from his work to support them both. However, when Mrs Patel realised that she would have to decide whether her daughter would have either a local or general anaesthetic (because of the high levels of distress and anxiety) before the stitches then she became more anxious and insisted that the nurse wait until her husband arrived. When Mr Patel did arrive he cuddled Roshi and held onto her hand while she had three stitches inserted in her forehead under local anaesthetic. However, Roshi was distraught and cried throughout the whole procedure despite the healthcare staff considering it a relatively minor procedure.

The Patel family is a close knit family and Mr Patel works as a dentist in a local practice while his wife stays at home to care for Gabe and the other two children. Soha, the eldest child, is 14 and has been doing well at school; she would like to move into a business career when she finishes her education. Mr and Mrs Patel are, however, becoming worried about Soha's health. She has started going out with friends at the weekend and Mr Patel is sure that he can smell cigarettes and alcohol on her breath. Furthermore, her diet appears to have deteriorated so that she prefers to eat chips and burgers and is only having small portions of fruit and vegetables (certainly not achieving her five portions a day). Her parents are worried about her because it appears that she is developing a range of poor health habits. They are also worried since Soha experiences epileptic seizures and has done so since the age of 11. Her complex partial seizures are occurring on a weekly basis and occasionally (perhaps every 6–8 weeks) she has a secondary generalised tonic-clonic seizure. Not surprisingly, her parents are worried about her health behaviours and the consequence it has on both her epilepsy and her long-term health.

Soha does not see what all the fuss is about and wants to be left alone as she says it 'is my life anyway' and feels that her behaviour is perfectly adequate and like the rest of her friends. There is certainly more family strife at the moment – in previous years the family got on extremely well and the Patels were a model of family life.

Why is this relevant to nursing practice?

This case study has relevance to nursing practice on a number of different levels. The nursing of children offers a unique challenge – it cannot simply be seen as dealing with small adults. Furthermore, the stage of development of the child influences the nature of the issues that may arise, the presentation of the form of problem, and the nursing intervention and psychological care that will have to be implemented. The case study highlights such issues: Gabe is aged 11 months and is at one stage of development. Roshi, the middle child, is five years of age and can be viewed as in another stage of development. Finally, Soha is in her teens and in the middle of adolescence. According to some psychological theories each of the Patel children is in a different stage of social, cognitive and individual development. Although the specific description of the nature of this development may differ between theories, it is apparent that children's understanding of health changes over time and that the age of the child impacts on the approach that the nurse should take.

Think about this

Consider the three ages of the Patel children. What sorts of health behaviour and understanding of health and illness would you expect from them?

3.1 Introduction

At the last national census there were just under 15 million children in the UK, accounting for almost a quarter of the population. Consequently, all nurses will come across children, either during their education, their practice or their personal life. Although there may be some nurses who feel that working with children is not for them, how children develop and are raised can have a long-term impact on how they may behave as adults. Therefore, all nurses – whether they work directly with children or not – need to have an understanding of how children develop and how this process has been characterised.

However, development is not just about children. Development is a continuous process which progresses in differing aspects throughout our lives. Hence, we need to explore how we develop in childhood, adolescence, adulthood and in older age. This chapter will explore development across the lifespan and how psychological theory can be applied to these different stages, and how this theory can be applied within our nursing practice.

Key message

Development occurs across the lifespan – from childhood through to old age.

This chapter will start at the beginning – with the newborn and how psychologists, such as Jean Piaget, have attempted to describe how children develop over their early life. The theories of Vygotsky and Erikson will subsequently be explored. Again, these will look at why they are relevant to your education and your clinical practice, not just if you are working in child health, but also if you are working in adult or mental health or with those who have learning disabilities.

The remainder of this chapter will then explore adult development before looking at older age, followed by death, dying and the grieving process.

3.2 Piaget's theory of cognitive development

Until the 1930s, children were considered to be small versions of adults. It was assumed that children thought in the same way as adults, but were incapable of behaving as adults due to their inexperience of the world. Although the flaws with this proposal may now seem obvious, this notion characterised many of the ideas surrounding child development at that time.

Jean Piaget (1896–1980), a Swiss psychologist, was instrumental in developing a theory of cognitive development that fundamentally challenged this perspective. Piaget rejected the behaviourist idea that children simply learned through a process of reward and punishment (see Chapter 2); rather, he argued that children develop progressively through a set of qualitatively different stages. At certain periods of the child's development, their way of thinking advances into completely new areas, allowing them to become more elaborate and sophisticated in their capabilities. These transitional points can be characterised into four invariant and universal stages:

0–2 years: sensori-motor stage

2–6 years: pre-operational stage

7–12 years: concrete operational stage

12+ years: formal operational stage.

Piaget argued that a child has to progress through these stages to become capable of understanding information in certain ways. Furthermore, in order for a child to progress through each transitional stage, Piaget suggested that they would have to be cognitively mature. Piaget suggested that these stages have to be progressed through in a set order and no stage can be left out. According to Piaget these stages are seen as universal, occurring in the same sequence for all children, irrespective of their social or cultural background. However, the theory does accept that the timing of each stage can be influenced by environmental or biological factors and an increase in the capacity of working memory (Keenan, 2002; Lowe *et al*., 2009). How can we define these stages, and how were they demonstrated and what do they mean for you as a nurse?

Key message

Children are not simply mini-adults. They have to progress through many stages in order to become capable of understanding information as adults do.

Quick check

What are Piaget's key stages?

The sensori-motor stage

The sensori-motor stage is the first of Piaget's stages and lasts for the first two years of life. During this time infants explore themselves, the environment and the relationship between these. Infants rely on using their physical sensory abilities, such as seeing, touching, listening and sucking, in order to explore their environment (i.e. sensory perceptions and motor activities, hence the sensori-motor stage).

In this stage infants develop important understandings. Cognitive structures begin to organise and behaviours become more intentional (Riddick-Grisham and Deming, 2011). They begin to appreciate that the external world is separate and distinct, and that an object can be moved by a hand (they grasp the concept of causality). Furthermore, they develop the notions of displacement and events. Also, during the latter period of the sensori-motor stage children make an important discovery: the concept of 'object permanence'.

Object permanence is the awareness that an object continues to exist even when it is not in view. For example, infants will lose interest in a toy when it has been covered by a cloth or hidden by a piece of paper (see Figure 3.1). When an infant has developed object permanence (by about eight months of age), when a toy is covered the child will actively search for the object, since they appreciate that the object continues to exist despite being out of sight.

This is important if we discuss the reactions of the child to their parents. Before the development of object permanence, children will usually recognise and respond to their mother (usually by the third day of life). However, when they are left by their mother they will not show any signs of distress since she is 'out of sight and out of mind'. However, when a child has developed object permanence and the mother leaves the child then they will become upset and show some form of **separation anxiety**. This is because the child now appreciates what they have lost – mum! However, there has been more recent research which indicates that object permanence occurs earlier than suggested by Piaget. It is also been suggested that the development of object permanence is more closely related to separation than previously reported (Charles and Rivera, 2009).

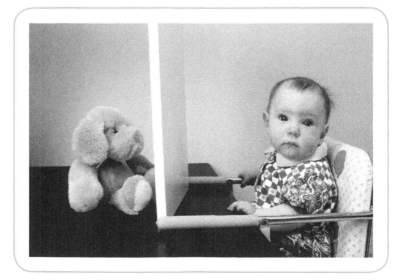

Figure 3.1 Object permanence

Source: Science Photo Library/Doug Goodman

Quick check

What do children use to explore their environment during the sensori-motor period?

Key message

During the sensori-motor stage, children become aware of their surroundings and the permanency of them. This leads to them developing separation anxiety when left by their primary caregiver.

The pre-operational stage

Piaget's second stage of cognitive development occurs between the ages of two and six years. At this stage children begin to use symbols such as language to represent their earlier sensori-motor abilities. Although children are still unable to understand concrete logic at this stage, they are now accomplished at using concrete symbolism (have the ability to use an object to represent something, a stick as a gun for example). Furthermore, one of the key elements of this stage is that children are still **egocentric**, and are therefore unable to take the point of view of others.

In order to test his theory, Piaget developed the three mountains task (Piaget and Inhelder, 1956); see Figure 3.2. In the task, a child is shown a scene of three model mountains which are all different colours. One has snow on top, one a house and the other a red cross. The child is allowed to explore the model and then asked to sit on one side while a doll is placed at a different location. The child is then shown ten pictures of different views of the model

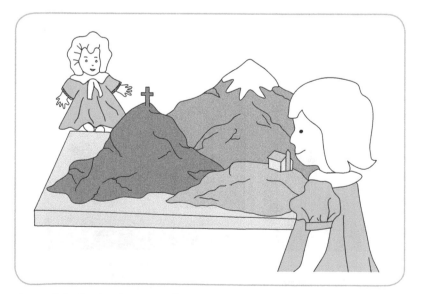

Figure 3.2 The three mountains task

and asked to select which one represents how the doll views it. Piaget and Inhelder concluded that children at the age of four were unable to recognise a perspective different from their own, always selecting the picture which matched their own view of the model. Six-year-olds showed some awareness but still often chose the wrong picture. However, children of seven and eight years consistently chose the picture that represented the doll's view, supporting Piaget's suggestion that children under the age of seven are egocentric, i.e. they fail to understand that what they see is relative to their own viewpoint. However, research has indicated that if the child is given the opportunity to walk around the three-dimensional model they do find it easier to complete the task. For this reason it is essential that when explaining procedures to a child a nurse should use concrete rather than abstract language. For instance, Kean (2010) examined how children constructed their experiences of visiting a critically ill family member in an intensive care unit. Kean found that children tended to speak about intensive care on a concrete level, focusing on the environment.

Key message

During the pre-operational stage, children can use objects to represent things.

Quick check

What can children do during the pre-operational stage which they cannot do at an earlier stage?

Think about this

Considering Piaget's stages, how would you have dealt with Roshi during her time at the hospital?

The concrete operational stage

The concrete operational stage is the third stage of Piaget's theory of cognitive development and usually occurs between the ages of seven and 12. This stage is characterised by an ability to think logically and organise thoughts in a coherent manner: however, children are not yet able to think in an abstract fashion or in hypothetical terms and are unable to combine information systematically to solve problems (Maynard and Thomas, 2009). One main characteristic of this stage is the loss of egocentric thinking and the child begins to think about others and develops an appreciation that their actions can have an impact on others as well as themselves.

Another group of experiments devised by Piaget were the tests of conservation, where children were shown two identical containers with an equal amount of liquid in them (see Figure 3.3). The liquid from one container was then transferred into another different shaped container in front of the children. They were then asked to hold the container which they thought had the most liquid: the children would consistently hold the cup which appeared to be the fullest despite the fact that they had previously watched the same amount of liquid

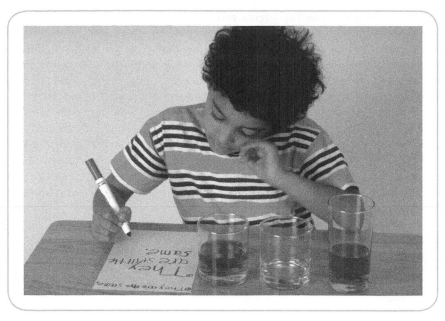

Figure 3.3 Piaget's conservation of volume task

Source: Laura Dwight/Corbis

being poured into the different shaped cup. Piaget conducted many experiments concerning conservation including mass, volume and weight, discovering that very few children had the ability to understand conservation before the age of five. However, at this stage, children are able to comprehend conservation tasks (i.e. the ability to understand that a certain amount of substance remains the same after its appearance changes) and are able to grasp the concept of reversibility (i.e. the ability to see physical transformation and imagine reversing this transformation, cancelling out the change).

Key message

The concrete operational stage is characterised by an ability to think logically and organise thoughts in a coherent manner.

Quick check

What would the child in the concrete operational stage be unable to comprehend about their nursing care?

The formal operational stage

The fourth and final stage of cognitive development begins at approximately 12 years of age and continues into adulthood. The formal operational stage is characterised by an ability to think in abstract terms, the ability to formulate hypotheses and deduct testable inferences.

Piaget suggested that while it is possible to achieve such abstract thinking, many people never reach this stage of cognitive development. During this stage, children begin to develop the ability to address abstract problems and are able to understand the finer meanings of death and dying (Linebarger *et al.*, 2009).

Think about this

How does an understanding of Piaget's theory help us appreciate children's understanding of health and illness at different ages?

Despite the impact of Piaget's research on cognitive development, it has not escaped criticism. Apart from the fact that Piaget based his observations on his own children, his work has recently been criticised for the lack of consideration given to contextual factors. For instance, Piaget neglects to acknowledge the view that children develop within a complex system of relationships and that these are affected by multiple levels of their environment (Carey, 1985). It has also been argued that Piaget's experiments were often too complex and unfamiliar for children and lacked in ecological validity. For instance, the three mountains experiment is unrelated to some children, who are not from mountainous countries, as this is not a normal experience for them. Subsequent research suggested that when experiments used objects which were more familiar to children they were able to see things from another's perspective at a much younger age than predicted by Piaget (Donaldson, 1978; Yoshida *et al.*, 2009). However, Piaget's theory has had a substantial impact on developmental psychology and has been the fundamental underpinning theory of child development for a number of years.

Application to practice

From our knowledge and understanding of the above stages, we can recognise that children within differing stages will appreciate health and illnesses in different ways. Previous research has linked Piaget's stages of cognitive development to children's beliefs about illness (Bibace and Walsh, 1980; Varkula *et al.*, 2010), Rickles *et al.* (2010; 299) explain that 'it is very likely that children form beliefs and attitudes about health, moreover, these attitudes and beliefs should change as children gain more experience and develop more skills at interpreting what they observe'. It is therefore important to develop age-appropriate interventions to assist children in their understanding of health, illness and treatment. This would relieve the unnecessary fear, guilt and anxiety that children often display when in a healthcare setting (Myant and Williams, 2005).

✦ **Pre-operational stage (2–6 years):** at this stage children are seen as having limited logic and are highly egocentric. Consequently, children's beliefs about illness are vague and often contain elements of fear and superstition. For example, at this stage they cannot grasp the finality of death.

✦ **Concrete operational stage (7–12 years):** at this stage children begin to understand that ill-health and death have biological causes. Myant and Williams (2005) report that children begin to recognise the risks (in the short term) of their own behaviour and the impact that this may have on their illness/health. In contrast, the long-term outcomes of their behaviour are less understood (Eiser, 1997). However, by the end of this stage, children begin to understand that death is final and they start to understand their own mortality.

During the past few decades there has been a gradual shift from viewing children as passive recipients of health information and healthcare to viewing them as active partners whose competence and information needs should be considered by healthcare professionals (Rickles *et al.*, 2010). Coyne (2006) reported on children's, parents' and nurses' views on the consultation with children in hospital and their participation in care. Results suggested that parents believed that children should be involved in the decision-making process, enhancing and promoting children's self-esteem. Children also indicated the need to be involved in the consultation process in order for them to understand their illness and prepare themselves for procedures. Children's views and opinions were, however, underused. Nurses held conflicting views on the involvement of children in decisions: for some nurses the child's involvement was dependent upon the child's cognitive maturity. Coyne suggested that a health professional's communication is a reflection of their recognition of a child's cognitive abilities rather than their actual competence to understand. Coyne concluded that it is important for nurses to examine their choices about whether to involve children in their care or not and to make explicit decisions with clear criteria for their involvement or otherwise.

Key message

Children should be involved in their care: the extent of their involvement should be determined by the child's cognitive development.

Quick check

Describe each of Piaget's stages of cognitive development.

3.3 Attachment

Attachment refers to the strong, long-lasting emotional bond that is evident between a child and their primary caregiver. Close relationships with the mother (or other primary caregiver) are essential for a child's successful development (and indeed survival in humans) and consequently studies of attachment (and separation) have been reported. The early studies of attachment were largely associated with a behaviourist approach. Behaviourism viewed the attachment process as occurring due to the mother providing essential reinforcement for the child in terms of food and comfort. However, a classic animal experiment by Harlow (1959) suggested that this was not adequate in explaining the process. During this experiment, Rhesus monkeys showed a preference for soft physical contact with an inanimate object even if it did not deliver milk. Hence, this study suggested that children do not only want to be attached to their mothers simply because of the mothers' ability to feed them – they gain more from the relationship in terms of comfort and attachment.

Key message

Infants get more from their interaction with their mothers than simply nourishment.

However, the name most associated with early studies of attachment is Bowlby (1969) who noted that babies exhibit a number of behaviours that have a survival value as they ensure that the parents (or caregivers) will support their basic needs. For example, crying, babbling and smiling signal needs, or clinging and non-nutritional sucking support approach behaviour. Bowlby's theory is based on an interactional model which, as the name suggests, proposes that attachment is dependent on the interaction between both the mother and the child, and not solely on an infant's or mother's behaviour. Therefore, mothers who are depressed may be unable to adequately respond to a child's needs which may, in turn, influence the child's subsequent behaviours. For example, Hennessy et al. (2009) suggested that early maternal separation and other disruptions of attachment relations are known to increase risk for the later onset of depressive illness. Equally, a child who may be pre-term may be unable to elicit the signalling behaviours needed to gain a response from an adult. Situations such as these can significantly influence the relationship formation between a parent and their child. Bowlby noted that attachment between a child and their primary caregiver acts as a template for subsequent social and intimate relationships. Hence, failure to develop this initial bond may damage the ability of a child to develop strong relationships in adult life. This is shown in a recent longitudinal study conducted by Zayas et al. (2011) who suggested that early maternal care giving predicts later adult attachment patterns with peers and partners.

Between the ages of seven months and one year, Bowlby noted 'separation anxiety' in babies where they became very distressed in the absence of their mother (or primary caregiver). At this point, a baby may also become very wary of any strangers who may approach them and show evident protests if they come too close to them, such as crying and evidently seeking closer proximity to their caregiver. Consequently as a result of Bowlby's emphasis on the detrimental effect of separation on children's mental health and various studies concerning separation (notably the seminal studies of Robertson and Robertson 1967–73), preceding the 1960s, the healthcare system altered in order to accommodate and encourage caregivers to stay with their child for the duration of their admission to hospital. Furthermore, recent research has indicated the importance of family-centred care within a hospital setting in reducing anxiety and gaining the best possible outcomes for younger and older children's recovery (Moorey, 2010; Bee, 2006).

Think about this

What do Bowlby's studies suggest for the care of children with a chronic illness, particularly those who require considerable time in hospital? How does this alter with the age of the child? Considering Bowlby's theory, can you explain Soha's behaviour? When considering Roshi in the hospital, how should a nurse deal with her behaviour?

Attachment types: secure, ambivalent and avoidant

Research observed that, in some cases, the way that children reacted when separated from their primary caregiver would differ. As a result, a series of experiments was conducted that explored the different types of attachment and how these may affect separation. Mary Ainsworth conducted a series of classic experiments concerning the nature of attachment and **stranger anxiety**. These were known as the 'strange situation experiments' (Ainsworth *et al.*, 1978; Ainsworth, 1985). During these experiments the child and their parent were taken into an unfamiliar room full of toys. They would then progress through a range of episodes such as: the arrival of a stranger who would speak to the parent, the parent leaving the room and the child with the stranger, and finally, the parent being reunited with the child. From these observations, it was concluded that children could be assigned to one of three classifications of attachment:

✦ **Secure attachment** – The child was ready and willing to explore their surroundings while using their mother as a safe base and was friendly to the stranger. However, when the mother was absent this willingness declined and the child showed some distress. In the reunion episodes the child was eager to be close to their mother or positively interact with them from across the room if they were playing.

✦ **Ambivalent attachment** – The child tended to be wary of the stranger and in the presence of the parent. The child protested intensely at the parent's absence and was ambivalent on their return, both seeking closeness and appearing angry with them.

✦ **Avoidant attachment** – The child tended to continue exploring the room throughout the episodes, avoiding physical and emotional intimacy with the parent. The child appeared to be unaware of the parent's absence and avoided them on their return. The child can also be comforted as easily by the stranger as by the parent.

It has been identified that parents of securely attached children are more accessible and far more positively responsive to their child than those parents who had ambivalent or avoidant attachments (Ainsworth, 1985). Hence, it is evident that an important prerequisite for the formation of a secure attachment is that of parental warmth.

So how does this affect our nursing practice? Well, due to the apparent differences in attachment types and the way that children respond to a stranger (i.e. an unknown nurse), it is important that when treating a child the nurse asks them for their permission and explains (at the appropriate level) the procedure (Moorey, 2010). This will help the child feel less threatened, and more at ease with the nurse.

3.4 Ecological systems theory

Although not a stage theory, another theory that we need to address is that of Urie Bronfenbrenner's (1917–2005) ecological systems theory. This theory views a person as developing within a system of relationships which are surrounded and affected by multiple layers of the environment. This theory identified different aspects or layers of the environment that influence children's development, including the microsystem, mesosystem, exosystem and the macrosystem (see Figure 3.4):

✦ **The microsystem** – the innermost layer of the environment that consists of interactions and activities in the person's immediate surroundings.

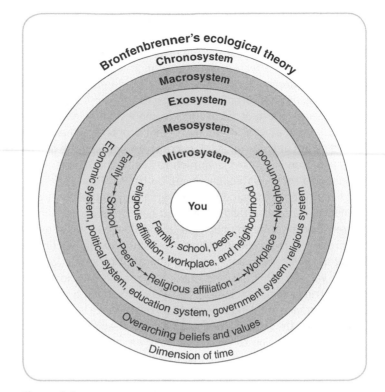

Figure 3.4 Bronfenbrenner's model

+ **The mesosystem** – the second layer encompassing connections between microsystems, e.g. a child's academic progress at school depends on parental involvement in school life.
+ **The exosystem** – social settings that do not contain the developing person but affect their development, e.g. extended family members, flexible work schedules, etc.
+ **The macrosystem** – the outermost layer consisting of cultural values, laws, customs of society and resources.

How these groups or organisations interact with the child will have an effect on how the child develops; the more encouraging and nurturing these relationships and environments are, the more advantageous the child's development will be. Furthermore, all relationships are bidirectional (i.e. how a child acts or reacts to people in the microsystem will affect how they treat the child in return and vice versa). Each child's special genetic and biologically influenced personality traits, what is known as temperament, affect how others treat them. For example, a friendly child is more likely to elicit positive reactions from an adult, while an irritable child may be met with impatience or even punishment from an adult (Crockenberg and Leerkes, 2003).

Think about this

Using Bronfenbrenner's theory, could you explain why Soha is behaving the way she is with no consideration for her health? Can you think of how her behaviour could be dealt with and possibly changed?

According to Bronfenbrenner's model, the best way to get a valid picture of a child's functioning is to observe that functioning in the context of normal routines and familiar settings. He reminds us that everything we do, believe or understand takes place in a particular social and cultural context and is affected, directly or indirectly, by that context. Thus a child's health is affected by environmental factors ranging from family lifestyle choices and cultural norms to airborne pathogens. Bronfenbrenner's model provides healthcare professionals with an excellent framework to promote improvement and maintenance in relation to their patient's health. Bryans *et al.* (2009) suggested that Bronfenbrenner's framework appears to offer a promising means of building on the current strengths of the health visiting service to further develop a 'person-in-context' approach to health improvement that is mindful of and responsive to multiple, inter-related influences on health. First, it is imperative that nurses recognise that health is not understood in a universal way, rather there are cultural and social beliefs that influence our understanding of good health. As parents are the seekers of help for their children then their beliefs must be acknowledged. Sometimes the functioning of children with chronic health conditions may be explained by the function and structure of the family, their cultural beliefs, etc. and so a full clinical history must account for such issues. Furthermore, the value of other systems outside the family should be remembered and the importance of referring a family on to other services should not be dismissed lightly. Another example of the importance of taking an ecological perspective is for the child in hospital – for the majority of children, the hospital ward is a new and unaccustomed microsystem. We need to consider how they are going to react and have an awareness of the needs of the child (and the family) in this environment. Clearly, involving the parents in the child's care will be important here (Moorey, 2010) but the degree of involvement will differ from family to family depending on the child's age, cultural customs and so on. Finally, it is important to remember that the family is about more than a child and their parent(s); the role of siblings, grandparents and other family members may also need some consideration

Key message

We need to consider the child and the whole of their environment when treating or interacting with them.

3.5 Vygotsky's socio-cultural theory of development

Lev Vygotsky (1896–1934), another notable theorist of cognitive development, viewed development as a continuum, with no upper age limit or discrete stages. He proposed the socio-cultural theory of cognitive development which indicated the importance of social interaction and social context on development. Vygotsky argued that children are capable of learning from others when the distance between the actual developmental level of the child and potential developmental level a child could reach with some adult help is relatively small. He referred to this concept as the **zone of proximal development** (ZPD). Essentially, Vygotsky suggested that children learn at one small step at a time when given help and guidance. For instance, when children acquire language they significantly enhance their ability to participate in dialogues, thus further enhancing their understanding and management of valued competencies within their culture (Winsler *et al.*, 2009). As well as this, when proceeding through school they gain and discuss academic experiences and concepts which significantly enhance their reflexivity, reasoning and problem-solving (Kozulin, 2003; Bodrova and Leong, 2007).

Peer mentoring usually occurs between an older, more able pupil and a pupil with slightly weaker skills. Bruner (1983) developed this further and suggested the concept of **scaffolding**, an interactive process where the more knowledgeable teacher alters the amount of support and guidance required by the child on the basis of the child's responses. In doing so, the teacher enables the child to gradually achieve and develop. The zone of proximal development and scaffolding concepts have both been highly influential within the field of health education, specifically in the development of peer mentoring programmes (Reis *et al.*, 2010).

Think about this

How can knowledge of Vygotsky's socio-cultural theory of development be applied to nursing? How would a self-help group for children help with their understanding of their condition?

Vygotskian theory is advantageous to nurses as it provides them with a framework in which to work that allows them to increase children's understanding and knowledge of health-related procedures and behaviours within an array of settings. We know from Piagetian theory that there is a stage-related progression in children's use of logic and their interpretation and understanding of health or illness concepts and that this links partly to the child's age. However, that does not mean that a four-year-old should not have the medical procedures they are about to undergo explained to them. Rather it means that the explanation will need to be given in terms and language the child can understand (Moorey, 2010; Kean, 2010). As Eiser (1989) notes, children will constantly seek to make sense of the world on the basis of their current knowledge and experience. It is therefore essential that children are given information which they *are* capable of grasping completely, in order to diminish the potentially frightening and harmful effects of illness or hospitalisation. Vygotsky reminds us that there is a social aspect to learning and that children do best when taught by more knowledgeable others who scaffold their understanding, and link explanations to experiences and knowledge within the child's own world (cf. Greenfield, 2004). Therefore, it is essential that, as a nurse, when you give a child an explanation, you must not only take into account their age and developmental stage but you must also consider their life experiences (Kean, 2010). This is essential in enabling them to advance from novice to expert in their understanding of their own illness. Additionally, Drew (2006) suggested that children will often feel uncomfortable and distressed when discussing their illness in front of those who are close to them for fear of upsetting them. Therefore, the nurse should not only take into consideration the needs and understanding of the child, but their families as well in order to ensure that they each have complete understanding of the issue.

However, although Vygotsky's theory emphasises the importance of social experiences, it is not the only factor contributing to development. Although he does recognise the importance of other biological factors contributing to development, he completely neglects to discuss the importance of these in relation to cognitive change.

3.6 Erikson's theory of personality development

Erik Erikson (1902–94) proposed an alternative theory of child development. In contrast to Piaget and Vygotsky who emphasised cognitive development, Erikson explored personality development. He proposed eight stages in human personality development, beginning in infancy and continuing into late adulthood (see Table 3.1). Each stage is characterised by psychological crises which the individual must resolve in order for a successful adult personality to emerge. According to Erikson, the success of these resolutions and subsequent 'normal' development must be understood in relation to an individual's cultural situation. For example, in the 1940s, Erikson discovered that newborn infants of Yurok Indians were deprived of milk from breastfeeding for the first ten days after birth and were fed a form of soup. Although this may seem unreasonable and cruel it is seen as essential within their cultural situation as they live in an environment where food was not largely available to them.

Think about this

How can Erikson's theory be applied to Soha and how she has grown up with her epilepsy?

Quick check

What are Erikson's stages?

Erikson's theory focuses on the importance of social and emotional development to children's responses to what is happening to them when they are ill or in hospital. Understanding this model can be advantageous for a nurse when attempting to understand and interpret a child's behaviour. For example, a young child who is ill may not fully understand what is happening or why they are in hospital. Providing explanations aimed at their level of understanding using what we know from Vygotsky may help this somewhat. However, children's behaviour may sometimes be at odds with their apparent comprehension and it may be that their social and emotional development holds the key to this. Take for example a 30-month-old child with asthma who is in hospital with a viral infection, suffering from respiratory distress. Oral prednisole has been prescribed as it is known to reduce disease severity and symptom duration for such cases. The nurse is confident that she has been able explain the importance of taking the medicine, yet still the child refuses. Taken at face value, this may appear to be a clear case of a toddler being deliberately difficult. However, according to psychosocial theory this child is in the second of Erikson's stages of personality development and so is striving for autonomy. Refusal to take the proffered medicine may be seen as an attempt to show autonomy. For example, Beach and Proops (2009) suggested that children may have differing levels of autonomy, sometimes making them competent to make medical

Table 3.1 Erikson's theory of personality development

Stage	Period of development	Description
Trust versus mistrust	Birth–1 year	Warm, responsive area provides infants with a sense of trust and confidence that the world is good. Mistrust occurs when infants have to wait too long to be comforted and they are handled harshly.
Autonomy versus shame and doubt	1–3 years	Using their recently acquired mental and motor skills, children want to be able to decide for themselves. Autonomy is achieved when parents allow a level of independence and do not shame or force the child.
Initiative versus guilt	3–6 years	Through make-believe and creative play, children can develop a sense of ambition and curiosity. Too much control on behalf of the parent is thought to induce excessive guilt.
Industry versus inferiority	6–11 years	At school, children develop the ability to work with others and achieve success. Inferiority develops when negative situations at home or school generate feelings of incompetence.
Identity versus role confusion	Adolescence	The adolescent questions their identity and role in society. Exploring values and vocational goals will enable the adolescent to develop a personal identity and positive behaviours.
Intimacy versus isolation	Early adulthood (18–40)	Young adults focus on developing intimate relationships. Failure to achieve basic trust earlier in life may result in an inability to form close relationships as an adult.
Generativity versus stagnation	Middle adulthood (40–65)	In middle adulthood, there is a focus on establishing a successful career and child-rearing.

Failure to resolve these crises results in an absence of accomplishment. |
| **Ego integrity versus despair** | Late adulthood (65+) | During this stage, adults reflect on their life. Those who feel that their life has been worthwhile will experience integrity. Those who feel that their life has been wasted will experience despair and fear death. |

decisions for themselves and other times not. Furthermore, children may refuse treatments that parents desire them to take. Therefore it is important that rather than insisting and getting cross with the child, attempts are made to allow the child to take the initiative, in order to mitigate future harmful effects on the child's developing ego.

However, Erikson's perspective is no longer evident within the mainstream views of human development. This could be explained by its strong commitment to clinical approaches, which therefore neglects other relevant and influential methods. Furthermore, it has been postulated that many of the ideas presented in his perspective (i.e. psychosexual stages and ego functioning) are too ambiguous, resulting in an inability to test its validity (Crain, 2005; Thomas, 2005).

Key message

Adolescents are not always being truculent, their behaviour is indicative of them striving for autonomy.

3.7 Adolescence – storm and stress

As we mentioned at the outset, rarely do psychologists agree and nowhere is this clearer than in adolescence research. In recent years there has been a dramatic growth in research which has created divergent beliefs and a plethora of psychological theories. Numerous views of the adolescent phase of development have emerged, principally the idea of adolescence as a period of 'storm and stress' (Arnett, 1999; Ayman-Nolley and Taira, 2000; Casey et al., 2010). In 1904 Hall proposed that adolescence is a period of psychological turmoil, essentially a period of storm and stress. This, according to Hall, comprised three specific characteristics: mood disruption, conflict with parents and engagement in risk-taking behaviours (Mancini and Huebner, 2004). Risk-behaviours may include: sexual risk-behaviours (i.e. Henrich et al., 2011), adolescent pregnancy and fatherhood (i.e. Miller et al., 2001) and, violent perpetration and victimisation (i.e. Matjasko et al., 2010). Hall also suggested that evolution occurs when organisms pass on their characteristics from one generation to the next, not in the form of genes but in the form of experiences and acquired characteristics (Arnett, 1999). Consequently, the development of the adolescent period, according to Hall, could be associated with some ancient period in evolution that was 'difficult'. This legacy was then passed down from one generation to another and manifested itself as storm and stress in the development of the adolescent period.

Arnett (1999) proposed an alternative view, a modified view of adolescence that incorporates the roles of individual differences and cultural variables. Subsequently, contemporary thought on the issue of storm and stress rejects the notion that it is a universal and inevitable process. Arnett proposes that not all adolescents experience storm and stress, rather adolescence is a period when storm and stress is *more likely* to occur. Consequently, it is important to consider the impact of individual differences and culture upon the development of storm and stress.

Research adopting Bronfenbrenner's model has identifed the important role of family, peers and teachers in socio-emotional development during adolescence (Chen and Farruggia, 2002; Kindermann, 2011; Liddle and Hogue, 2000; Miller *et al.*, 2001). Parental warmth, conflict and establishing autonomy are vital factors in emotional development; absence of parental warmth, whether physical or verbal, may result in symptoms of storm and stress. Furthermore, conflict in, and a desire to, establish autonomy during adolescence have also been found as a source of storm and stress (Greenberger *et al.*, 2000). Peer relationships represent a further dimension to the social context of development and have been reported as important for adolescent psychological well-being in different cultures (Greenberger *et al.*, 2000; Steinberg and Morris, 2001).

Think about this

What does this mean for your nursing practice when treating an adolescent?

3.8 Putting theories into action

Adolescence is a transitional developmental period between childhood and adulthood. In this stage development can have considerable biological, psychological and social role changes, and probably more of such changes than any other stage of life except infancy (Lerner *et al.*, 1999). Adolescence is a key time for the development of positive health behaviours (e.g. diet and exercise), along with the emergence of health risk behaviours (e.g. unsafe sex practices, smoking and drug use (O'Cathail *et al.*, 2011)). Thus, the period of adolescence is the most appropriate time in developing positive health behaviours efficiently and preventing bad behaviours from flourishing.

From the work of Bronfenbrenner we can note the importance of others who are involved with an adolescent including the family, peers, school and work environments – all of which offer the opportunity for preventative interventions. However, some of those listed may be more indisposed to interventions than others. For instance, microsystems, such as peer groups, can influence adolescents' development by encouraging the adoption of risk-taking behaviours such as irresponsible sex, drug use and drinking (Muuss, 2006). Furthermore, an adolescent's microsystem and a mesosystem can support or oppose each other. A divergent relationship could potentially form between two microsystems, consequently causing problems and risks in adolescent development which could lead to the adoption of risk-taking behaviours (Muuss, 2006). Nevertheless, some studies have suggested that improving peer relationships may prove beneficial in improving health behaviours (Steinberg and Morris, 2001); for example, recruiting non-smoking adolescents to act as health educators/promoters amongst their smoking peers (Garrison *et al.*, 2003).

When attempting to define target interventions it is important to select appropriate age ranges because of the developmental changes that occur throughout childhood. For example, it could be argued that smoking/obesity, etc. prevention should be directed towards 11- and 12-year-old children and their families for several reasons. First, the body image of children of this age is more malleable as are attitudes towards eating and illness (Bissell and Hays, 2011; Robinson *et al.*, 2008). Hence, although adolescents may struggle with a negative body image and unhealthy eating patterns, the body image of younger children may be more flexible, with prevention being more likely to succeed (Kater *et al.*, 2000). Second, from the age of 11 or 12, children become more autonomous in their health-related self-management behaviours (Pradel *et al.*, 2001). In terms of Piagetian cognitive developmental theory, at the age of 11 or 12 children are entering the 'formal operational' stage (Piaget, 1972) and are developing the skill of abstract thought. Consequently, children at this cognitive stage can begin to imagine the potential consequences (both positive and negative) of a specific health behaviour which, as a result, allows them to take more control of their behaviours.

Additionally negative consequences of poor health behaviour may be too far in the future for a pre-formal operational child to imagine (e.g. imagining long-term lung cancer or heart disease as a consequence of smoking). Gough *et al.* (2009) suggested that young smokers downplay the health risks associated with smoking and believed them to be a youthful phenomenon, which would cease upon entering adulthood. Children may therefore need some concrete and immediate examples for them to consider before they will make their change in behaviour. To deal with this the nurse could ask the child to provide personally relevant examples to ensure they understand the concepts being important to children at this age, such as body image (e.g. smoking gives you bad skin and makes you smell when kissing).

3.9 Working with older adults

As mentioned previously, development is not simply about childhood – development occurs across the lifespan. Much of psychology and that discussed in this text concerns adult development (e.g. how we change and react to circumstances – see Chapter 2); there is another period of significant change – old age.

All nurses, from whichever branch and whatever speciality, need to have an understanding of issues surrounding the care of the older adult. The UK population is ageing, with the 2001 Census estimating that 11 million older people (over pensionable age) are living within the UK. Hence, at some stage in your professional career, you will most likely interact with an older adult.

However, the question that we must try to answer is: what is an older adult? And what do we mean by 'old'? A simplistic response would be to suggest that it is anything over the retirement age (currently 65 years). However, the proportion of people aged over 65 years is substantial and it can be seen that the population is ageing. Currently, 17 per cent of the population is represented by people 65 years and over, with the fastest population increase in those aged 85 and over (Population Trends, 2011). These figures are set to rise in the future as life expectancy has been seen to have increased consistently over the last several decades, which is most likely to be due to the increase in the provision and standards of healthcare. It is estimated that the number of people aged 65 and above will increase by 15 per cent and the number of people aged 85 and above will increase by 27 per cent by 2015 (Department of Health and Care Service Improvement Partnership, 2005). According to

Jones (1993), everyone over retirement age is seen as forming a strange homogenous mass, with limited abilities, few needs and few rights:

What other section of the population that spans more than 30 years in biological times is grouped together in such an illogical manner? . . . As a consequence, older people suffer a great deal . . . As for experience and wisdom, these qualities are no longer valued . . . They are devalued by the community, as well as by their owners.

Therefore attempting to define the 'older adult' as anybody aged over the retirement age is compounded with difficulties – a 65-year-old may have completely different needs and expectations from an 84-year-old. Hence, some have suggested that we divide those aged over 65 into three groups:

✦ young-old (65–80)

✦ old-old (80–90)

✦ very old/oldest old (90+).

Key message

The 'elderly' cannot be considered a homogenous group.

Think about this

How would you expect a young-old to think and behave in comparison to an old-old, or oldest-old? What specific needs would you envisage for each of the groups?

Consideration has also been given in relation to what one might consider to be 'old'. Kastenbaum (1979) suggested that there were at least four 'ages of me'.

Kastenbaum's (1979) ages of me questionnaire

✦ My chronological age is my actual age, dated from the time of birth.

✦ My biological age refers to the state of my face and body. In other people's eyes, I look as though I am about . . . years of age. In my own eyes, I look like someone of about . . . years of age.

✦ My subjective age is indicated by how I feel. Deep down inside, I really feel like a person of about . . . years of age.

✦ My functional age, which is closely related to my social age, refers to the kind of life I lead, what I am able to do, the status I believe I have, whether I work, have dependent children and live in my own home. My thoughts and interests are like those of a person of about . . . years of age, and my position in society is like that of a person of about . . . years of age.

Source: Kastenbaum, R., *Growing Old – Years of Fulfilment*, 1st edn, © 1979.

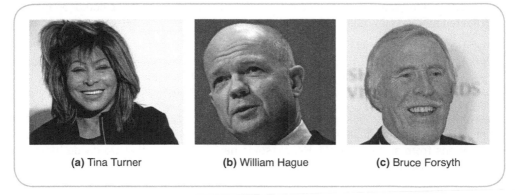

(a) Tina Turner   **(b)** William Hague   **(c)** Bruce Forsyth

Figure 3.5 How old are these people?

Source: Getty Images: (a) Miguel Villagran/Staff; (b) Christopher Furlong/Staff; (c) Dave Hogan/Stringer

Look at the celebrities in Figure 3.5. Can you try and guess how old each of them is? Do they act as you would expect somebody of that age to act? How do you think they should act? How would you expect a 40-, 50-, 60-, 70-, or 80-year-old to act? Is there a stereotypical way you think older people should behave?

Just as it is inappropriate to think of all old people as acting and behaving in a similar way to Tina Turner or Bruce Forsyth, it is also inappropriate to think of the older person as doddery, fragile and cognitively impaired. Yet many people continue to hold this view. For instance, when an Ageism Survey was carried out by Age Concern (2006), of the 1,843 people interviewed about their perceptions of the elderly, it was found that: 'One in three respondents said that the over-70s are viewed as incompetent and incapable' (Age Concern, 2006: 3). We all (whether we are nurses or not) have to avoid stereotyping people according to their age. However, this is particularly important for those in the caring professions since it can lead to a **self-fulfilling prophecy**: where 'If you expect older people to be dependent, and therefore consequently treat them as if they are dependent, and encourage them to respond as if they were dependent, eventually they may indeed become more dependent. Low expectations will necessarily lead to under-achievement' (Slater, 1995: 17). More recently, Coudin and Alexopoulos (2010) suggested that the mere activation of negative stereotypes can have broad and harmful effects on older individuals' self-evaluation and functioning, which in turn may contribute to the often observed dependency among older people. Similarly, Adler (2000) reports on a number of studies that demonstrate that stereotypes can affect how the elderly think about themselves in ways that can be detrimental to their mental and physical health. Furthermore, Ruppel *et al.* (2010) discovered that due to stereotypes people have the propensity to under-diagnose certain illnesses such as depression. This was due to health professionals misattributing depressive symptoms as being caused naturally due to the person's age.

Stereotypes of older people – the elderly – are more deeply entrenched than (mis)conceptions of gender differences. It is therefore not surprising that people are overwhelmingly unenthusiastic about becoming 'old' (Stuart-Hamilton, 1997).

Key message

Stereotypes of the elderly can be widely inaccurate.

What views do you hold of the elderly?

Look at each of the following statements (taken from Schaie and Willis, 2002) and say whether they are true or false (the answers are at the bottom of the box*):

1. Most people over 65 are financially insecure.
2. Rarely does someone over the age of 65 produce a great deal of work of art, science or scholarship.
3. The shock of retirement often results in deteriorating physical and mental health.
4. Old people are not very interested in sex.
5. Old people get rattled more easily.
6. Old people should be active to keep their spirits up.
7. Old dogs can't learn new tricks.
8. In old age, memories of the distant past are clear and vivid, but memories of recent events are fuzzy.
9. Women live longer than men because they don't work as hard.
10. Elderly patients do not respond well to surgery.
11. Most old people become senile sooner or later.

*All are false except 6 and 8.

Odell and Holbrook (2006) suggest that care that should be provided for older people requires special expertise. This is due to the following reasons:

✦ Physiological ageing alters the presentation of disease and effects of medication.
✦ Incidence of depression, dementia and delirium become increasingly common.
✦ Pre-existing conditions can make self-care more difficult.
✦ Social support for successful discharge requires complex organisational skills.

Key message

When interacting with an older adult, do not expect them to act in a stereotypical 'old' manner. Treat them as an individual.

3.10 Cognitive changes in adulthood

Cognitive Impairment is defined as a slight impairment in cognitive function with otherwise normal function in the performance of activities of daily living (Prabhavalkar and Chintamaneni, 2010). There are a number of losses which are associated with **cognitive impairments**. Hall (1988) divides these into four losses. These are:

✦ **Intellectual loss** – loss of memory, loss of sense of time and loss of expressive and receptive language abilities.
✦ **Affective/personality loss** – loss of affect, antisocial behaviour and paranoia.
✦ **Planning loss** – loss of ability to plan activities and functional loss.
✦ **Low stress threshold** – decreased ability to tolerate stress.

Until relatively recently it was commonly assumed that intellectual capacity peaked in the late teens or early twenties, levelled off, and then began to decline fairly steadily during middle age, declining rapidly within old age. However, these cross-sectional studies were methodologically weak. Furthermore, several studies have indicated that at least some people retain their intellect well into middle age and beyond (Bosma *et al.*, 2003). Nevertheless, this evidence does seem to suggest that there are some age-related changes in the differing types of intelligence and aspects of memory.

In terms of intelligence, there is some indication that older people's IQ score deteriorates as they increase in age. Physiological changes related to the ageing process can have a serious effect on the brain's functioning which, in turn, can have an impact on intellectual performance (Beinhoff *et al.*, 2009). Therefore, it can be argued that the primary cause of intellectual deterioration in elderly people is the natural slowing of a person's nervous system processes (Stuart-Hamilton, 2007).

As well as intellectual deterioration, several aspects of an individual's memory appear to decline with age. As we age our memories of recent events tend to become less precise and less specified (Glisky *et al.*, 2001), and for some individuals memories such as declarative, non-declarative, working memory and remote memory become worse. This may affect the ability to live safely without assistance (Shagam, 2009). Memory is the ability to store, retain and recall information and experiences. A possible explanation that could explain memory deterioration could be the declined effectiveness of our information processing system (Stuart-Hamilton, 2007). Research conducted using recall tests has suggested a pronounced difference in memory recall, with older adults performing significantly lower (see Old and Naveh-Benjamine, 2008 for a meta-analysis of the research). Conversely, research concerning recognition tests has presented very small differences between younger and older individuals, with many of the differences often disappearing altogether (Luo and Craik, 2009). Nevertheless, evidence does seem to suggest that elderly people's memories do deteriorate for more recent events. This is seen particularly in elderly individuals with cognitive impairments where they seem to have more difficulty recalling events from later on in life but are able to recall events from their youth and early lives (Cuetos *et al.*, 2010).

Key message

Cognitive change is evident with increasing age.

Quick check

List the cognitive changes associated with ageing.

3.11 Social changes in late adulthood

Cumming and Henry (1961) suggested a social disengagement theory (SDT) to account for an individual's relationship with society, claiming that: 'Many of the relationships between a person and other members of society are severed and those remaining are altered in quality.' This disengagement involves the mutual withdrawal of an individual from society (through compulsory retirement, children leaving home, death of a spouse and so on). It is suggested that as an individual increases in age they become more solitary, retreat into the inner world of their memories and become emotionally disengaged. As far as society is concerned, the individual's withdrawal is part of an inevitable move towards death – the ultimate disengagement.

Think about this

In the light of SDT, are retirement homes a good thing?

Maintaining close relationships with others is often a significant factor in determining whether older people feel a sense of belonging within the social system. This may become important with age, because individuals withdraw from society both behaviourally (e.g. forced retirement) and attitudinally (attributing diminishing powers, abilities and qualities to older people). Hence, there is a need for both relatives and friends to ensure a positive older age experience. Overall, individual adaptation to old age on all levels has been shown to be related to the extent and quality of friendship and social networks that older people may hold (Donnelly and Hinterlong, 2010). Recently research has suggested that when older people participate in social networking sites they have the potential to reduce loneliness (Ballantyne *et al.*, 2010).

Think about this

How could you increase the friendship network of an elderly patient living alone?

In contrast to the SDT is the activity theory. This suggests that it is the ageist society that withdraws, against the wishes of most people. The withdrawal is not mutual.
Optimal aging requires several things:

✦ Continuing activity, including the maintenance of activities adopted in middle age.

✦ Replacing employment work with some form of substitute during retirement.

✦ Discovering substitutes for spouses or friends who may have passed on.

✦ Maintaining some form of role. Elderly individuals often assume many different roles within society.

Key message

Whatever theory you consider accurate, it is important for the older adult to engage in social activities.

3.12 Dementia

While it can be said that decreases in memory and numerous other cognitive abilities may be attributed in part to a normal age-related decline, where this is not the case and it can be seen that cognitive functioning of an individual falls below that of other individuals with a normal ageing decline, there is a possibility that such cognitive impairments may instead be a symptom of early neurodegenerative illness such as dementia (Cargin *et al.*, 2006). Dementia has been defined as 'an acquired global impairment of intellect, memory and personality' (David, 2009: 8). According to the Diagnostic and Statistical Manual of Mental Disorders IV (DSM-IV) a diagnosis of dementia requires impairment in memory, which can be defined as impaired ability to learn new information and to recall previously learned information. The diagnosis should also include impairment in at least one more area of cognitive function, such as language, executive functioning, impairment in motor activity and impairment in recognition. The diagnosis also should include a clinical course which is characterised by gradual onset and continuing decline (American Psychiatric Association (APA), 2000). It is estimated that approximately 24 million people across the world are living with dementia, and around 820,000 of these are living in the UK (Luengo-Fernandez *et al.*, 2010). This condition is found to affect around 1 in 20 individuals over the age of 65 and increases substantially to 1 in 5 for individuals over the age of 85. Furthermore, this figure is posited to double every 20 years (Ferri *et al.*, 2005). In comparison, there are approximately 18,500 people under the age of 65 with dementia living in the UK (Burgess *et al.*, 2006). There are many types of dementia, which can be differentiated into four categories (Alzheimer's Society, 2011), including:

+ **Frontotemporal dementia** – concerned with problems located within the brain's structure, particularly within the frontal and temporal lobes. Diagnosed in approximately 8–15 per cent of cases.

+ **Dementia with Lewy bodies** – small abnormal structures which develop inside nerve cells and lead to the degeneration of the brain's tissue. Diagnosed in approximately 10–15 per cent of cases.

+ **Vascular dementia** – caused through the diminishment of brain cells due to a lack of oxygen. This is caused by a cerebrovascular disease. Diagnosed in approximately 10–20 per cent of cases.

+ **Alzheimer's disease** – onset of this particular form of dementia is subtle but leads to progressive neuronal damage which, in turn, leads to memory loss, decreased cognitive functioning and disorientation. Diagnosed in approximately 50–60 per cent of cases.

As we can see, the most common form of dementia is Alzheimer's Disease, accounting for more than half of all cases. Dementia is a result of a decline in executive brain functioning, whatever the cause, and is usually diagnosed using a variety of clinical skills and evidence acquired through personal history, psychological assessment and brain scans (Burns and Hope, 1997), distinguishing age-related memory loss from that due to a disease process such as dementia especially in its early stages.

Think about this

What impact does dementia have on physical and mental well-being? How will this impact on the individual patient and their carer?

Key message

The rates of dementia in the UK are increasing. There are four categories of dementia: Frontotemporal dementia, dementia with Lewy bodies, Vascular dementia and Alzheimer's Disease. Alzheimer's Disease accounts for over half of all cases of dementia.

One of the main characteristics of dementia is cognitive impairment. Nurses should be aware that dementia care is no longer seen as a collection of deficits, where there is no hope for a patient. Instead, nurses should involve the patient as actively as possible, as well as utilising their strengths and abilities (Burgess *et al.*, 2006). The quality of life of a patient can be improved through the initiation of adequate communication and specialised individualised care. Adapting communication levels so that it is slow and simple will help a patient with dementia feel at ease (Turk and Turk, 2009). However, this does not mean (of course) the use of patronising language, just that it has to be adapted to your patient. Similarly, as we noted above, it is essential that you view dementia appropriately and not in a stereotypical manner, as this may influence how a patient feels and the satisfaction they gain from the care they receive.

Due to the psychological, social and behavioural disturbances related to dementia, an elderly person who is suffering with dementia will be significantly more dependent in comparison to an individual without dementia. Everyday activities can be disrupted by dementia (Aretouli and Brandt, 2010; Roper *et al.*, 1983; Shagam, 2009), thus there is a significantly higher need for support even in relation to basic everyday tasks. An additional concern is that the individual with dementia (especially in the early stages of the disease) may become angry and frustrated with both themselves and people around them due to their inability to be independent. Hence, there is a need for the nurse to understand that this may occur and be equipped with an understanding of how best to deal with the situation.

It has been discovered that elderly patients tend to be treated for their 'present illness', while pre-existing illnesses are ignored. For example, Hellzen *et al.* (2003) found that elderly patients who had a diagnosis of long-term schizophrenia as well as suffering from dementia tended only to be treated as a schizophrenic patient alone. As well as this, dementia needs to be distinguished from other conditions which it may overlap with or have some similarity with; these include delirium and depression, which can improve with appropriate treatments (Adams, 1997: 188).

Key message

It is essential that you take into account all past and present diagnoses of a patient in conjunction with their dementia.

When conversing with a patient, the nurse should aim to involve them in a conversation about themselves, rather than just discussing their present illness. The **person-focused approach** is very much dominant here, in which one of the aims is to maintain personhood in the face of failing mental powers (Kitwood, 1997).

Bush (2003) suggests that the focus should be on the person with dementia as an individual, not their diseased brain, on the person's emotions and understanding, not memory losses, and on the person within the context of marriage or family and within a wider society and its values. These can be attained with core values that stem from the humanistic approach (Suri, 2010):

+ **Congruence:** What the nurse verbally states should also be displayed via the non-verbal channel or in actions.

+ **Unconditional positive regard:** Should be demonstrated by caring for an elderly patient without any conditions or constraints on the relationship.

+ **Empathic understanding:** The nurse should attempt to understand how the elderly patient feels, thinks and perceives their symptoms as well as the environment around them.

Think about this

What does the person-centred approach mean in practice? Discuss with colleagues and come up with some concrete examples.

Communication with a patient with dementia

The importance of effective communication with dementia sufferers has grown with the increasing prevalence of the degenerative condition (Wang *et al.*, 2011). If caregivers ignore or fail to respond to these messages, more irritable or aggressive behaviours may result.

Feil (1996) suggests that **validation therapy** is the process of communicating with a disorientated older person. This is achieved by validating and respecting the person's feelings, in whatever context is real to that person at that time, even if it may not connect with the present reality of the hospital setting.

According to Morton's (1997, 1999) **pre-therapy**, there are a number of principles that can be beneficial for nurses who are caring for an elderly patient with impairments. The technique consists of the following reflections:

+ **Situational reflections:** used to strengthen contact with the world, and relate to facts, situation, people, environment and events.

+ **Facial reflections:** the nurse states the emotion that is apparent in the client's facial expression.

+ **Word-for-word reflections:** coherent communication or meaningful sounds are repeated by the nurse in an attempt to support communicative contact.

+ **Body reflections:** the nurse mirrors the posture or movements of the patient or reflects them via verbal description.

According to Iliffe and Drennan (2001), concentrating on effective communication with a patient who has dementia is the key to both understanding and resolving behaviour disturbances. Underlying all of these approaches is the emphasis on enhancing the quality of life for the elderly patient by keeping them actively involved. One of these approaches is to focus and utilise the positive resources within and surrounding the elderly patient. This apparent link between positive attitude and the enhancement of positive health is regularly publicised in the media.

Therefore it is critical as a nurse to learn and apply appropriate communication strategies and skills with dementia patients (Wang *et al.*, 2011).

Key message

An individual with dementia needs to be actively involved in their care in order to positively enhance their health and quality of life.

Quick check

Give some tips on how best to communicate with a person with dementia.

3.13 Death and dying

The final stage of our development – or ending, to be more accurate – is death. Death comes to all of us and it will be a common experience for many nurses throughout their professional career. The loss, through death, of loved ones (bereavement) can occur at any stage of life. The psychological and bodily reactions that occur in people who suffer bereavement (whatever form it takes) are called grief. The observable expression of grief is called mourning. We have to recognise that grief can begin before the actual death, and those dying can also grieve for their own death. Nurses have a crucial role to play in helping patients with a terminal illness (along with their friends and families) to come to accept their condition (Porter, 2010). This being said, emotional work will therefore form an important part of the critical care nurse's job. The significance of death, breaking bad news and interpersonal relationships are sources of emotional stress for the critical care nurse caring for the family of the critically ill. Therefore unless appropriately supported and managed, emotional work may lead to occupational stress and ultimately burnout (Stayt, 2009; see Chapter 5 for more information about burnout).

Key message

Death is inevitable. You need to be prepared for your involvement in bereavement and the grieving process for both a patient, and their family and friends.

3.14 Children's understanding of loss

When exploring children and their understanding and way of dealing with loss (infants up until early adolescence), it becomes apparent that there are enormous differences dependent on their stage of development (Rickles *et al.*, 2010: 301; Traeger, 2011). This can be understood in terms of children's cognitive stage development (as highlighted earlier on in this chapter). As a result, the way a nurse communicates with a child who is faced with issues such as loss, grief and death will need to differ accordingly. Table 3.2 illustrates the different grief reactions a child may exhibit depending on their stage of development. Furthermore, it highlights the potential input from a nurse or healthcare professional in supporting a child.

Table 3.2 Grief and developmental stages

Age	Understanding of death	Behavioural/ expression of grief	What can the nurse do when caring for a child who is grieving or is terminally ill?
Infants	Do not recognise death.	Separated from mother – sluggish, quiet and unresponsive to a smile or a coo.	Awareness by nurse that even though infant does not recognise death they are still affected by the lack of presence of the significant other.
	Feelings of loss and separation are part of developing an awareness of death.	Physical changes – weight loss, less active, sleep less.	
2–6 years	Confuse death with sleep.	Ask many questions: How does she eat?	Death here is associated with something that is mystical, magical and peaceful so make sure that your answers reflect this.
	Begin to experience anxiety by 3.	Problems in eating, sleeping and bladder and bowel control.	Giving the chid via non-verbal communication as much security as possible, i.e. comfort, attention, love.
		Fear of abandonment.	
		Tantrums.	
3–6 years	Still confuse death with sleep, i.e. is alive but only in a limited way.	Even though the child may have seen the deceased buried they still ask questions.	Answer acknowledging that concept of death up until about 5 is associated with something magical and peaceful, i.e. daddy is with the angels like you saw him in your dream.
	Death is temporary, not final.	Magical thinking – their thoughts may cause someone to die.	From 5 and thereon this begins the process of change to being associated with something that is scary and painful – hence afraid of the dark during the latter phases of this age group.
	Dead person can come back to life.	Under 5 – trouble eating, sleeping and controlling bladder and bowel functions.	
		Fear of darkness.	

(Continued)

Table 3.2 Grief and developmental stages (*Continued*)

Age	Understanding of death	Behavioural/ expression of grief	What can the nurse do when caring for a child who is grieving or is terminally ill?
6-9	Curious about death.	Ask specific questions.	Communication here should take into account the child's comprehension of death, which has changed from something that is magical and painless to something that is painful and destructive.
	Death is thought of as a person or spirit (skeleton, ghost, bogeyman).	May have exaggerated fears.	Even if a parent has protected the child from the subject of death, children will have an understanding from peers, education and the most influential source – the media.
	Death is final and frightening.	May have aggressive behaviours (especially boys).	
	Death happens to others, it won't happen to me.	Some concerns about imaginary illnesses.	
		May feel abandoned.	
9 years and older	Everyone will die.	Heightened emotions, guilt, anger, shame.	Guilt is a predominant feeling when grieving at this stage. You will need to take this into consideration.
	Death is final and cannot be changed.	Increased anxiety over own death.	Encourage the child to talk as much as possible and work though the guilt. Closing up over a long period of time may result in reference to a counsellor. Peers as a support network are highly beneficial here.
	Even I will die.	Mood swings.	
		Fear of rejection, not wanting to be different from peers.	
		Changes in eating habits.	
		Sleeping problems.	
		Regressive behaviours (loss of interest in outside activities).	
		Impulsive behaviours.	

(*Continued*)

Table 3.2 Grief and developmental stages (*Continued*)

Age	Understanding of death	Behavioural/ expression of grief	What can the nurse do when caring for a child who is grieving or is terminally ill?
9 years and older		Feel guilty about being alive (especially related to death of a parent, sibling or peer).	

Source: Partly adapted from National Cancer Institute, U.S. National Institutes of Health
http://www.cancer.gov/cancertopics/pdq/supportivecare/bereavement/Patient/allpages/

Think about this

How would you communicate with a child who is grieving for themselves, or their mother? Imagine the child is three years old, six years old, nine years old and 12 years old. How does this relate to Piaget's cognitive developmental stages previously outlined?

3.15 Models of grief

According to Archer (1999), a widely held assumption is that grief proceeds through an orderly series of stages or phases with distinct features. Traditional models have one main commonality, the need for grief work, which is described as 'an effortful process that we must go through entailing confrontation of the reality of loss and gradual acceptance of the world without the loved one' (Stroebe, 1998).

Parkes' (1972, 1986) four-stage model describes the phases of bereavement and in turn the grief work that one faces within this process (as displayed in Table 3.3).

The model is very much stage-like; however, the emphasis is on some sort of grief work, with the end result being adjustment to life without the deceased. One way nurses can use this model is also to apply it to terminally ill patients, with the end goal being acceptance of the illness. For example, many recent studies have focused on understanding anticipatory

Table 3.3 Parkes' phases of grief (1972/1986)

Phase	Reactions, emotions in each phase
One	Initial reaction: shock, numbness or disbelief.
Two	Pangs of grief, searching, anger, guilt, sadness and fear.
Three	Despair.
Four	Acceptance/adjustment. Giving a new identity.

grief in terminally ill patients (Cheng *et al.*, 2010). After all, patients who have been diagnosed with a terminal illness will go through exactly the same grieving process as someone who has lost a loved one and is grieving (Drew, 2006).

Key message

Grief can be seen as a process of stages, each of which has to be worked through in order to complete the process.

Another prime example of a similar stage-like model is that of Kübler-Ross' (1969) five-stage bereavement model, as shown in Table 3.4. This model has provided a framework for caregivers and nurses when working with individuals who are experiencing personal loss. Kübler-Ross was one of the first researchers to study patients and their families from the diagnosis of a terminal illness up until death. It was only after Kübler-Ross' research that more emphasis was given to palliative care and the importance of quality of life even if a patient will die (cf. Devi, 2011; Melin-Johansson *et al.*, 2010). Also, after the development of this pioneering work death and terminal illness were no longer regarded as a taboo subject, and thus it changed nursing/palliative care forever.

Quick check

List Parkes' and Kübler-Ross' stages of grief.

Table 3.4 Kübler-Ross' model (1969) – the five-stage model

Stage	Example	Explanation
Denial and isolation	'No, not me' or 'It can't be me – you must have the results mixed up.'	During this stage there is constant denial of the new status when a patient or family are told. Denial acts as a buffer system allowing the patient to develop other coping mechanisms. It can also bring isolation and the patient may fear rejection and abandonment in suffering, and feel that nobody understands what the suffering is like.
Anger	'It's not fair – why me?'	This is the stage whereby anger is taken out on practitioners such as nurses (and also doctors, relatives or other healthy people). Typical reactions are, 'because of you (the nurse), I can't go home and pick my children up from school' or 'because of you (the nurse) I have to take time out so you administer pain to me', or 'it's okay for you, you can go home at the end of the day'. Also there is a shift from the first stage from 'no it can't be me, it must be a mistake', to 'oh yes it is me, it was not a mistake'.

(Continued)

Table 3.4 Kübler-Ross' model (1969) – the five-stage model (*Continued*)

Stage	Example	Explanation
Bargaining	'Please God let me . . .'	This is an attempt to postpone death by doing a deal with God/fate/hospital. At this stage, people who are enduring a terminal illness and looking for a cure or 'a bit more time' will pay any price and will usually get manipulated at this stage. It is not uncommon for patients who have never been religious now to turn to religion – almost bargaining again – 'if I pray you will grant me another extra couple of days'. The problem is that even when the couple of extra days are granted, these are never enough, the patient wants more.
Depression	'How can I leave all of this behind?'	This time is very much a quiet, dark and reflective period, very similar to someone actually experiencing depression. During this stage, the dying patient does not want reassurance from a nurse, but at the same time does not want to be ignored. During this time family members of the dying patient begin the five-stage model so are very much attempting to be proactive, i.e. in denial that the family member is going to die. They may even become angry at the patient for 'giving up'. The dying patient during this stage would like people around them to be quiet, and this is where nurses can make a difference. All they want is someone to be present who does not question and is not angry. There will be questions the patient will ask and they need to be answered honestly (especially because they don't have to pretend to be strong away from the family). In addition to this, the patient during this stage would also like the nurse to anticipate questions.
Acceptance	'Leave me be, I'm ready to die.'	A stage where the individual is neither depressed nor angry. The individual has worked through feelings of loss and has found some peace. During this stage the patient has let go and is ready to go. Also within this stage, family members are very much angry or questioning why the patient is at peace when they still want to change the status of the patient. The patient, however, has begun the process of letting go during the depression stage and has finished this process of acceptance. They are ready to move on.

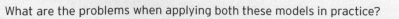

Think about this

What are the problems when applying both these models in practice?

Research in Focus

Gibson, F., Aldiss, S., Horstman, M., Kumpunen, S. and Richardson, A. (2010) Children and young people's experiences of cancer care: A qualitative research study using participatory methods. *International Journal of Nursing* **47**, 1397-1407.

Background

Previous research has the propensity to consider only the views of parents in relation to children's cancer care services. Due to this there has been very little research concerning the ability of children's cancer services in actually meeting the needs of the children they care for. Therefore this study aimed to explore the views of children and young people in relation to their cancer care. Furthermore, it also aimed to develop a conceptual model of communication and information sharing.

Methods

Participants: Thirty-eight participants were recruited from three Principal Cancer Treatment centres in the UK. Participants were at different stages of their treatment – on treatment, ending of treatment, and up to 18 months following treatment, and were split into three groups dependent on age: 4–5 years, 6–12 years and 13–19 years.

Measures: Age-appropriate, participatory-based techniques were assumed in data collection over a six-month period. These techniques included interviews and activity days, draw and write methods, and the use of play and puppets.

Results

Some findings confirmed previously reported issues concerning young children's inability to discuss their preferences, their views on the importance of being within familiar environments and having parental support for all ages. Furthermore, new findings discovered that older children were worried about parents and their tendency to lead any communication with health professionals, and that all children worry about their symptoms and the permanency of them. The area which children differed dramatically in preferences was in relation to communication and information sharing. Thus, a conceptual model of communication roles of patients, their parents and the healthcare professionals was proposed in order to illustrate communication patterns. This model posits that 4-12-year-olds tend to reside in the background when sharing information with health professionals until they gain autonomy. At this point they move into the foreground with their parents taking their place in the background and assuming a supportive role. This model may enable younger children to acknowledge their ability to discuss their preferences. Furthermore, parents and professionals can adapt it in learning to concentrate on their supportive roles rather than leading communication pathways.

Implications

This contributes to nursing practice within a cancer setting by offering a perspective on the preferences and needs of children and young people who are receiving cancer care.

→

It was discovered that the predominant difference of preferences was in relation to communication; therefore it is essential to consider these differences and the implications of these differences when communicating and sharing information with children and young people.

3.16 Conclusion

Psychology has attempted to highlight and explain an individual's development from birth through to our eventual death. Many studies have indicated that cognitive abilities, behaviours and social interactions differ across the lifespan. Knowledge of these differences is essential in enabling and assisting the nurse in approaching and having the ability to relieve patients of any concerns that they may have.

Think about this

Can you identify any stages of development across the lifespan? Do these stages affect an individual's level of understanding? How do you think the ages of Mrs Patel's children will affect their understanding of health and illness?

3.17 Summary

+ Development is not just about childhood, it is about changing and developing continuously throughout our entire life.
+ Children are not simply small adults.
+ Piaget proposed a stage theory – children progress through a set of qualitatively different stages.
+ Piaget's theory included the following stages: the sensori-motor stage (0-2 years), the pre-operational stage (2-6 years), the concrete operational stage (7-12 years) and formal operational stage (12+ years).
+ Attachment ensures that children get more from their mothers than simply nourishment.
+ John Bowlby noted that babies showed separation anxiety when their mothers are absent.
+ Bronfenbrenner developed the ecological systems theory to explain how everything in a child and all levels of their environment affects how a child grows and develops.
+ Vygotsky emphasised the importance of the social context on development, specifically the influence of social interaction.
+ Erikson proposed eight stages in human personality development, beginning in infancy and continuing into late adulthood.

+ The older adult population is ageing, but the 'elderly' cannot be considered a homogenous group.

+ Stereotypes of older people (the elderly) are deeply entrenched and can be widely inaccurate.

+ There are a number of cognitive losses and impairments associated with ageing.

+ There are social changes associated with ageing.

+ A significant characteristic of dementia is cognitive impairment.

+ The person with dementia needs to be actively involved in their care.

+ The loss, through death, of loved ones (bereavement) can occur at any stage of life.

+ The psychological and bodily reactions that occur in people who suffer bereavement (whatever form it takes) are called grief.

+ Grief can be seen as a process of stages, each of which has to be worked through.

Your end point

Answer the following questions to assess your knowledge and understanding of psychology across the lifespan.

1. If a child shows secure attachment, what behaviour will they exhibit when a parent leaves them in an unfamiliar environment?

    (a) Be ready and willing to explore their surroundings.
    (b) Be clingy with the parent.
    (c) Show anger towards the parent.
    (d) Try to reconcile with the parent.
    (e) None of the above.

2. What is adolescent egocentrism?

    (a) The adolescent's belief that friends are more important than family.
    (b) The adolescent's preoccupation with him- or herself.
    (c) The adolescent's desire to start romantic relationships.
    (d) The adolescent's ability to think at the formal operations stage.
    (e) None of the above.

3. Which factor(s) have been identified as critical to maintaining positive mental and physical health in late adulthood:

    (a) having grandchildren
    (b) retirement
    (c) social support
    (d) (a) and (b)
    (e) (a), (b) and (c)?

4. Identify the correct statement from those given below, with respect to peer influence in adolescence:

    (a) Adolescents tend to choose friends who have markedly different interests to their own.

→

(b) Adolescents tend to choose friends who have similar interests to their own.

(c) Adolescents invariably report that peer pressures have a major influence on their behaviour.

(d) Causation exists between friends' behaviour and adolescents' choices and actions.

(e) None of the above.

5. According to Erikson, what stage of psychosocial development is prominent during adolescence:

(a) trust vs. mistrust

(b) identity vs. role confusion

(c) autonomy vs. shame and doubt

(d) initiative vs. guilt

(e) none of the above?

Further reading

Baillargeon, R. and DeVos, J. (1991) Object permanence in young infants: Further evidence. *Child Development* **62**, 1227-1246.

Baltes, P.B. and Mayer, K.U. (1999) *The Berlin Ageing Study: Ageing from 70 to 100.* Cambridge, UK: Cambridge University Press.

Bee, H. (2006) *The Developing Child.* 11th edition. Addison Wesley: London.

Brooks, A.M. (1985) *The Grieving Time: A Year's Account of Recovery from Loss.* Garden City, NY: Dial Press.

Dunkle, R.E., Roberts, B. and Haus, M.R. (2001) *The Oldest Old in Everyday Life: Self Perception, Coping with Change, and Stress.* New York: Springer.

Graff, M.J.L., Vernooij-Dassen, M.J.M., Zajec, J., Olde-Rikkert, M.G.M., Hoefnagels, W.H.L. and Dekker, J. (2006). How can occupational therapy improve the daily performance and communication of an older patient with dementia and his primary caregiver? A case study. *Dementia* **5**(4), 503-532.

Kean, S. (2010) Children and young people visiting an adult in intensive care unit. *Journal of Advanced Nursing* **66**(4), 868-877.

Kozulin, A. (ed.). (2003) *Vygotsky's Educational Theory in Cultural Context.* Cambridge, UK: Cambridge University Press.

Kübler-Ross, E. (1969) *On Death and Dying.* New York: Macmillan.

Meins, E. (1997) *Security of Attachment and the Social Development of Cognition.* Hove: Psychology Press.

Schucksmith, J. and Hendry, L.B. (1998) *Health Issues and Adolescents: Growing Up and Speaking Out.* London: Routledge.

Wang, J.J., Hu, C.J. and Cheng, W.Y. (2011) Dementia patients: effective communication strategies. *Journal of Nursing* **58**(1), 85-90.

Weblinks

http://www.simplypsychology.pwp.blueyonder.co.uk/attachment.html
Attachment. This site contains detailed information on all of the main attachment theories. There is also a video of Harlow's experiment of attachment in Rhesus monkeys.

http://www.dementialink.org
Dementia Link. This site provides useful information and support for patients, carers and health professionals.

http://www.alzheimers.org.uk
Alzheimer's Society. An up-to-date link providing useful information regarding dementia.

http://www.compassionatefriends.org
Compassionate Friends. This website offers support for those who have experienced the death of a child.

http://www.piaget.org
Piaget. This site is all about Jean Piaget, the influential developmental psychologist.

http://www.srcd.org
Society for Research in Child Development. This website contains all the latest news and developments in the world of child development, including links to interesting journal articles.

Check point

Your starting point		Your end point	
Q1	D	Q1	A
Q2	C	Q2	B
Q3	B	Q3	C
Q4	D	Q4	C
Q5	B	Q5	B

Chapter 4

Social processes

Learning Outcomes

At the end of this chapter you will be able to:

✦ Understand the relative contribution of verbal and non-verbal communication in conveying messages

✦ Appreciate the role of 'attitudes' in influencing our behaviour

✦ Understand how to influence and modify attitudes

✦ Persuade people to change their attitudes to healthcare and consequently their behaviour

✦ Understand how groups affect a person's ability to conform to a particular health regime

✦ Understand how adherence to advice can be improved

✦ Realise how the concepts of power and status influence our willingness to conform to healthcare.

Your starting point

Answer the following questions to assess your knowledge and understanding of social processes in nursing.

1. Which of the following is true of Milgram's (1963) study of obedience? The study found that:
   (a) Quite ordinary people taking part in a laboratory experiment were prepared to administer electric shocks just because an experimenter told them to do so.
   (b) Participants believed that the shocks they administered would not harm anyone.
   (c) Apparently pathological behaviour may not be due to individual pathology but to particular social circumstances.
   (d) (a) and (b).
   (e) None of the above.

2. What were the conclusions drawn about ordinary people based on Milgram's famous study of obedience?
   (a) People will engage in high levels of destructive obedience when faced with strong situational pressures.
   (b) People will engage in low levels of destructive obedience when faced with strong situational pressures.
   (c) People's personality is the strongest determinant of obedient behaviour.
   (d) People will challenge authority figures when they become distressed by their commands.
   (e) (c) and (d).

3. Which one of the following statements about social support is true?
   (a) Social support in a broad social network impacts positively on health and stress.
   (b) Social support in small groups helps one resist pressures to comply with an outside majority or to obey an immoral authority.
   (c) Both (a) and (b).
   (d) Neither (a) nor (b).
   (e) Social support has no impact on health.

4. A change in behaviour or belief as a result of real or imagined group pressure is:
   (a) compliance
   (b) conformity
   (c) acceptance
   (d) reactance
   (e) none of the above?

5. Attribution theory:
   (a) was initiated by Leon Festinger
   (b) considered how individuals manage to infer the 'causes' underlying the behaviour of others, and even their own behaviour
   (c) became influential because it was instantly accessible to the average researcher in North America
   (d) was backed up by a large bank of research
   (e) is none of the above?

Case Study

Jenna is a 21-year-old who has mild learning difficulties. She is admitted to hospital after her social worker finds her collapsed at home where she lives with her flatmate. Jenna has great difficulty communicating her emotions verbally and her friends and family usually rely on her non-verbal behaviours to recognise how she is feeling.

While at the hospital, Jenna is examined by Poppy, a newly qualified nurse who has been assigned to Jenna. Poppy finds that Jenna is severely underweight and is suffering from exhaustion. Furthermore, when Jenna is asked a few questions to get some more information about her and her family history it becomes apparent that she has recently taken up smoking. Although she knows it is bad for her health, she feels that it helps her reduce her worries. During Jenna's examination her social worker recognises Jenna's non-verbal signals and determines that she is very anxious and distressed by the procedures and the possibility of being admitted to hospital.

While Poppy is attending to Jenna, the social worker tells Poppy that Jenna is very distressed by the procedures that are being carried out. Poppy acknowledges this and, in order to reduce any anxiety, tries adapting her own non-verbal communication skills in a way that will reassure Jenna.

After many tests, it is confirmed that Jenna may have an eating disorder which is getting progressively worse and is also affecting her day-to-day living. Poppy thinks that there are some underlying issues which may be perpetuating Jenna's bad eating habits and suggests that it may be advantageous to Jenna if she gained some support from either a counsellor or a support group. However, Jenna gets extremely aggravated at this suggestion and claims that she can look after herself without any more help. Poppy then goes on to try and persuade Jenna of the positive aspects that this support would have on her health and well-being.

Why is this relevant to nursing practice?

This case study demonstrates the relevance of social processes at a number of different levels. First, all of us work and live in a social world, irrespective of our age, our sex, ethnicity or intellectual ability. We all communicate with others through a variety of different ways and the nurse has to appreciate these fully both so they can understand what another person is saying (or perhaps not saying) and so they can communicate effectively with others. However, social processes are not just about communication, they include anything that involves an interaction with others. In this chapter we will explore some of these and demonstrate the relevance to nursing practice.

Think about this

Consider Jenna's initial contact with a hospital – what sort of interactions will she have? How will this make her feel?

4.1 Introduction

Interacting and communicating with others is a significant part of the nursing profession. By the laws of probability there will be some nurses who will never talk or interact with people but they will be very few in number. The focus of this chapter will be on all other nurses who do interact with others surrounding them. These may be your friends, your medical colleagues, your nursing colleagues, other professions or, looking back at the case study, your patients and clients. The aim of this chapter is to explore the social processes involved in our interactions and to examine how they may influence the relationship that you form with others. Furthermore, we will determine how and why knowledge of this relationship can assist you with your practice.

To begin with we will look at the importance of **non-verbal communication** (NVC) and how this can be beneficial in any kind of social interaction, whether it be between nurses and members of the public, between different healthcare professionals, or even between friends and family. This is important, since some studies suggest that almost three-quarters of any message are conveyed by non-verbal communication. This means that a message and the importance of that message is significantly influenced by how we may convey it rather than what we actually say.

We will then move on and explore the concepts of **attitudes** and **cognitive dissonance**, which are important in all areas of healthcare. We will also need to explore **persuasion**, and the concepts of **conformity** and **obedience**. How are these related to health and social status? How are these issues and further issues of **power** and **status** related to the work of the nurse? How are these related to the concept of compliance (or adherence or concordance) to health? And, how can we manage and increase client empowerment?

Finally, we will then turn our attention to **stereotyping** and the impact it can have on our nursing practice.

Think about this

+ List all of the people you interact with in your work.
+ What type of relationship do you have with these people?
+ What type of techniques do you use to try to alter their behaviour?
+ What sort of techniques do they use on *you*?

4.2 Non-verbal communication (NVC)

When trying to convey a message to another individual, we can adopt a number of strategies. The most obvious one is to just say something. For instance, if someone were to ask, 'Have you done your assignment?' the meaning of this sentence would be clearly understood by the recipient, wouldn't it? Well, just with this simple message there can be numerous interpretations depending on the non-verbal messages one might present. For example, if we look

Table 4.1 Non-verbal communication

Face	What would the message be?
Happy	Are you joking?
Serious	Get on and do your assignment!
Angry	Haven't you done it yet?
Sarcastic	You're not going to do your assignment are you?
Worried	You are going to lose marks doing it this late.

at each of the 'faces' in Table 4.1 and try to imagine that the simple question had been asked by each 'face' – what would the message say? Would the message change depending on the face that said it?

Non-verbal communication (NVC) refers to any form of behaviour which conveys a message, distinct from written or verbal language. These include facial expressions, communicative gaze and eye contact, body movements and posture (proxemics – communicative use of personal space), arm and hand gestures, and various body movements (kinesics) (Coleman, 2009). NVC is a more subtle form of communication in comparison to speech, and therefore it can often be hard to determine. Nevertheless, non-verbal behaviour is considered important for successful communication (Andre *et al.*, 2011; Zolnierek and DiMatteo, 2009). Argyle (1988) suggests that the non-verbal component of communication is five times more influential than the verbal aspect.

Key message

When trying to convey an important message, it is important to take into consideration not only what you say but how you say it.

In order to adopt effective communication, it is essential to present clear messages, and interpret and respond to a message in an appropriate way. In any nurse dyad both parties reveal a great deal about themselves through the use of NVC. For this reason it is essential that all nurses have an understanding of this concept (Casey and Wallis, 2011; Curtis *et al.*, 2011; Jootun and McGhee, 2011).

Let's look at an extreme example. If you were telling a patient that they had a life limiting condition, it is unlikely that you would do it laughing. Similarly, you would not do it crying wholeheartedly. These reactions would both be inappropriate. A professional manner would be essential when in this particular situation. But, of course, the NVC required in a professional setting may differ according to the setting. Hence, a nurse will have to have the ability to communicate appropriately and also understand the recipient's NVC.

Nishizawa *et al.* (2006) discovered that when student nurses communicated with each other, they adopted significantly less non-verbal communicative behaviour than qualified nurses. The authors posited that training programmes should be implemented in order for student nurses to improve both their own non-verbal skills and their understanding of patients' and clients' NVC.

Think about this

Have a conversation with a friend about any problems you are experiencing with your nurse training. During the conversation ask your friend to show empathy using verbal and non-verbal communication. Note any non-verbal forms of communication that your friend uses. Now change roles and repeat the task.

Through the use of NVC we can express either confidence or nervousness which can impact on the confidence of our patients, clients and colleagues. It also provides information about one's feelings and intentions (whether someone likes us or not). We can use NVC to transmit a whole range of different emotions, attitudes, directions, and guidance. Indeed any message can be enhanced (or damaged) by NVC. For example, Zolnierek and DiMatteo (2009) suggested that NVC in a medical care setting is highly correlated with better adherence. The authors illustrated that there was a 19 per cent greater risk of non-adherence among patients whose physicians communicate poorly than among those whose physicians communicate well. Hence, the ability to use and understand NVC appropriately is essential when conversing and interacting with our patients and others whom we may come into contact with.

So what exactly is it?

NVC covers a considerable range of activity from the subtle intonation in a person's voice to the more obvious facial expressions (e.g. grimacing) and hand gestures (e.g. shaking a fist) (Casey and Wallis, 2011). Table 4.2 illustrates a range of non-verbal messages and how they can be related to your practice.

Quick check

List the key areas of non-verbal communication.

From the information presented in Table 4.2 how important are NVC in your day-to-day work? Research has explored the use of NVC in nurses. For example, Caris-Verhallen *et al.* (2001) reported that nurses use mainly eye gazes, head nodding and smiling as a means to establish a good relationship with their elderly patients. What is important to note is that the NVC (like any form of communication) should change depending on the situation and the person you are talking to. For instance, due to the cognitive impairment evident in individuals with dementia, their abilities to communicate effectively may be limited. In turn, this inability may affect a nurse's ability to understand and cater for their patients' needs. In a situation such as this, it is essential that the nurse shows sensitivity towards their patient and encourages them to communicate in a way most appropriate and comfortable for them (Jootun and McGhee, 2011; Smith *et al.*, 2010). Furthermore, the way you communicate may also need to vary depending on what message you are trying to convey and in what situation. Eye gazes and eye contact are considered the most important and useful, in conveying information, of the NVC skills assumed by nurses. However, too much eye contact can make a client/patient feel embarrassed and uncomfortable. Conversely, a lack of eye contact can

Table 4.2 Non-verbal communication

Non-verbal communication	Description	Related to nursing practice
Eye contact	The visual sense is dominant for most people, and therefore especially important in non-verbal communication.	Eye contact is key when giving important information – this could be good or bad news over a diagnosis for example.
Facial expression	Universal facial expressions signify anger, fear, sadness, joy and disgust.	Think about your facial expression when changing a dressing – do you want to show anger or disgust?
Tone of voice	The sound of your voice conveys your moment-to-moment emotional experience.	Tone of voice is of key importance when, for example, trying to reassure somebody with depression.
Posture	Your posture – including the pose, stance and bearing regarding the way you sit, slouch, stand, lean, bend, hold and move your body in space – affects the way people perceive you.	When a client/patient is telling you important information, leaning forward will make you appear interested.
Touch	Finger pressure, grip and hugs should feel good to you and the other person. What 'feels good' is relative; some prefer strong pressure, others prefer light pressure.	When telling patients distressing information, touch can be a powerful communicator.
Timing and pace	Your ability to be a good listener and communicate interest and involvement is affected by timing and pace.	When your client is telling you key elements of their mental health you will need to ensure your interventions are appropriately timed.
Sounds that convey understanding	Sounds such as 'ahhh, ummm, ohhh,' uttered with congruent eye and facial gestures, communicate understanding and emotional connection. More than words, these sounds are the language of interest, understanding and compassion.	These minimal encouragers can help the patient/client pass on more information.

be unnerving and worrying. Therefore, it is essential that you are able to use and adjust these skills appropriately.

Another area in which NVC plays an essential role is in pain behaviours (for more information see Chapter 7).

Key message

Eye contact is important when conveying a message. However, remember that too much can be unnerving for an individual.

An acronym that has been posited as useful when engaging in NVC is SOLER (Egan, 2002). It suggests that when engaging with a patient we should:

+ **S** – **S**it facing our patient
+ **O** – keep our posture **O**pen
+ **L** – position ourselves **L**eaning slightly forward
+ **E** – establish and maintain **E**ye contact
+ **R** – keep our posture **R**elaxed.

As well as our body movements, we need to consider the paralinguistic features of NVC. These are our way of speaking and the characteristics of our voice, which can be explained as (McCabe and Timmins, 2006):

+ Volume – the need to determine whether it should be loud or soft.
+ Intonation and pitch – the need to determine what frequency is suitable for the meaning we are trying to convey.
+ Rate of speech – the speed at which we speak can reflect our emotions and attitudes.
+ Tone of voice – the need to consider volume, intonation and rate of speech in conjuction in order to convey different messages.
+ Conversational cues – we need to be aware of how to use these in order to show our interest and our agreement or disagreement.
+ Choice of words – the need to consider these and how we emphasise certain words as this can indicate the degree of our interest.

Nurses need to take all of these into consideration when trying to convey a particular message to their patient in a way that is appropriate and understandable to them.

Another distinct aspect of NVC is touch. Touch is considered a particular type of NVC and can be particularly beneficial in a therapeutic setting. Five discrete categories of touch were identified by Jones and Yarbrough (1985):

+ positive affect (e.g. to show appreciation)
+ playful (e.g. to show humour)
+ control (e.g. to draw attention)
+ ritualistic (e.g. greetings)
+ task-related (e.g. nurse taking a pulse).

Two of the five categories that are used widely within nursing practice are positive affect – to communicate reassurance and nurturance – and task-related touch – the use of touch to accomplish tasks such as pulse taking or bathing a patient. Touch has been linked to the phenomenon of caring which in turn fits the concept of nursing practice. Therapeutic touch when used appropriately can be used to convey warmth, empathy and comfort. Reynolds (2002) reported on the usefulness of therapeutic touch when used appropriately in nursing children with cancer.

As postulated by Gleeson and Higgins (2009) touch can also be effective in mental health nursing; however it is only considered therapeutic to patients if used judiciously, with effective interpersonal skills. It is also suggested that nurses need to both be sensitive to the individual's needs and honour their personal space and cultural background.

Think about this

Where and when would you use each of the categories of touch in your practice?

Again, it is important to know when and with whom to use touch. The use of touch by nurses in adult patients has been shown to have differing effects depending on whether they are on males and females (and also whether the nurse was male or female). For instance, Gleeson and Higgins (2009) carried out a study exploring nurses' perceptions of touch; they suggested that male nurses had concerns that touching female patients would be misinterpreted as a sexual advance. The authors also suggested that male nurses would protect themselves by using touch in a cautious and minimal manner, and only in a public space, where others could view the interaction. Furthermore, Whitcher and Fisher (1979) carried out a study where both males and females were touched by a nurse during a pre-operative interaction. Although brief and 'professional' this had a significant effect on post-operative physiological and psychological questionnaire measures. The female patients who had been touched reported less fear and anxiety and had lower blood pressure readings than patients who had not been touched. Unfortunately, the reverse was noted in male patients – they were more anxious and had higher blood pressure. Additionally, research has illustrated that these sex differences may reflect more general status differences: people who initiate touch are thought to have higher status than those who receive touch. When the person touching is clearly higher in status than the recipient, it has been demonstrated that men and women react in a positive way to being touched (Fuller *et al.*, 2011).

Key message

Stop and look – you can learn more from what people do than from what they are saying.

Although difficult, NVC can be learned and can be developed over the course of your training. Ishikawa *et al.* (2010) developed a programme for teaching NVC skills to try and examine whether it would improve awareness and performance of NVC. The authors concluded that the programme was effective in increasing awareness of NVC, but it was not sufficient to change actual performance. Additionally, Levy-Storms (2008) identified that therapeutic communication techniques including NVC skills such as eye contact, affective touch and smiling, can all be taught. Furthermore, effective use of these skills can benefit quality of life for nurses, individuals with learning disabilities and older adults.

Think about this

Considering Jenna in the case study from the beginning of this chapter, what types of non-verbal communication would you use in order to reassure and calm her whilst performing the procedure? What non-verbal behaviours would you expect her to display?

Quick check

What is the meaning of the following facial expressions?

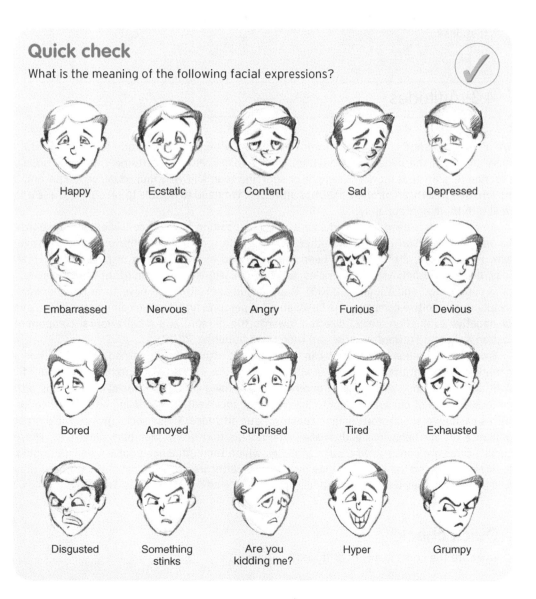

Happy   Ecstatic   Content   Sad   Depressed

Embarrassed   Nervous   Angry   Furious   Devious

Bored   Annoyed   Surprised   Tired   Exhausted

Disgusted   Something stinks   Are you kidding me?   Hyper   Grumpy

Think about this

Discuss the types of NVC that would be useful in the following situations:

+ telling a mother her child has cancer
+ discussing medication issues with a young woman with schizophrenia
+ trying to develop cooking skills in a young man with learning difficulties
+ helping an old man with his continence
+ telling a 14-year-old her mother has died in an accident
+ telling a couple that the ultrasound scan of their unborn child is perfectly normal.

What type of NVC would you expect the individual patient/client to exhibit in the above situations?

4.3 Attitudes

We all have a range of attitudes. Some of these may be benign (attitude towards a certain make of pencil sharpeners or serviettes), others may create an extremely warm or hostile reaction (e.g. attitudes towards religion or sporting teams). Every individual, be it a parent, a patient or a healthcare professional, has attitudes. We need to be able to recognise these and deal with them appropriately.

An attitude has been described as a learned disposition to react consistently in response to an object, person or issue in either a favourable (positive) or unfavourable (negative) way. Furthermore, attitudes have been characterised as an enduring organisation of feelings, beliefs and behaviour tendencies directed towards socially significant objects, events or groups (Hogg and Vaughan, 2008). Many argue that attitudes have three components, including a cognitive component (a belief about a person), an affective component (a positive or negative evaluation feeling directed towards the person) and a behavioural component (action is directed towards the person) (Hogg and Vaughan, 2008).

From the definition provided, it can be seen that attitudes are learned – they are not a genetic component that come with us when we are born – we learn them throughout our life. Attitudes are formed as a result of **observational learning** during our social interactions with various aspects of our environment. Child-rearing, socialisation, schooling and identification with a particular social group help to construct our attitudes. These social groups wield great influence on our behaviour and create social norms that group members adhere to. These social norms are constructed around attitudes which then influence people's understanding, their reactions and the decisions they make. In a healthcare setting a patient's attitudes may well affect how they understand and follow healthcare advice (Nixon and Aruguete, 2010).

Quick check

What are the components of attitudes?

For example, take an individual who has been trying to give up smoking for some time but has been unsuccessful in their attempts. After some time, they decide to discuss their attempts with a practice nurse and it becomes apparent that their attitudes are being influenced by family and friends. This illustrates how an individual and their family's attitudes can have an influential role in their behaviour (see Chapter 7). Furthermore, the effectiveness of the treatment that is suggested – nicotine replacement therapy (NRT) – to help individuals give up smoking can also be influenced by attitudes (Nixon and Aruguete, 2010), for example, if they believe there is a possible risk of addiction to nicotine as a detriment of NRT or that NRT 'was worse than smoking'. Therefore, the attitudes of significant others, and an individual's own attitudes, have a major impact on their decision and progress in their feat to quit smoking (Halterman *et al.*, 2010).

Key message

Attitudes of both the individual and significant others can have a key impact on the success of treatment.

This explains that attitudes can impact on health from many different directions – the attitudes of the smoker's family have impact upon the support they provide for the individual and consequently the individual's ability to succeed. Similarly, the individual's own attitude towards NRT is impacting on the use of appropriate interventions and (probably) the success of the intervention. Therefore we need to understand an individual's attitudes in order to determine and predict how their behaviour may be affected. Similarly, if we can succeed in changing their attitude then we may also be able to change their behaviour.

Unfortunately, it is not this simple, and some people have reported that there is no relationship between attitudes and behaviour. For example, Gregson and Stacey (1981) found only a small correlation between attitudes and self-reported alcohol consumption. Furthermore, the authors discovered that there was very little beneficial impact of changing attitudes on the changing of one's behaviour. Similarly, Dave *et al.* (2009) found a limited relationship between attitudes towards fast food and unhealthy consumption. As a consequence of these and many other studies it has been posited that overt behaviour and attitudes are not directly associated with one another. For instance, the link between them has been found to be promoted and disrupted by a number of conditions (Smith and Stasson, 2000) and the consistency of attitude-behaviour is dependent on:

✦ how accessible an attitude is to the individual

✦ how the attitude is expressed – privately or within a group setting

✦ how much an individual may identify with a group.

Therefore, it seems that we cannot always determine how an individual may behave only by considering the attitudes they hold. We also need to take into consideration whether the context or other people may have an influence on an individual's behaviour.

So, why spend time on this concept if it is a complete waste of time? Well, the use of attitudes has been developed further within health psychology in looking at 'social cognition models' that can help predict behaviour. For example, it has been demonstrated that a person's beliefs and attitudes about medication can predict treatment adherence (Beltran *et al.*, 2007; Munson *et al.*, 2010).

These models are explained further in Chapter 5 and demonstrate the value of attitudes within healthcare practice and how these are essential to alter behaviour and improve health. However, what we also have to explore are nurses' attitudes – does the attitude held by a nurse impact on their behaviour and actions? Although nurses do participate in professional training, they are still humans who hold their own attitudes (Byrne *et al.*, 2005). Therefore, as a nurse, you need to acknowledge that you have your own views and attitudes in order to avoid the potential influence that these may have on your professional practice. Furthermore, you need to be aware that your colleagues, peers and seniors also have their own attitudes and views.

Nurses also have attitudes that may influence how they provide care for patients (Albers-Heitner *et al.*, 2011; Kang *et al.*, 2011; Matziou *et al.*, 2009; Schafer *et al.*, 2011). Attitudes towards people with mental illness are generally negative in the general population. These negative attitudes manifest themselves in the form of bias, distrust, fear, embarrassment, anger, stereotyping and avoidance. Unfortunately, due to these attitudes, the way a nurse cares for a patient can be influenced by these manifestations. Moreover, these attitudes may also result in many nurses avoiding a profession within mental health practice (Schafer *et al.*, 2011). Additionally, nurses' negative attitudes towards disabled people are well documented, explaining that they do not exhibit the essential sensitivity and appropriate attitudes towards them. Recent research has examined nurses' attitudes towards disabled children and illustrates these negative attitudes and that these negative attitudes can act as barriers to the rehabilitation process (Matziou *et al.*, 2009).

Think about this

How you would you improve Jenna's attitude towards her bad eating habits? How would this differ when trying to change an elderly adult's attitude towards taking their medication for hypertension?

Cognitive dissonance

As explained, attitudes may be positive and we can use these to change the behaviour of our colleagues and our clients. However, what about when attitudes collide? What happens when we have two different views on certain behaviours or towards a certain belief? According to Festinger (1957), there is a pressure for one to be consistent, thus **cognitive dissonance** occurs when one becomes aware of inconsistencies in their cognitions (thoughts, attitudes and beliefs). Dissonance can be defined as a motivational state which results when our behaviour is inconsistent with the attitudes we hold (Stone and Cooper, 2001). This apparent dissonance will create psychological tension within an individual (Cooper, 2007), which will then pressure them to remove or reduce the inconsistency. Therefore, health-related messages that conflict with an individual's normal behaviour may cause a sense of dissonance. One clear example of this is in individuals who smoke (e.g. Radsma and Bottorff, 2009) – they may have one piece of information suggesting that smoking is unhealthy, but they will also have conflicting information (that they get pleasure from smoking). These pieces of information are inconsistent, resulting in cognitive dissonance.

People seek harmony in their attitudes, beliefs and behaviour, and because dissonance is unpleasant psychologically they make every effort to reconcile and resolve their conflicting thoughts. Furthermore, as the dissonance becomes stronger their motivation to resolve it also becomes stronger. Festinger (1957) compared dissonance to hunger, arguing that when either occurs humans are motivated to reduce or eliminate it.

Think about this

Consider Jenna's smoking habit and the cognitive dissonance that she exhibits due to it. How will she try to resolve this dissonance? How can this be both positive and negative? How can the nurse use cognitive dissonance to support change in behaviour?

There are three strategies which can resolve dissonance (Cooper, 2007; Taylor *et al.*, 2003; Simon *et al.*, 1995); first, the individual can revoke the behaviour in some form. However, these behaviours are often resistant to change. Another strategy a person may adopt is through rationalisation or denial which allows them to keep their current attitudes and behaviour. For instance, in the case of the adverse health effects of smoking, people may search for evidence that supports one side of the argument or attack the credibility of the information given. Furthermore, the greater the dissonance, the stronger the pressure to reduce it and one way people may attempt to do this is by avoiding the information to begin with. If the information can be avoided then behaviour change is likely to be very difficult. The final strategy, and usually the one adopted most often, is for the individuals to change their attitudes.

Think about this

Think of a time you have experienced cognitive dissonance during your training. How have you tried to resolve this?

Quick check

What is cognitive dissonance?

4.4 Stereotyping

Related to attitudes are stereotypes. Stereotyping involves classifying people according to personal attributes associated with a particular social group or category (Taylor *et al.*, 2003). Stereotypes are often based on characteristics such as age, gender, personal appearance, ethnic origin or national or regional characteristics: they are never a representation of what the person is actually like as an individual.

Nurses, like the general public, may be influenced by the stereotyping of individuals (Brown, 2006; Simpson and Fothergill, 2004). Furthermore, research has suggested that nurses also have to be aware that there are stereotypes of them that are held by the public. For instance, male nurses have to be aware of their professional, legal and ethical responsibilities as they, in particular, tend to face problems in their practice due to the stereotypes which are related to their gender (Gleeson and Higgins, 2009; Prideaux, 2010). There is also a widely held view that nursing is not an intellectually demanding or challenging job which is the result of media representations of nurses (Cabaniss, 2011). Because of this, it is important that you have an awareness of this concept so as to avoid any interference with the development of a good therapeutic relationship between nurse and patient. Stereotypes are usually focused on the negative aspects associated with a particular group, therefore they tend to be considered by many as the central component of prejudice and discrimination (Arkon *et al.*, 2011).

In healthcare, personality types and diagnostic categories are determined through the use of scientifically reliable measures and are usually used to assist in the medical or psychological treatment of patients. However, this type of stereotyping can have negative implications when allowed to take precedence over a patient's personalised medical plan. Nurses have the propensity to bring, often unintentionally, their own biases into their professional practice which can significantly influence the care that is administered to the patient (Brown, 2006).

Rosenthal and Jacobson (1968) demonstrated the damaging nature of stereotypes in their classic experiment regarding the **self-fulfilling prophecy**. The researchers went into a school where they maintained they were there concerning the evaluation of a newly designed IQ test on the students. However, unknown to the teachers, they randomly labelled the students 'clever' or 'ordinary' and made sure the teachers accidentally overheard the names of the students who had done well. On returning at the end of the academic year, the researchers discovered that students labelled 'clever' had made greater gains than the students labelled 'ordinary'. Observations indicated that students labelled as clever received more attention, encouragement and positive praise from the teacher than the 'ordinary' students. The result became known as the 'Pygmalion effect'. This research highlights the significant implications of stereotyping and the self-fulfilling prophecy on patients and the care that they receive from nurses within the healthcare setting.

Think about this

Mandy was a student nurse who had just begun a placement on a surgical ward. John was a patient who had come into hospital for a hip replacement operation. The staff-nurse had told staff that John was diagnosed with schizophrenia and 'may act peculiar' as his hospital notes stated that he suffered from auditory hallucinations. How would you feel if you were in the same scenario as Mandy? Discuss any anxieties and fears you may have about schizophrenia.

It is important that nurses develop a frame of reference, which includes awareness of their feelings and reactions to certain mental and physical health issues that could possibly be stigmatising. It is essential for you to be aware of and familiar with the implications of stereotyping so that these concepts do not interfere with the delivery of professional personalised care.

4.5 Persuasion, conformity and compliance

We have discussed how one's behaviour and attitudes are related. We also need to consider how we could change or develop our attitudes and behaviour to promote health for example. Within the nursing profession, there will be situations where a nurse may have to persuade an individual to do certain things. These may range from the mundane – getting your colleagues to make you a cup of tea – to the more important – getting somebody to change a dressing or to help you move somebody in an appropriate way. This persuasion may be on an individual basis or on a group basis: you may want to persuade your team that you all need to move in a certain direction or change process and policy.

This section will explore the various concepts in relation to persuasion, compliance, authority and power and how we may use these to get others to do what we want them to. Health and social care is one area where changing one's attitudes and behaviours are essential in promoting healthy habits (Shahar *et al.*, 2009). For example, we want individuals to have a negative attitude towards smoking which would then be reflected in an individual's behaviour. As well as this we also want individuals to have positive attitudes towards certain healthy behaviours, such as having immunisations, engaging in regular exercise. However, for these attitudes to have a positive effect on an individual's health, we want them to be adopted and translated into action.

Persuasion

Persuasion is the process by which an attitude change is brought about. Usually persuasion takes the form of a message that contains arguments for and against a particular attitude and is targeted towards a particular audience (Hogg and Vaughan, 2008).

Persuasive communication was first systematically examined after the Second World War by exploring Hitler's (mis)use of communication and how the Cold War developed and was perceived within the USA (Hovland *et al.*, 1953; McGuire, 1986). Hovland and colleagues (1953) found that in order for effective persuasive communication, resulting in attitude change, four distinct variables are important in the act of persuasion; attention, comprehension, acceptance and retention. Based on their research concerning the communicator, the communication and the audience, the authors developed a model concerning effective persuasive communication (see Table 4.3).

Quick check

What are the key factors involved in communication?

The source of communication (who): the communicator

The first thing we need to take into account when considering persuasion is the communicator, who is trying to convey the message. There are a number of factors associated with the communicator of a message, which significantly impact the audience's acceptance of the message they are trying to convey. These variables are highlighted in Table 4.4.

Table 4.3 Factors involved in persuasive communication

Factors	Process	Outcome
Source (the sender)	Comprehension	Perception change
✦ credibility		
✦ attractiveness		
✦ similarity		
Message (the signal)	Attention	Opinion change
✦ order of arguments		
✦ one- vs. two-sided arguments		
✦ type of appeal		
✦ explicit vs. implicit conclusion		
Audience (the receiver)	Acceptance	Action change
✦ persuadability		
✦ initial position		
✦ intelligence		
✦ self-esteem		
✦ personality		

Table 4.4 Communicator factors important in communication

Key factor	Comment
Source **Perceived credibility**	Audiences are mostly persuaded by communicators who are highly credible. For instance, the more credible the source, the more powerful the message and the more likely we are to act on it. Unless the recipient views the message as bizarre – then we tend to question the credibility of the source. Subsequent research has indicated that credibility has two separate components, namely, trustworthiness and expertise.
Source **Perceived attractiveness** **or likeability**	Attractive and popular message senders are more likely to have an impact (Roskos-Ewoldsen and Fazio, 1992). Take the adverts on television – a large majority of the actors are attractive.
Source **Perceived similarity** **(reference groups)**	We tend to be persuaded more easily by people or groups who are similar to us or who we identify with: for example a member of your peer group should be more persuasive than a stranger. However, there are some subtle differences in this. When the query is one of taste or judgement then similar sources are better accepted. When the issue concerns a matter of fact then dissimilar sources do better.

Think about this

(?)

So exploring these factors how can we ensure that our message is received and is acted on? The factors outlined in Table 4.4 are important and relevant to our discussion. How can you, as a nurse, improve your credibility and your attractiveness? What about similarity with your patients? How can this influence your practice?

Key message

Credibility, attractiveness and similarity of the message sender are of key importance when attempting to persuade.

Although all these factors are important within the persuasion process we need to be aware that these may vary depending on who the target audience is. For instance, we can assume that each of these will be different when presenting to a younger or an older audience. This was shown in a recent study examining impressions of, and memory for, positively and negatively framed healthcare messages that were presented in pamphlets to 25 older adults and 24 younger adults. This study suggested that older adults relative to younger adults rated positive pamphlets more informational than negative pamphlets and remembered a higher proportion of positive to negative messages (Shamaskin et al., 2010). The educational level of the audience may also be an influential factor. For instance, research has suggested that individuals who are well educated have more of a propensity to carefully consider the issues and content within a message, whereas individuals who are less educated are more influenced by superficial aspects of the message such as the attractiveness of the communicator (Petty and Cacioppo, 1986). This may have implications for promoting health due to the unwelcome messages coming from professional purveyors, thus healthcare professionals need to assume more innovative ways of advertising healthy behaviour and lifestyles.

The message itself (content)

So far we have spoken about the communicator – the person sending the message. Now we need to move on and consider the actual message which is trying to be conveyed. Surely this is the most important component of the trilogy? In order for a message to be conveyed to the target audience in an effective and successful manner the sender needs to ensure that the receiver understands the message and, importantly, is able to act upon it. Therefore, we need to consider what characteristics of a message are important and influential in order to strengthen our messages and practice.

Several message variables have been found to be important when endeavouring to convey a message. At the easiest, repetition is both important and necessary. In order for a message to be understood and recalled it helps if the message is repeated often. Indeed, research by Arkes et al. (1991) suggests that simple repetition of a message makes it appear truer to the recipient. Repeating the message appears to influence how it is stored and accessed in an individual's memory (see Chapter 5); consequently it is better remembered and, ultimately, acted upon. However, it has been found that repetition is not always successful and may only promote attitude change to a certain point (Ko *et al.*, 2010; Cacioppo and Petty, 1979). This may be due to the increased levels of tedium that may occur with time, and therefore gaining a negative reaction to the message. Indeed, Adams and Neville (2011) reported that individuals who were repeatedly told a health promotion message they felt was not relevant were negative towards the message and started to ignore it the more it was repeated.

One way that many have tried to influence behaviour is through fear. Indeed, fear has been used extensively to try to change health-related behaviours. But of course, such messages can become too fearful and this may have negative consequences. For example, a nurse may visit a school and give a talk on the 'evils of smoking' and try to use fear to get the message over. Similarly, in the 1980s gravestones and the grim reaper were used to try to get the message over about AIDS. More recently, we have pictures of diseased lungs to try to stop smoking behaviour, and pictures of people dying in cars to try to stop people drink-driving. But does this work? Early studies have indicated that there is an inverse-U effect (e.g. Janis, 1967; McGuire, 1969). Keller and Block (1995) argue that using fear at a low level in a message may not be enough to motivate the patient to attend to the message and spell out the harmful consequences of the behaviour. However, a very frightening message may arouse so much anxiety in the patient that they are unable to grasp the content of the message and process the information needed to change the behaviour (Sengupta and Johar, 2001). But what is a fearful message? This obviously differs depending on the nature of the message and the audience it is being presented to. The fear response may be heightened in children, but certain teenagers may need a more fearful message, especially if they have become desensitised. Many researchers now assume an expectancy-value framework (Chiang *et al.*, 2011; Wentzel and Wigfield, 2009). This enables them to understand the impact of fear on persuasion by considering the nature of the feared event, the person's perceived vulnerability and the perceived effectiveness of the recommended measures (Taylor *et al.*, 2003). This approach has been largely adopted in relation to health communications concerning the use of condoms, adopting health diets and quitting smoking (Gibbons *et al.*, 2009; Taylor *et al.*, 2003). However, fear alone does not always result in a change of behaviour. For example, Kim *et al.* (2009) examined an education programme for mass communication to encourage young children to learn and develop healthy behaviours against all types of influenza using messages containing fear and humour. Results suggested that at post-tests a significant behaviour change or improvement of health practices were not apparent for fearful or humorous messages.

It has also been argued that the message can sometimes be too powerful to achieve its purpose. A highly emotional message can interfere with the effective systematic processing of the message, resulting in the person avoiding it altogether due to the anxiety it causes (Witte and Allen, 2000). For example, nurses found that parents of overweight children find being told that their children are overweight difficult to deal with and experience denial, defensiveness and excuses about their children being overweight as common reactions (Edvardsson *et al.*, 2009). Similarly, Brown and Locker (2009) investigated the idea that emotive imagery used in health promotion advertising can facilitate a defensive response that adversely affects risk perception. In this study 100 student drinkers were either shown a printed message accompanied by images designed to maximise emotional distress or the same message presented using less emotive images. The findings suggested that the more emotive messages produced more denial and defensiveness and consequently the messages were avoided. Both of these studies explain that emotive images may trigger defensive avoidance responses that reduce risk estimated in some audience populations.

Framing a message in a certain way can influence whether a message is accepted by a patient and leads to a change in attitude and behaviour. When used successfully it can be a useful tool in persuasive communication. Rothman and Salovey (1997) carried out a review of how to promote health-related behaviour and found that message framing was an important determinant. The authors suggested that when the behaviour is in relation to detecting an illness, such as breast self-examination, the message is best framed in terms of preventing loss. Whereas, if the behaviour aims to lead to a positive outcome, such as taking exercise, the message should be framed in terms of gain. Therefore, when trying to get a particular message across to our patient, which is in terms of a serious illness, we need to identify whether we should consider both sides of the argument or whether only one side should be expressed, and the more appropriate should be focused on. Although some may be better persuaded by an informed, two-sided argument, others may become confused by these but better persuaded by a single-sided argument.

Think about this ?

Thinking back to Jenna, how do you think a fearful message could influence her bad eating habits? Would using fear tactics work in the case of an individual with learning difficulties? Would you have to adapt the level of feeling in order for it to be appropriate?

Think about this ?

Do fear-arousing messages enhance persuasion? How fearful can a health-related message be to be effective? Think about these audiences: what level of fear could you use?

+ Getting children to brush their teeth.
+ Getting teenagers to use condoms with their partners.
+ Getting older individuals to wear safe slippers when at home.
+ Getting individuals with schizophrenia to take their medication.
+ Getting your colleagues to change your rota.

The audience (whom?)

The third element in effective communication is the audience – the recipient of a message. Your audience may differ in the way they respond to an argument, therefore it is essential to understand the differing characteristics that may be apparent in your target audience. We have to be extremely careful when discussing particular issues with our audience and be aware of how the audience may have an impact on the presented message. Early researchers, Lumsdaine and Janis (1953), posited that when dealing with patients who are fairly intelligent but oppose the argument, you need to present each side of the argument. Conversely, if the patient is already favourably disposed towards the argument and has a lower intelligence level it is more appropriate to present only one side of the argument. However, a number of problems arise from this observation. What do we mean by intelligence? Does this mean that we should treat less intelligent people unfairly and not give them all aspects of the information? These are a number of points for discussion. Nevertheless, when deciding how to present information, you need to consider relevant aspects in relation to your target audience (Hutson, 2008). For example, when conversing with a colleague your language and tone may differ from when you are discussing an issue with a patient. Pettigrew and Donovan (2009) studied the role of motivation and ability in older audiences' interpretations of mental health promotion messages. In this study older individuals were asked to share their thoughts and feelings about the content and style of a series of mental health messages. The authors suggested that older individuals desired to exhibit compliance, showed the importance of perceived personal relevance and showed sensitivity to the tone of the message. As well as this, the way in which you present information to your client or patient will differ according to what you understand of their background. Therefore, you need to consider not only intelligence but their gender, age, self-esteem, social class, culture and their **medical literacy** (Hutson, 2008; Lachlan *et al.*, 2009; Rhodes and Wood, 1992; Keys *et al.*, 2009).

Think about this

You are giving the following messages to a client with paranoid schizophrenia, a medical consultant and the author of this book. How would your communication change when:

+ telling them about a drug regime for heartburn
+ developing a healthy lifestyle
+ telling them about a new system for entering your secure building
+ inviting them to a party?

Key message

You need to change your message depending on the audience and in accordance with their attributions and characteristics.

The channel of communication

The final comment has to be on the channel of communication. The most effective medium for conveying a message is direct communication from person to person, whether this be from nurse to patient or from client to consultant. However, written communication needs considerable processing. Hence, this form of information can be highly advantageous to persuasive communication when presented in leaflets or information booklets (Shaddock, 2002). Leaviss (2010) postulated that usability of health information leaflets can influence the effect of frame on intentions to follow the health promotion advice. However, when writing leaflets and guidance notes, you have to ensure that you provide material in a suitable format and at an appropriate level for the audience (Shamaskin *et al.*, 2010) (see Table 4.5 for tips on how to improve written communication).

Table 4.5 How to improve written communication

Desirable feature of the message	Psychological packaging feature(s) likely to help	Physical packaging feature(s) likely to help
That it is noticed	Verbal symbols: 'Warning', 'Danger' Graphic symbol and novelty	Highlighted by use of: colour, border, space, font type and size
That it is legible		Contrast Size of type Avoid text all in capitals Spacing
That it is read	Ensure high readability Use short words Use familiar words Short sentences Avoid negatives Specify vulnerable groups Personalise wording and content Vary wording and content	High legibility
That it is understood	Ensure high readability Explain technical terms Use active rather than passive sentences Be specific in any instructions Use headings wherever possible	High legibility
That it is believed to be true	Cite sources for the message who are likely to be seen as high in: ✦ credibility ✦ expertness ✦ attractiveness	
That it is believed by its target audience	Explicitly mention target groups Deal with counter-propaganda	
That it is remembered if necessary	Ensure high readability Use repetition Use specific/concrete statements Use explicit categorisation Use primacy effect	Highlighting parts of the message which need to be remembered

Conformity and compliance

We now move on to exploring how we can change people's behaviour through **conformity**, **obedience** and **compliance**. These three elements are all linked and provide an important foundation for understanding the relationship between the nurse and client/patient and with colleagues.

Conformity

Conformity is the first element to be discussed and can be defined as a social influence which involves a person's attitude and behaviour yielding to social or group norms and values (Hogg and Vaughan, 2008). Conformity affects our attitudes and behaviours and can affect a patient's adherence to healthcare advice. For example, Bazillier *et al.* (2011) found that children's healthy eating was affected by motivation to conform to friends' and parents' norms. Similarly Mahalik and Burns (2011) suggested that gender role conformity was important to predict young men's health behaviours.

The most famous study performed using conformity was undertaken in the 1950s by Asch (1952). He aimed to investigate how people are affected by group pressure to conform to a particular behaviour. Participants were told that they were taking part in a task that involved visual judgement. During the task they were shown a line on a piece of card. Participants were then asked to match the line with one of three lines on a separate card. Unknown to the participant they were put in a room with a number of confederates (i.e. people who were not participants but worked for the researcher) who had been told to select the incorrect line. In Figure 4.1, the confederates were asked to say that line A in the comparison list was exactly the same length as the standard, despite the fact that the obvious correct answer is line B.

It was discovered that 50 per cent of the participants conformed to the majority, selecting the same incorrect line as the confederates. Only 25 per cent remained independent of the group pressure and selected the correct line.

> ## Think about this
>
> The Asch study was conducted in the 1950s. Do you think the same thing would happen these days? Do you think nurses conform? The last time you were on a ward, was there an occasion where you conformed because you thought you had to?

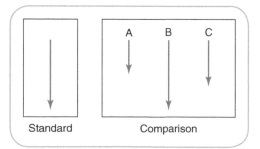

Figure 4.1 Asch's presentation of lines

Many studies have explored the Asch effect and some have suggested that it was a 'child of its time'. However, there is considerable research evidence that confirms it is both a consistent effect and one that can be observed across various situations, cultures and times (e.g. Takano and Sogon, 2008; Hollins and Bull, 2008). For instance, Mori and Arai (2010) recently replicated Asch's study finding that the minority of women participating conformed to the majority group confirming Asch's results.

But what relevance has this for nursing? Do you think it has an impact on you? Well, if we think of the example provided in the following box – a case from professional practice – what would you do in this situation?

Professional practice issues

In professional practice, a third year student nurse (Colin) was on a placement on a geriatric ward. During the placement he observed that patients were not being turned on a regular basis as recommended in his training and as he had observed on other wards. When he pointed this out to a more experienced nurse she became agitated and informed him that this was a very busy ward and they had their own way of doing things. He took this to a team meeting and all of his colleagues also reported that this was the case. The student nurse was in a minority of one and hence had a dilemma: would he conform to the majority and compromise the quality of patient care or would he seek advice from his practice facilitator and upset the rest of the team?

It has been posited that, particularly for nursing students, the need to conform can be strong (Levett-Jones and Lathlean, 2009). Many lack confidence because of their inexperience and feel discourteous when pointing out concerns to more experienced and qualified colleagues. Sometimes roles within a team and any available knowledge are ambiguous and difficult to determine. Nursing students tend to have a desire to fit into the team they are part of, and therefore, sometimes, this desire can impair their judgement (Levett-Jones and Lathlean, 2009). However, the patients' needs must *always* take priority over the group norms and it is essential that nurses are aware of this.

Quick check

What is conformity?

Compliance

Compliance is generally viewed as the degree to which medical advice is followed in order to reach a therapeutic goal (Kelly, 1995). At this stage, we need to consider the term compliance and whether this term is appropriate. The terms 'compliance' and 'adherence' are synonymous and are often used interchangeably. Compliance was the dominant term which was frequently used during the early stages of research. This research tended to investigate the patient and whether they followed their practitioner's instructions appropriately. Haynes *et al.* (1979) defined compliance as: 'The extent to which the patient's behaviour (in terms of taking medication, following diets or other lifestyle changes) coincides with medical or health advice.'

The term compliance implies that the patient will follow the nurse's orders without any questions, is always in a less informed position, and that a failure to comply is the fault of the patient (Donovan and Blake, 1992; Van Hecke et al., 2009). This term has been heavily criticised in nursing literature for its paternalistic view of the health professional-patient relationship, in which the patient is perceived to be passive and expected to obey the clinician's orders (Snelgrove, 2006). Many nurses feel uneasy about the label, due to the large extent to which it lays blame on the patient (Russell et al., 2003). Consequently, the term 'adherence' was employed, but again this was criticised and more recently the term concordance (i.e. alignment of the patient's and the nurse's views – a partnership) is preferred (e.g. Ekman et al., 2007). In this chapter we will use these three terms interchangeably (although we prefer the term concordance) depending on the nature of the research being reported.

Think about this

What sort of factors do you think might cause non-compliance with the medical advice given for the treatment of hypertension?

Research has shown that when patients feel that they are actively involved in their treatment, adherence levels to treatment increase. Therefore the term concordance has been introduced by some in healthcare to represent a shared understanding between healthcare professionals and patients about their care, treatment and management (Ogden, 2007).

Key message

People do not always follow medical and nursing advice.

Compliance is considered to be a determinant of patient well-being. However, as already mentioned, many patients do not comply with the healthcare advice given (Ibrahim et al., 2010). Therefore we have to pose the question: what are the factors that influence compliance with medical advice? The principal reasons that have been identified for poor compliance include adverse effects, forgetfulness, changing priorities or schedules and confusion about dosing regimens (Ibrahim et al., 2010). An example of this is in the case of an elderly patient who has many medical problems requiring complex drug regimens, finds it difficult to take the numerous medications multiple times each day and needs help from a nurse to remember to take these medications (Latif and McNicoll, 2009). Other reasons for poor compliance may be poor motivation, pain, discomfort, lack of knowledge and understanding and unwillingness (Van Hecke et al., 2009). The relationship between the patient and the healthcare provider has also been considered.

Phillip Ley (1981, 1989) developed the **cognitive hypothesis model of compliance**. According to this model, patient compliance can be predicted by:

✦ patient satisfaction with the process of the consultation

✦ understanding of the information provided during the consultation

✦ the retention and recall of this information.

Think about this

What aspect of the nurse–patient consultation would result in patient satisfaction?

A study investigating the role of some of the factors highlighted by Kreuter *et al.* (2000) showed that increased patient education can lead to higher rates of 'conformity' and better health outcomes. Patients' ability to recall the information that the nurse has conveyed to them is influenced by a multitude of factors such as anxiety, the primacy effect (the tendency for the information that is presented first to be remembered), medical knowledge, intellectual level and the importance of the statement (Shorney, 2004). This will be explored in further detail in Chapter 5.

Quick check

✦ Describe the three variables that Hovland and associates (1953) suggest are important in the communication of persuasion.

✦ Explain how the concept of conformity can affect a patient's willingness to reduce the amount of alcohol they consume.

✦ In a group, discuss some of the factors that may influence an adolescent patient's willingness to continue taking insulin for juvenile rheumatoid arthritis.

4.6 Power and status and its influence on obedience

As highlighted above, the concept of compliance or adherence can be influenced by the principles of persuasion. Furthermore, it can also be influenced by the amount of power a person is perceived to have. Power is the capacity of one person to influence another individual to do what they would like while resisting the attempts of another to influence them; influence is power in action (Hogg and Vaughan, 2008). The degree of power one individual has over another depends on the level of imbalance in the relationship and on how much power one person is perceived to have by another (Hogg and Vaughan, 2008).

Raven (1965) identified six bases of social power that people can access in order to persuade others: reward power, coercive power, informational power, expert power, legitimate power and referent power (Hogg and Vaughan, 2005):

✦ **Reward power** – give or promise of rewards for compliance.

✦ **Coercive power** – a threat of punishment for non-compliance.

+ **Informational power** – a belief that the influencer has more information than oneself.
+ **Expert power** – the certainty that the influencer has generally greater expertise and knowledge than oneself.
+ **Legitimate power** – the belief that the influencer is recognised by a power body to make decisions and direct.
+ **Referent power** – a respect or identification with the source of influence.

Think about this

How can the bases of social power be applied to nursing? Which of these could be adopted, and how, in dealing with Jenna and her resistance at accepting support?

Power is implicit in all social relations including the nurse–patient relationship (Ashmore, 2010; Oudshoorn, *et al*., 2007). Historically, nurses' approach to providing care for patients has been using the expert model of care. This approach tends to reinforce an unequal power base, with the nurse acting as an authoritative expert who expects total compliance from their patients without question. Obviously this has now changed, and there is more of a partnership approach to nursing practice (Hand, 2002; Carter, 2009).

The concept of power and obedience to authority was famously demonstrated in the 1960s by an experiment undertaken by Stanley Milgram. Within this study, participants were members of the general public who were given money as an incentive for their recruitment. When they arrived at the prestigious Yale University for the study they were introduced to another 'volunteer' who was actually a confederate of the researcher. It was explained to the participants that they were taking part in a study concerning learning and were then asked to draw lots with the confederate. This was to ascertain who would be the 'teacher' and who would be 'pupil'. However, the lots were fixed so that the real research participant always took the role of 'teacher'. The pupil (confederate) was then taken into an adjacent room and strapped to a chair in full view of the participant (teacher). The teacher (participant) was then taken back to their room where they were given their instructions. They were provided with a set of questions to present to the pupil and for every question they answered incorrectly they were to administer an electric shock. The shocks increased in 15 volt increments all the way up to 450 volts, where 450 volts was marked red for danger. The results were astounding: 26 out of 40 participants continued as instructed by the experimenter right up to the administration of 450 volts. This was despite the audible shouts and screams that could be heard from the adjacent room (where the pupil was supposedly strapped to the electric chair).

This study demonstrates that symbols of authority can result in unquestioning obedience to authority. The fact that the study was carried out at a very prestigious university in the pursuit of scientific knowledge by lab-coated scientists demonstrates how power and status influence our decision to obey. This led to a variety of hypotheses related to the medical and nursing profession. Can the power of the nurse or medical consultant be increased by wearing a uniform – the 'white coat' – and carrying the stethoscope around the neck? Ask yourself whether this is a useful position for the practitioner or the patient/client.

Think about this

As a newly qualified nurse Sara had been instilled with the ideal of client-driven practice during her training. After several weeks working on a long-term care ward for the elderly she became aware that nursing practice on this ward was not client-driven. Many of the patients who asked to use the toilet were often left for long periods of time before evacuation and patients were often left in wet incontinence pads for cost-cutting reasons. What should Sara do? Should she speak to the staff nurse about her concerns?

Sara was right to show concern over the way that patients were being treated. This treatment is wholly unacceptable. Not only are nurses using excessive power to control patients wishing to use the toilet, they are also demonstrating a form of economic power over patients by leaving them in wet incontinence pads. Sara should speak to the staff-nurse over her concerns. It is important that she uses the skills that she has learnt during her training to ask questions and question the cost to patient care when asked to comply with such practice.

It is important that nurses have a proper understanding of the meaning of power and how it fits in with a client-empowering approach to nursing (Sheehan, 1985). This will enable them to recognise their responsibility and regulate their exercise of power appropriately. In general practice, negative power is only exercised in certain situations and when in a patient's best interest, for instance when there are concerns that something untoward may happen to them (Palviainen *et al.*, 2003).

Think about this

How do you think these six power bases apply to the nurse–patient relationship? What about different types of patient/client – a depressed man, a psychotic woman, a middle-aged man with Parkinson's disease, a child with cancer? What about other forms of relationships – the nurse–doctor relationship, for example, in a psychiatric ward, in an ENT clinic or in an operating theatre?

Research in Focus

Efstathiou, G., Papastavrou, E., Raftopoulous, V., and Merkains, A. (2011) Factors influencing nurses' compliance with the standard precautions in order to avoid occupational exposure to microorganisms: A focus group study. *BMC Nursing*, **10** (1), 1–12.

Background

Due to the occupational exposure to micro-organisms within nurses' working environment, a nurse may acquire an infection at some point during their career. Previous research has indicated that nurses' compliance to the Standard Precautions guidelines (to protect healthcare professionals from exposure to micro-organisms) is significantly →

lower than what is necessary. In addition, the occurrence of exposure to micro-organisms (i.e. needle-sticks etc.) among nurses is very high. Therefore, this study examined the factors which contribute to nurses' compliance with Standard Precautions in order to avoid the potential of occupational exposure.

Methods

This study assumed a focus group approach to explore the relevant issues. These included four groups (N = 30) of nurses in order to elicit their perceptions and view of the factors which influence their compliance with the Standard Precautions.

Results

The result identified a number of factors which influenced nurses' compliance with the guidelines. For instance, they indicated that emergency situations, a lack of protective equipment, a heavy workload, patients' discomfort with the equipment, and no nursing personnel implementing the guidelines, were all barriers making compliance extremely difficult. Furthermore, many nurses indicated that when a nurse gains so much experience, following some of the guidelines is unnecessary. Some nurses also indicated that it was often difficult for them to change their behaviour towards something even though they knew it was wrong.

Conclusion

The authors concluded that in order for nurses to adapt and change their behaviour, there is a need for them to have an understanding of how these factors may influence their compliance with the Standard Precautions. Furthermore, this understanding will facilitate the implementation of programmes which promote preventative actions in order to avoid occupational exposure.

4.7 Conclusion

Human beings are social animals and benefit from social interaction. These social processes can influence the relationship that individual nurses have with their patients, clients and colleagues. Nurses have to be aware of the influence that aspects of non-verbal communication, conformity and compliance can have on encouraging health promotion in their patients. However, they also need to be aware of power and status and how these can be detrimental to the practice of the client-empowerment approach. Therefore, it is essential that you consider and appreciate these concepts in order to understand and influence your patients' behaviour while regulating your exercise of power appropriately. This knowledge can be highly advantageous in assisting you with your professional practice.

Think about this

Looking back at the interaction between Jenna, the nurse and the social worker, what social processes were involved? How could the nurse communicate effective health-promoting messages?

4.8 Summary

+ Non-verbal channels of communication are important for the good development of the patient-nurse relationship.

+ Negative attitudes need to be replaced with more positive attitudes through the use of learning, direct experience and persuasive communication.

+ Cognitive dissonance is a process by which individuals are motivated to implement attitude change when they feel anxiety due an unbalance in their cognitions.

+ For affective persuasion Hovland *et al.* (1953) identified these steps – attention, comprehension, acceptance and retention.

+ People may conform to social groups in order to validate their opinions and obtain social approval and acceptance.

+ Compliance with healthcare is influenced by a multitude of factors. Ley's (1981) cognitive hypothesis model of compliance identified that compliance is a mixture of patient satisfaction, understanding of the information given and ability to recall the information given during consultation.

+ Obedience to authority happens in healthcare. Nurses must recognise their responsibility and regulate the exercise of power.

+ Stereotyping and labelling can interfere with the delivery of personalised care.

Your end point

Answer the following questions to assess your knowledge and understanding of social processes in nursing.

1. What is cognitive dissonance?

    (a) When a person experiences inconsistencies in their cognitions.
    (b) A form of non-verbal communication.
    (c) An attitude towards others.
    (d) A cognitive attitude towards medication.
    (e) A way of understanding the person.

2. Which of the following is true?

    (a) Accurate predictions of specific behaviour can be derived from people's specific attitudes.
    (b) Attitudes formed as a result of direct experience are poor predictors of behaviour.
    (c) The more general the attitudes involved, the greater the accuracy in predicting particular behaviours.
    (d) The best conclusion is that attitudes do not predict behaviour.
    (e) None of the above.

→

3. Whether a teenage girl will actually undergo a vaccination is best predicted by the _____; how someone reacts to a beggar who approaches them on the street is best predicted by the _____.

   (a) theory of planned behaviour; attitude to behaviour process model
   (b) attitude to behaviour process model; theory of planned behaviour
   (c) theory of planned behaviour; theory of planned behaviour
   (d) attitude to behaviour process model; attitude to behaviour process model.

4. A nurse who is trying to persuade someone will be better able to produce an attitude change if (s)he:

   (a) speaks rapidly and does not deliberately set out to persuade
   (b) speaks slowly and does not deliberately set out to persuade
   (c) speaks normally and deliberately sets out to persuade
   (d) uses a lot of gestures
   (e) does all of the above.

5. A message that emphasises the costs of not eating breakfast is _____; a message that emphasises the benefits of eating breakfast is _____.

   (a) generally effective; generally ineffective
   (b) generally ineffective; generally effective
   (c) positively framed; negatively framed
   (d) negatively framed; positively framed
   (e) none of the above.

Further reading

Aronson, E. (2008) *The Social Animal* (10th edn.). New York: Worth/Freeman.

Eagly, A.H. and Chaiken, S. (1997) *The Psychology of Attitudes*. Fort Worth, TX: Houghton Mifflin Harcourt.

Chesney, M. (2003) Adherence to HAART regimens. *AIDS Patient Care and STDs* **17**, 169–177.

Cacioppo, J.T. and Petty, R.E. (1986) *Central and Peripheral Routes to Persuasion: The Role of Message Repetition*. New York: Springer-Verlag.

Elwyn, G., Edwards, A., Kinnersley, P. and Grol, R. (2000) Shared decision making and the concept of equipoise: The competences of involving patients in healthcare choices. *British Journal of General Practice* **50**, 892–899.

Hutson, M. (2008) Know your audience. *Psychology Today* **41** (4), 27.

Rutter, D. and Quine, L. (2002) *Changing Health Behaviour*. Buckingham: Open University Press.

Simpson, P.F. and Fothergill, A. (2004) Challenging gender stereotypes in the counselling of adult survivors of childhood sexual abuse. *Journal of Psychiatry and Mental Health Nursing* **11**(5), 589–594.

Stone, J. and Cooper, J. (2001) A self-standards model of cognitive dissonance. *Journal of Experimental Social Psychology* **37**, 228–243.

Wong, N.C.H. and Cappella, J.N. (2009). Antismoking threat and efficacy appeals: Effects on smoking cessation intentions for smokers with low and high readiness to quit. *Journal of Applied Communication Research* **37** (1), 1–20.

Weblinks

http://www.spring.org.uk/2007/11/10-piercing-insights-into-human-nature.php
PsyBlog. This blog site gives a top ten list of the major social psychology research experiments. There is also information on non-verbal communication and relationships.

http://smokefree.nhs.uk
Quit Smoking with the NHS. If reading this book has inspired you to quit smoking, or maybe you'd like to help someone else to quit, this website will help you.

http://people.umass.edu/aizen/index.html
Icek Ajzen and the Theory of Planned Behaviour. This is the website of Icek Ajzen, the developer of the Theory of Planned Behaviour. There are lots of useful diagrams and articles to help you learn more.

http://www.experiment-resources.com/stanley-milgram-experiment.html
Milgram Experiment. A video and further resources on the (in)famous Milgram experiment.

http://www.helpguide.org/mental/eq6_nonverbal_communication.htm
Nonverbal Communication Help Guide. This site provides a useful guide to interpreting others and tips on how you can use this in your relationships every day.

Check point

Your starting point		Your end point	
Q1	D	Q1	E
Q2	A	Q2	D
Q3	C	Q3	A
Q4	B	Q4	C
Q5	B	Q5	D

Chapter 5

Perception, memory and providing information

Learning Outcomes

At the end of this chapter you will be able to:

✦ Be aware of the impact of perception on the interpretation of situations and information

✦ Understand models of memory and the various memory stores

✦ Appreciate models of attention and their relevance to nursing practice

✦ Understand the impact of knowledge, satisfaction and memory on adherence

✦ Be aware of a number of techniques for improving your own and your patients' memory

✦ Be aware of some of the conditions that can result in memory loss

✦ Be aware of a number of factors influencing adherence to treatment; and possible interventions to improve adherence levels

✦ Explore various cognitive models of health behaviour and how these can be applied to nursing practice

✦ Be able to understand the motivational interviewing approach to changing risky behaviour.

Your starting point

Answer the following questions to assess your knowledge and understanding of cognition, memory and information provision.

1. The original Protection Motivation Theory (PMT) claimed that health-related behaviours can be predicted by a number of components. But which of the following is *not* one of these:

   (a) response effectiveness
   (b) severity
   (c) susceptibility
   (d) self-efficacy
   (e) none of the above?

2. Based on the theory of planned behaviour, if the important people in your life want you to cut down on the amount of alcohol that you drink, what else needs to be in place in order for your alcohol consumption to change?

   (a) Personal belief that reducing alcohol consumption will be beneficial.
   (b) Perceive self to be capable of drinking less.
   (c) Subjective norms are in place.
   (d) All of the above.
   (e) (a) and (b).

3. What does rehearsal resemble:

   (a) echoic memory
   (b) acoustic interference
   (c) autobiographical stories
   (d) encoding
   (e) inner speech?

4. What is a 'chunk,' in short-term memory:

   (a) a partial memory, not complete
   (b) a single organised thing or item
   (c) a 'magic number' which aids retrieval
   (d) a hierarchy
   (e) a binary 'bit' of information?

5. Cued recall involves which one of the following:

   (a) bringing information to mind in response to non-specific cues
   (b) bringing information to mind in response to specific cues
   (c) identifying information provided at test time as having been encountered previously
   (d) responding differently to previously encountered information than to new information
   (e) none of the above?

Case Study

Noel is a 28-year-old man who works in the finance office for a large supermarket chain. Noel has been working in an office since completing his accountancy degree a few years ago. Noel always had a problem with his weight and he now tips the scales at 27 stones (over 160 kilos). He has found that a regular wage packet, limited exercise, regular nights out and access to a plentiful supply of food (he has a staff discount) means that his has put on considerable weight.

Noel is married and currently has a five-year-old son, Dave; he and his wife are trying for another child. His wife is also obese and they fear that their weight is getting in the way of them having another child. Their child, Dave, is rather chubby and takes a great delight in eating fish fingers and chips to the exclusion of most other food. Noel's wife is on medication to try and improve her chances of conception. She takes this regularly whereas Noel's reflux medication is rarely taken as prescribed.

Noel now finds that his regular diet of take-aways and pre-packaged meals with limited fruit and vegetables is leading him on a downward spiral. He used to play five-a-side football with 'the lads' but given his weight and since he becomes out of breath easily he has stopped playing, he merely turns up for the post-match drinking session.

Noel has been to the GP who fears for his health. However, despite the constant pleading by the GP to lose weight, Noel continues to put on weight. Furthermore, despite being on anti-reflux medication Noel is still suffering.

Why is this relevant to nursing practice?

This is relevant for a number of reasons. First, Noel is overweight (considerably) and it should be the responsibility of every healthcare professional to promote healthy lifestyles. So, how can the nurse do this? There are a number of models developed in psychology, and presented here (and others in Chapter 4) that allow for the healthcare professional to tailor their advice appropriately and to ensure the maximum chance of success. Furthermore, Noel has been advised to take medication but he fails to do so correctly. Whilst inconvenient and distressing in this example, in another case it may be more serious and even life threatening. So how can the nurse maximise the chances of success? How can they ensure that their patients/clients are true partners in the relationship?

Think about this

Consider Noel and his wife. Why does Noel not take his medication and yet his wife takes hers? What sort of factors might be involved here?

5.1 Introduction

This chapter will look at various cognitive processes – the way we perceive the world around us and what enables us to remember various activities. We will then move on and consider how we can combine these processes and apply them to our professional practice. Neisser (1967) coined the phrase 'cognitive psychology' and defined it as the study of how people learn, structure, store and use knowledge. In short, this is the branch of psychology that is concerned with the study of mental states and processes such as problem solving, memory and language. Furthermore, it considers the internal process which we draw on when perceiving our environment and how we conclude what actions are deemed most appropriate (Eysenck and Keane, 2010).

But why is this relevant to you? What use does this have in your professional career as a nurse? Well, although at first inspection hard-core cognitive psychology may not appear relevant to nursing, it has considerable uses which may underlie much of your professional practice. For example, patients' medication routine. How can this be enhanced? How can you as a nurse assist the patient with their medication programmes so adherence is maximised? What about dealing with the ward situation and how to treat people appropriately? What about out in the community with people with differing needs and expectations? Cognitive psychology explores memory – what it is, what can affect it and how it can be improved. The area of perception is also important – you need to be able to take a holistic view of the patient. A community psychiatric nurse needs to be able to explore the perception of the patient, the views of the family as well as the evidence-based practice you have amassed throughout your education. How successful the patient is in managing or recovering from an illness or state of ill-health will be determined to some degree by how much the patient retains and uses that information.

For example, look at the picture in Figure 5.1 – what do you see? You, as a student professional nurse, probably see a tool, an instrument, something that you may use frequently with your clients, or you may come across on a daily basis in your practice. But think again, what

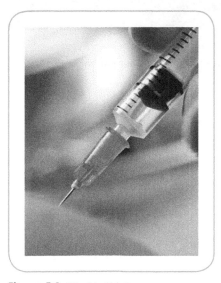

Figure 5.1 What is this?
Source: Getty Images/Image Source

would your patient see? Would they see a tool or something useful or something common, or would they be scared? What would they expect? They may not be as familiar with the equipment as you are. What would their reactions be?

Think about this ?

Consider the pictures in Figure 5.2. What do you think the psychological reactions would be to each picture from each of the following:

✦ a 16-year-old diabetic girl

✦ a 50-year-old chronic schizophrenic

✦ a six-year-old boy requiring a local anaesthetic

✦ a 22-year-old woman with learning disabilities requiring a contraceptive injection?

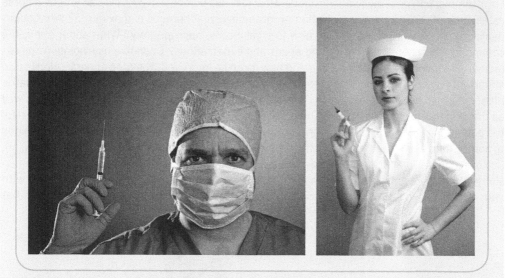

Figure 5.2 **What do you see? What does your patient see?**

Source: Getty Images: Juan Silva; Jupiterimages

This chapter will explore these mental processes and how they can have an influence in relation to your practice. To start with we will explore perception before moving on to memory – its definition and improvement.

5.2 Perception

Most of us will have come across the shapes outlined in Figure 5.3. But look at them again; is the one on the left a vase or two faces? Similarly the one on the right: two people may view the image as being a woman who is young, or an older woman; which do you see?

These two illusions highlight a big issue of importance in nursing: two individuals can perceive the same stimulus in vastly different ways, and these perceptions can influence how we

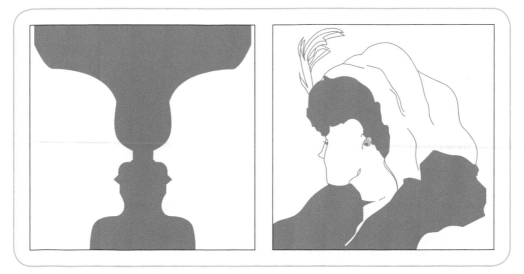

Figure 5.3 Perceptual illusions

think and feel about that stimulus (Lai and Chang, 2009; Tubbs-Cooley *et al.*, 2011). This issue penetrates all aspects of life: for instance, to a nurse a syringe is a medical tool, an everyday object which elicits little emotional response. For a patient with a phobia of needles these same stimuli appear exaggerated and produce feelings of fear and anxiety.

The way we perceive stimuli can affect both our emotional response and our memory for that situation – 'the needle was HUGE!' (Eysenck and Keane, 2010). Let us consider other relevant factors which may influence our recall of events.

Key message

People perceive things differently: what you see as normal and pain free may not be seen in the same way by your patients.

The visual process that has taken place when you look at those perceptual illusions in Figure 5.3 is referred to as the **top-down process**. According to Gestalt psychologists, the top-down approach is how perception works overall in that we strive to see things as a whole so that they are meaningful (Eysenck and Keane, 2010). In contrast to this, there is also the **bottom-up process**, which means that the shapes and colours are recognised alone and then the picture is built up. The process by which we structure the input from sensory receptors is based on the principle of perceptual organisation (Baron, 2001) which allows us to perceive shapes and forms from incomplete and fragmented stimuli. As humans we are all striving to have consistency – to fill in all the gaps.

Quick check

What are top-down and bottom-up processes?

The Gestalt principles of grouping include:

+ figure/ground
+ proximity
+ similarity
+ closure
+ continuity.

Figure/Ground

The vase shown in Figure 5.3 is an example of this tendency to pick out form. We don't simply see black and white shapes – we see two faces and a vase.

The problem here is that we see the two forms of equal importance. If the source of this message wants us to perceive a vase, then the vase is the intended *figure* and the black background is the *ground*. The problem here is a confusion of figure and ground.

Here is an example from practice:

+ a nurse appears with a hypodermic needle
+ the patient will focus on the needle
+ the nurse is rather attractive (or alternatively, rather unattractive) and is carrying a needle
+ there is now confusion of figure and ground (nurse and hypodermic) and consequently less focus on the hypodermic needle.

This is not to say that in order to overcome needle phobia there should always be an attractive nurse delivering the injection! Rather it is an example where two objects (nurse/hypodermic) can swap levels of importance.

Proximity

Items or individuals that are close together in space or time tend to be perceived as grouped together. Thus, if you want your patient to associate the treatment with the nurse or practitioner, put them close together. On the other hand, if you want them to perceive two ideas as associated, present them in close proximity but not both in view. For example, you may want to hide a hypodermic needle from sight so you, the nurse, are not associated with it.

Look at Figure 5.4:

+ When you look at (a) you see (a nurse + a nurse) + a bed;
+ When you look at (b) you see (a nurse + a bed) + a nurse.

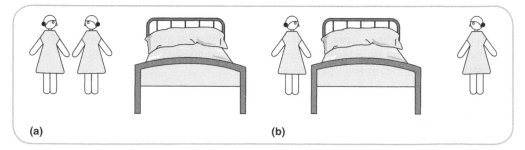

(a)   **(b)**

Figure 5.4 Example of proximity

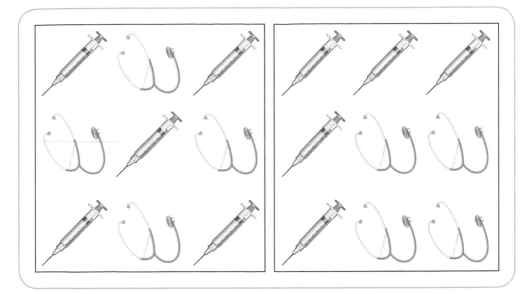

Figure 5.5 Example of similarity

Similarity

Things which are similar are likely to form 'Gestalten' groups. So in Figure 5.5, on the left you probably see an X of hypodermic needles against a background of the stethoscopes; on the right you may see a square of the stethoscopes, partly surrounded by hypodermic needles. So, if we want our patients to perceive the elements of our message as belonging together we should try to give them the same shape.

Closure

W A S H O   Perc ption

Look at this image. We can still read WASHO, see the square and read 'Perception' despite the missing information. It may be that your patients often prefer to be able to complete health messages themselves and there is some evidence to suggest that, for example, health promotion messages in which the general public are required to play an active role in completion of the message are retained for longer (although there is, of course, the danger that they may complete it wrongly!).

Continuity

Where figures are defined by a single unbroken line, they tend to be seen as an entity (see Figure 5.6). This principle is, of course, of particular importance in graphic design. Even something as simple as drawing a squiggle to link up apparently disparate elements on a page can be helpful in suggesting to the reader that they are parts of a whole. Remember – your

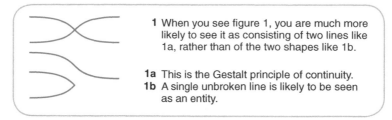

1 When you see figure 1, you are much more likely to see it as consisting of two lines like 1a, rather than of the two shapes like 1b.

1a This is the Gestalt principle of continuity.
1b A single unbroken line is likely to be seen as an entity.

Figure 5.6 The Gestalt principle of continuity

written messages are important and you can provide additional information to your readers by using graphic design.

Figure 5.7 shows another example of the continuity principle.

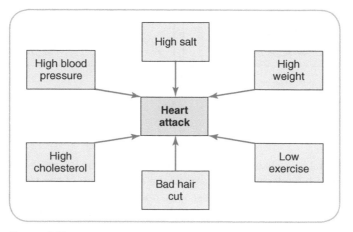

Figure 5.7 Continuity principles – items can be suggested to be linked even if bizarre!

Think about this

How can you use these laws of perceptual grouping in your practice?

Laws	Explanation	Your practice
Similarity	Tendency to perceive similar items as a group	
Closure	Tendency to perceive objects as whole entities despite the fact that some parts may be missing or obstructed from view	
Figure and ground	Tendency to look at the obvious figure	
Continuity	Tendency to perceive complete patterns in terms of similar shape	
Proximity	Things seen close together are seen as being associated	

Key message

There are several perceptual laws that can be incorporated into your practice.

Quick check

Name the Gestalt principles of grouping.

5.3 Memory

A cognitive process that plays a significant role in the day-to-day practice of nurses and patients is our memory. The importance of memory permeates all aspects of our lives – we would be little without a functioning memory. If we explore our professional activities then we can see we need to have a good memory. We need to recall the names of our colleagues and patients. We need to remember and recall what we have learned at university. We need to remember our patient's diagnosis, how to treat them, our daily routines, what has been discussed with a patient and how they are going to progress. It also has an important role for patients – understanding, decision-making and their ability to follow the treatment regime.

In this section the nature and processes of memory, as we currently understand it, will be outlined, and the implications of this knowledge for nursing practice will be discussed. Common problems in encoding and retrieving knowledge will be explored and the causes and impact of common patterns of memory loss will be outlined.

Key message

Memory is what makes us human and is involved in all our daily activities.

What is memory?

Memory is the ability to store, retain and recall information and experiences. Memory is commonly accepted as being made up of three central processes: encoding, storing and retrieving information. **Encoding** refers to the process whereby sensory information is transformed into a representation (e.g. some kind of chemical memory trace) suitable for storage. **Storage** refers to the process by which sensory information is retained within the memory system. **Retrieval** refers to the process whereby stored information is recovered. This is also known as 'recall' or 'remembering' (Eysenck and Keane, 2010).

Key message

Memory is made up of a process of encoding, storing and retrieving information.

What has this got to do with nursing?

As mentioned earlier, an important part of a nurse's role is to communicate with the patient, to help them understand their diagnosis, its implications for their daily lives, and the treatment options available to them (Bridgeman and Malinoski, 2009). How this is communicated to the patient will affect the way in which this information is coded, stored and subsequently recalled. It also has an impact on the patient's ability to cope with the behavioural and emotional consequences of their condition and on treatment decision-making. Similarly, there is an abundance of research to suggest that forgetting is of central importance in non-adherence to treatment plans and, in turn, this may affect patients' overall recovery and quality of life (Hommel *et al.*, 2011; Devonshire *et al.*, 2011).

How is memory structured?

Most psychologists agree that there are at least two distinct memory stores – short-term memory (STM) and long-term memory (LTM). Trying to remember a telephone number for a few seconds is a popular example of short-term memory as it illustrates two central features: STM holds a very small amount of information (it has a limited capacity); and for only a small period of time (it has a limited duration). LTM, on the other hand, can (in theory) last for a lifetime and is posited to have unlimited capacity. For example, you might recall your childhood memories or a gift you received on your birthday five years ago.

> ### Key message
>
> Memory has both a short-term and a long-term component.

Memory stores

Atkinson and Shiffrin (1968) developed one of the first systematic accounts of the structures and processes involved in human memory. They attempted to give us an explanation as to how information flows from one storage system to the next. The 'multi-store model' or 'dual process theory' postulates that memory consists of three distinct stores: a sensory store, STM store and LTM store – see Figure 5.8. According to the model, information from

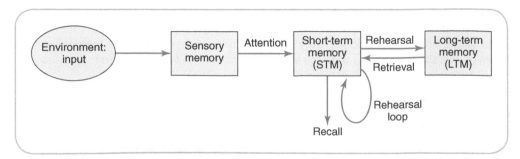

Figure 5.8 Multi-store model of memory

the environment is received by the sensory store. A small fraction of this information is attended to where it is processed further by STM. In turn, and only after sufficient rehearsal, information processed in the STM store is transferred to LTM. In addition to these distinct stores, the proposed system also contains transient control processes where rehearsal is the key element. It is posited that rehearsal is an essential function which, if neglected, will lead to the loss of information, and consequently forgetting. Therefore, the more the information is rehearsed, the stronger the memory trace will become.

Evidence supporting the distinction between short-term and long-term memory comes from Glanzer and Cunitz (1966). They carried out an experiment in which they presented participants with a list of words and asked for free recall (a memory test in which the words can be recalled in any order). When free recall occurred immediately after the list was presented there was evidence for a **recency effect**, meaning that participants typically recalled those items from the end of the list first and got more of these correct. There was also evidence of a **primacy effect**, meaning that the first few words in the list were also well remembered. Poorest recall was for those items in the middle portion of the list.

Think about this

Think about providing information on medical treatment to an individual with the following: anxiety disorder, moderate learning disabilities, angina, Parkinson's disease. What sort of aspects of memory should you take into account?

It was argued that the recency effect reflected retrieval from STM, whereas the primacy effect reflected retrieval from LTM. Glanzer and Cunitz tested this hypothesis by employing an interference task (counting backwards; the Brown-Peterson technique) between learning and recall. The idea was that if the recency effect does demonstrate STM, by preventing rehearsal the effect should disappear. Indeed, Glanzer and Cunitz found that counting backwards for only 10 seconds virtually eliminated the recency effect, but otherwise had no effect on recall. Further evidence for separate stores comes from studies investigating capacity, duration and encoding.

Key message

You can use primacy and recency effects in your practice: important information should be presented either at the start or end of a consultation.

Quick check

Draw the multi-store model of memory.

Sensory memory

Sensory memory is a basic form of storage, which retains very brief, literal copies of sensory information needed for STM. It is modality specific (i.e. information is held in the form in which it was received), has a large capacity for information (although only a fraction of this information is actually processed) and functions outside of awareness (Eysenck and Keane, 2010). According to the multi-store model there is a separate store for each sensory register, i.e. vision, hearing, smell, taste, etc. However, most research has concentrated on the **iconic store** (visual store) and the **echoic stores** (auditory store).

Think about this

How can your knowledge of sensory memory assist with your practice?

5.4 Attention

There is a considerable overlap between the areas of memory and attention. For example, Broadbent's (1958) filter theory of selective attention was in many ways the main precursor of the multi-store model. Broadbent argued that sensory stimuli from the environment gain access in parallel to a sensory buffer. One of the inputs is then selected (filtered) on the basis of its physical characteristics (e.g. familiarity, comprehensibility), while the other stimuli remain in the sensory buffer store for later processing. If the stimuli are not processed they are then filtered out. This filter is needed to prevent the limited capacity of STM from becoming overloaded. Once past the filter, the information is processed thoroughly.

Quick check

What inputs into the sensory buffer?

Information received within sensory memory can decay rapidly so it is important for you, as a nurse, to ensure that your patient is attending to the health information being provided. It is also important that the information is familiar and intelligible to prevent it from being filtered out. Understanding health information can be problematic when the information is complex or new; thus information should be conveyed to the patient using everyday examples and avoiding the use of medical jargon (Anderson *et al.*, 2011; Banja, 2007).

The number of **distractions** a patient encounters can also explain how much information is attended to (Lavie, 2010). Within the hospital setting there are many distractions such as busy wards and high levels of background noise; not to mention internal distractions such as pain, fear or anxiety. Using a slightly higher tone of voice and expressing interest while talking (Cherry, 1966), referring to the patient by name and acknowledging internal distractions are simple yet effective techniques which will focus the patient's attention (Haskard *et al.*, 2009).

Information that is delivered in a variety of different formats is more likely to be attended to. A simple way of delivering information in different formats is to use written material to complement verbal information. Indeed research suggests that complementing verbal information with written material can increase patients' attention, enhance comprehension and improve recall. Researchers have also highlighted the importance of using other aids to complement verbal information. For example, Scott *et al.* (2006) recommended aids such as consultation tapes and summary letters. The use of pictures in addition to verbal information has also proved helpful when recalling information, particularly for those who have low literacy skills (Houts *et al.*, 2006; Speros, 2011).

Think about this

What distractions were there in the environment when you were talking to your last patient? What influence did these distractions have on them and their recall of information? What could you do about it?

Short-term memory

The capacity of STM has been investigated using span measures. This is an assessment of how much information can be stored in memory at any one time. In a review, Miller (1956) found that the capacity of STM was seven plus or minus two items (7 ± 2 Magic number seven) and that this was irrespective of whether the items were numbers, letters or words. As seven words will always contain more than seven letters, one might think that a person should remember fewer words than letters. However, in his article Miller illustrated how **chunking** (i.e. integrating units of information) can be used to extend the capacity of STM and explain this phenomenon. Therefore, instead of only holding 7 ± 2 single items such as a digit or a letter, it can actually hold chunks of information such as 7 ± 2 words.

Think about this

When revising information for an examination, how could you use chunking to aid your revision?

Whenever we reduce a large amount of information into a smaller amount we are chunking: this not only increases the capacity of STM but also increases the likelihood that the information will be stored for longer. It also denotes a form of encoding, by imposing a meaning on otherwise meaningless letters or numbers. Obviously what constitutes a 'chunk' will depend on your personal experience. For example, 'NHS' is one chunk as long as you are familiar with the National Health Service. If you are not familiar with this then the abbreviation 'N H S' would constitute three chunks.

Key message

The shorter the chunks, the easier is it to remember the information. Chunking can help!

Time to try

Quickly read through the list of letters below, then cover the list and try to write the letters down in the correct order

S	A	V	A	O
R	E	E	E	G
U	R	S	Y	A
O	O	D	N	S
F	C	N	E	R

How many did you remember in the correct order? The likelihood is that you remembered about seven letters (plus or minus two). Now look at the letters again starting with F (bottom left-hand corner) and read upwards until you get to S and then drop down to C until you get to A and so on. Did you recognise the chunks? If you did you should have remembered all of the letters.

F O U R   S C O R E   A N D   S E V E N   Y E A R S   A G O

THIS SHOULD GIVE YOU 'FOUR SCORE AND SEVEN YEARS AGO'.

Making use of chunking techniques during a consultation can significantly improve patients' recall of health information. A nurse can 'chunk' a verbal consultation by breaking up information with open questions (Haskard, 2009). This will not only ensure that the patient understands the previous chunk of information, but will also highlight aspects of the consultation that the patient may not have understood (Speros, 2011). When chunking information it is important to consider that patients are more likely to remember the first thing and the last thing that has been stated (this is the primacy/recency effect discussed earlier in this chapter); thus nurses should endeavour to provide the most important 'chunk' of information at the beginning and/or end of the consultation.

Rote rehearsal (also known as maintenance rehearsal) is a technique which involves repeating information over and over again out loud. This technique is useful when communicating information that is complex or new. One way of applying this technique would be to ask the patient to repeat what has been said as well as referring back to important information throughout the consultation.

Key message

Get your patient to repeat the information – this can aid memory for the information.

Audio or video recording the consultation can also act as a method of rehearsal and in turn facilitates patient recall. For example, Thomas et al. (2000) found that approximately 80 per cent of patients who listened to an audio recording of their consultation rated it as useful or very useful. Likewise, Liddell et al. (2004) found that providing patients with an audio-tape reduced misunderstandings and improved comprehension. What is more, 24 per cent of patients reported hearing information not attended to during the consultation. Furthermore, Watson and McKinstry (2009) carried out a systematic review of interventions designed to enhance recall of medical information. Finding that written and tape-recorded instructions appear to improve recall in most situations, the authors also suggested that incorporating psychological theory may help in patient recall. In order for patients to adhere to healthcare advice, it is essential that they are able to recall the information after consultation. Recall of information has also been suggested as predicting patient satisfaction, and in turn, enhancing adherence to recommended treatment (Watson and McKinstry, 2009).

Therefore, it can be elucidated that rehearsing information can improve memory recall. Rehearsal or repetition seems to require some kind of inner speech, whereby we 'say' the information either overtly or mentally again and again to keep it circulating within STM. This suggests that STM may encode information acoustically (Hanley and Thomas, 1984).

According to Gibson *et al.* (2002), patient confusion often arises because health information is too complex or lacks clear relevance to the patient's situation. Thus, in order to prevent patient confusion the nurse should ensure that health information is brief, simple, is linked to patient goals and is, in short, patient-centred (Husson *et al.*, 2011). Attributing meaning to health information can lead to greater recall.

Think about this

What memory techniques can you use to improve memory for information in your patients?

Key message

Brief, simple and categorised information aids memory.

Long-term memory

LTM is often categorised into episodic and semantic memory (Tulving, 1972), explicit and implicit memory (Graf and Schacter, 1985), and declarative and procedural knowledge systems (Cohn and Squire, 1980). Episodic memory contains memories about specific experiences or events occurring in a particular place at a particular time. Semantic memory on the other hand contains memory for factual information about the world. Typical examples of semantic memory include knowledge about language, how to calculate percentages and the dates of the Second World War. 'Explicit memory is revealed when performance on a task requires conscious recollection of previous experiences' (Graf and Schacter, 1985: 501). The memory tests discussed earlier in this chapter (e.g. free recall) all involve the use of explicit memory. In contrast, 'Implicit memory is revealed when performance on a task is facilitated in the absence of conscious recollection' (Graf and Schacter, 1985: 501). A typical example of implicit memory would be being asked to write a list of the countries you have visited – you know the names of the countries not because you were instructed to learn them, but because you have learned them in the natural course of events. Finally, explicit memory depends largely on the declarative knowledge system, whereas implicit memory depends largely on the procedural knowledge system (Eysenck and Keane, 2010). Declarative and procedural knowledge systems are related to Ryle's (1949) distinction between 'knowing that' and 'knowing how'. An example of declarative knowledge is *knowing that* Paris is the capital of France, whereas an example of procedural knowledge is *knowing how* to ride a bicycle or how to tie a shoelace.

Quick check

What are the main categories of LTM?

The capacity of LTM is very large and generally considered to be unlimited (Eysenck and Keane, 2010); yet the truth is that no one really knows how much information LTM can store. However, it is likely that there is a physical limit in terms of the actual brain cells available, but it seems unlikely that we will ever reach this upper limit. Table 5.1 outlines the features of different forms of memory.

Table 5.1 Comparing short- and long-term memory

	Sensory memory	Short-term memory	Long-term memory
Duration	¼ to 2 seconds	Up to 30 seconds	Unlimited
Capacity	Large	7 ± 2 items	Unlimited

How long does LTM last? Because of the difficulties in measuring LTM, a precise estimate cannot be given. However, we do know that the elderly never lose their childhood memories and that many skills such as riding a bicycle are never forgotten (Cuetos *et al.*, 2010). Therefore, in theory, information can be held in LTM for several years, which may in fact span the individual's entire lifetime. Bahrick *et al.* (1975) produced a simple but clever demonstration of LTM using photographs from high-school year books. They asked 392 ex-high-school students of various ages to recall the names of people in their class. Researchers also showed them a set of photographs and asked them to identify individuals. Even after 34 years participants were able to name 90 per cent of photographs of their classmates, supporting the idea that LTM does indeed store information for a very long time.

Think about this

How can a nurse use STM and LTM in their practice? What are the differences in concepts and applicability?

5.5 Information presentation

Two theories which are particularly applicable when looking at how information is presented are the levels of processing theory and schema theory. These will be briefly outlined and recommendations for practice will be discussed in relation to their suggestions.

Schema theory

A theory that can explain a number of errors in the memory process, at both the encoding and retrieval stages, is termed a schema theory (Lin-Bing *et al.*, 2007; Li-Rong and Nian Yue, 2010). A schema is a mental script, which guides individuals and influences how they perceive and interpret events around them based on previous experiences. When we receive information, we locate it within a schema. Schema theory discusses the way in which information or memories are organised. The theory suggests that our knowledge of people or events is stored in an elaborate network based on our pre-existing knowledge of that event or person. Basically, individuals have slots in which to store information about different things. For example you may have a professional experience slot, a hospital slot and a treatment slot holding all the information you have about that person, situation or object. When no direct knowledge about that subject is available it is filled with anecdotal evidence from friends or the media, and this then provides a base from which to predict or interpret events involving that subject.

These structures aid us to carry on our everyday lives by providing a structure from which to understand and deal with the complex world around us; they also save a lot of cognitive effort. There are several types of schema, each of which assists us in different activities:

✦ person schemas (e.g. patient)

✦ self-schemas (e.g. about you)

✦ role schemas (e.g. nurse)

✦ event schemas (e.g. hospital).

This information is important since these structures may impact negatively on memory for medical information (Van Vlierberghe *et al.*, 2010). The pre-existing information you or your patient holds can impact on how information is interpreted and consequently on behaviour. For example, stereotypes (see Chapter 4) are a simple cognitive framework for dealing with whole groups of people, which can be perpetuated by inferences made from nursing uniforms (Alford *et al.*, 1995).

Quick check

List the different forms of schema.

Think about this

What is the general stereotype of nurses? How can this influence how you behave or are treated?

Launder *et al.* (2005) also suggested that this can cause problems when patients have pre-existing ideas about their medication, illness or their treatment and are given more (accurate) information. Moreover, information can be distorted to fit the current schema. The nurse should ensure that preconceived ideas and beliefs are explored fully with the patient before new information is provided, which also enhances patient-centred care (Price, 2006).

Key message

Information you give to your patient may be distorted based on what the patient thinks you are trying to tell them and their existing information.

Levels of processing model

Another theory that can add to our understanding of patients' memories in relation to health information is the levels of processing model (Craik and Lockhart, 1972). According to this model, it is the depth at which information is processed that is important in terms of how it is stored and subsequently recalled. Processing information according to its meaning produces stronger, longer-lasting and more elaborate memory traces than processing information according to its sound (phonemic processing) or physical appearance (shallow processing). Referring back to the initial models presented, short-term memory is that which is processed at a shallower level (e.g. acoustically), whereas long-term memory lasts longer as it is remembered in terms of its meaning. This therefore removes the need for separate storages, with information existing on a continuum in terms of its depth of processing.

This theory tells us of two methods when rehearsing information. Rehearsing material by simple rote repetition, or maintenance rehearsal, is classified as shallow. Rehearsing material by exploring its meaning and linking it to semantically associated words is called elaborative rehearsal and is classified as deep (Craik and Lockhart, 1972).

So, how can we use this information? How can this improve our own memory, and how can we use it with our patients? Providing health information within the context of the patient's everyday life is one way of enhancing meaning; this can be done, for instance, by linking prescribed medication to the patient's everyday routine. This theory also explains the success of mnemonic techniques for enhancing recall, a method discussed later in the chapter. Furthermore, we also need to explore (at each level) the understanding of the information to ensure that deep processing has occurred (Ragland *et al.*, 2003). There are a number of other methods for improving memory and we will explore these in more detail later in this chapter.

5.6 The role of cues

We have all had the experience of going somewhere, be it upstairs, to the kitchen, to a particular patient and then when getting there, forgetting why we had gone, so we backtrack either physically, returning to where we were, or mentally. What was I thinking about that reminded me to do this? These are great examples of the role of cues in memory recall. It may be that you have experienced situations in which a patient was doing well with their treatment plan but upon returning home failed to adhere to the plan and returned to hospital.

Think about this

How can you use cues in your practice to get the following individuals to take their medication:

✦ a 45-year-old with chronic schizophrenia

✦ a 24-year-old with epilepsy

✦ a person with pre-senile dementia

✦ a 16-year-old with diabetes?

It is important to provide patients with cues to act that not only occur within the hospital setting but can be transferred to the home setting. Cues can be extremely helpful in elderly individuals. For instance Cochrane (2010) examined the use of autobiographical memory cues as cognitive support for memory, and suggested that autobiographical cues may be effective for improving everyday memory performance in healthy older adults and patients with mild stages of Alzheimer's Disease. So why is it that cues work so well? Levels of processing theory would suggest that cues are the meaning to which meaningless activities such as doing an exercise or taking a pill are attached. By putting this information within a meaningful situation such as a daily routine, it is recalled better. If we look back at schema theory, cues can be explained as the activation of a network of information for which the action is a part. For instance, Park *et al.* (1992) report on how external cues can be used with older adults to improve their memory for treatment and hence increase medication adherence.

Key message

Cues can aid recall and improve adherence to treatment.

5.7 The role of perceived importance

It sounds obvious, but information is less likely to be remembered if the patient considers it to be unimportant. For example, if a patient does not understand the implications or importance of not taking their medication at particular intervals then they are less likely to remember and subsequently do not adhere to this routine (Baroletti, 2010; Katic *et al.*, 2009; McHorney and Gadkari, 2010; Zikmund-Fisher *et al.*, 2009). The role of perceived importance in memory encoding and recall has been displayed in a number of research studies. Kessels (2003), based on the work of Ley (1979), highlights the importance of information in memory. If the importance of the information is stressed then it was discovered that there would be an improvement in adherence to treatment. For example Zolnierek and DiMatteo (2009) carried out a meta-analysis finding that when information is communicated well by medical staff then patients will consequently improve adherence to treatment.

Key message   🔑

Stressing the importance of a message can improve adherence to treatment.

5.8 Mnemonic aids

'i' before 'e' except after 'c'. Mnemonics are a well-known way of aiding memory and work by pairing a meaningless stimulus, such as the type of drug used to treat a particular condition, with a meaningful stimulus, something already in the long-term memory, such as a daily routine or journey. If we return to the levels of processing theory, you can see that this technique works by attaching meaning to new information providing a deeper memory trace and as such results in a more memorable piece of information. There is a lot of support for the success of these techniques, particularly in teaching children with learning disabilities (Goll, 2004; Scruggs *et al.*, 2010), those with emotional or behavioural disturbance (King-Sears *et al.*, 1992), or dementia patients with memory and communication difficulties (Smith *et al.*, 2010). Some further examples of mnemonic aids are presented in Table 5.2.

Think about this   ?

Consider the various topics you need to revise for your study. Think of some mnemonics to help you do this.

5.9 Compliance, adherence and concordance to treatment

Within this chapter we have considered various cognitive processes – perception, attention and memory – from a very technical perspective. However, these come together when the patient is attempting to follow information from the nurse or other healthcare professionals. This used to be termed 'compliance', but was re-termed 'adherence' during the 1980s. However, both terms suffer from the implication that it is an authoritarian relationship – the nurse or healthcare professional telling the patient what to do (see Chapter 4). Consequently, the term 'concordance' is now used within the literature to indicate more of a partnership approach: 'The patient being an equal partner, supporting the ethos of shared decision-making between patient and health professional rather than more traditional paternalism' (Weiss and Britten, 2003). This concept has been examined in several recent studies, which all elucidate that there should be a shared decision-making between the patient and the healthcare professional (Latter, 2010; Sahlsten *et al.*, 2009; Wills, 2010).

Table 5.2 Mnemonic use in nursing practice

Mnemonic principle	Definition	Example in practice
Elaboration and the keyword mnemonic	Converting names into meaningful words or even making words active.	The 12 cranial nerves: 'Obviously Our Overseas Travelling Tourists Are Finding Very Good Value At Hotels'
		Olfactory nerve (I)
		Optic nerve (II)
		Oculomotor nerve (III)
		Trochlear nerve (IV)
		Trigeminal nerve (V)
		Abducens nerve (VI)
		Facial nerve (VII)
		Vestibulocochlear nerve (VIII)
		Glossopharyngeal nerve (IX)
		Vagus nerve (X)
		Accessory nerve (XI),
		Hypoglossal nerve (XII)
Association	Giving meaning to a word or name which then must be attached to something.	Take for instance the need to take certain medication on specific days. You could use the name of the drug as a clue, say amoxicillin, a must until the weekend. If the name of the pill is too long or complex then using the colour or shape of the medication is another memory trick. Yellow pills could be bananas, blue could be blueberries, etc.
Story system	Advantage over the link system is that the flow of the story will allow the remainder of the list to be retrieved whereas the link system will lose all the information if one link has been lost.	I walked into the house and saw my bowl of fruit – my yellow bananas – and then I went into the kitchen and got my blueberries . . .
Loci system	Based on the principle of mentally positioning things to remember in a well-known room.	Visualise your tablets in your bathroom so you remember them always.
Rhyming word peg	Rhyming meaningful words or numbers with established words.	To the tune of 'Row, row, row your boat' to assist in remembering the characteristics of DNA:
		We love DNA, Made of nucleotides, A phosphate, sugar and a base, Bonded down one side.
		Adenine and Thymine, Make a lovely pair, Guanine without Cytosine, Would be very bare.

Key message

Compliance, adherence and concordance refer to the same thing, but concordance is the most appropriate term: it emphasises the partnership between the patient and the nurse.

Therefore, compliance and adherence refer to the cooperation of a patient in following medical advice about treatment, whereas concordance takes into consideration the needs and desires of the patient (Snowden, 2008). Another distinction that has to be emphasised is intentional versus unintentional non-adherence. For example, on some occasions the patient will not follow the advice given since it was not explained properly, or it has been forgotten. In this case, it can be classified as unintentional non-adherence. For example Unni and Farris (2011) suggested that beliefs in medicine were a significant predictor of forgetfulness and carelessness in taking medication in older adults. In contrast, there are occasions when the patient makes an active choice not to take the medication as instructed.

Think about this

Why would a patient choose not to take their medication as indicated?

There are low levels of adherence to many forms of medication and this has a significant impact on the expenditure of the health service. Snowden suggests that non-adherence alone costs the NHS some £6.8 billion in the UK. However, more important on an individual basis is the potential significant impact on the patient. For example, estimates of non-adherence to medication for unipolar and bipolar disorders range from 10 to 60 per cent with a median rate of 40 per cent (Lingam and Scott, 2003). Similarly, some 20 to 70 per cent of headache sufferers are not using medication optimally and 40 per cent do not keep appointments (Rains *et al.*, 2006). In cross-sectional studies published from 1980 to 2001, around 18-22 per cent of renal graft recipients were found to be non-adherent to immunosuppressants (Gremigni *et al.*, 2007). Additionally rates of non-adherence in inflammatory bowel disease have been suggested to be around 40 per cent (Lakatos, 2009).

It is not just in physical health that there are issues, but also in mental health. Cramer and Rosenheck (1998) report that in people with schizophrenia the average rate of non-adherence is 42 per cent. More recently, Novick *et al.* (2010) examined 6731 schizophrenic patients finding that 71 per cent were adherent to antipsychotic medication and 29 per cent were non-adherent over the three years they were examined. Non-adherence rate were found to be significantly associated with an increased risk of relapse, hospitalisation and suicide attempts. Furthermore, McAllister-Williams *et al.* (2006) and Berk *et al.* (2010) suggest that low adherence is becoming a major concern for individuals with bipolar disorders.

Consequently, non-adherence results in a number of negative consequences: reduced positive recovery on the part of the patient, with frequent relapses, high frustration levels and wasted time on the part of the healthcare professional and significant costs to the health service. In the next section of this chapter we will look at the possible causes of non-adherence and will then turn to possible psychosocial interventions for improving adherence levels.

Key message

Non-adherence can be costly both to the taxpayer and the individual patient.

5.10 Causes of non-adherence

The causes of non-adherence are complex, where the patient–practitioner relationship, treatment regimen and other disease-related factors play a key role (Lakatos, 2009). A useful model for exploring non-adherence is based on the work of Phillip Ley who presented a cognitive model of compliance (1981, 1989). According to this cognitive hypothesis, patient adherence can be predicted by patient satisfaction, understanding, and memory (recall) (see Figure 5.9).

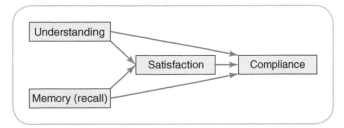

Figure 5.9 The cognitive hypothesis model of compliance

Think about this

How do you think you can influence (either positively or negatively) patient satisfaction?

In terms of patient satisfaction there are three elements (Wolf *et al.*, 1978):

+ **The cognitive aspect** – satisfaction with the amount and quality of the information provided by the healthcare professional.
+ **The affective aspect** – the extent to which the patient feels that that the healthcare professional listens, understands and is interested.
+ **The behavioural aspect** – the patient's evaluation of a healthcare professional's competence in the consultation.

Quick check

What are the components of non-adherence according to the cognitive hypothesis model?

However, the major focus of this chapter is on the other two factors: understanding and memory. Any setting where treatment is being offered can be a highly anxious and distressing environment (remember the perceptual point we highlighted at the outset of this chapter). Consequently you will want to reduce anxiety and concern. Hence, if treatment is completed in a more relaxed setting (e.g. at home) then there is a better chance of any recall.

There are different ways in which the nurse can provide instructions for treatment, and the method will influence how likely a patient is to remember them. For example, the more oral and written information you can provide a patient, the more likely you are to enhance their adherence (McDonald *et al.*, 2002; Watson and McKinstry, 2009). This is because information that is received by more than one sense is more likely to be registered within memory and retained for a longer period of time (see above). Furthermore, Morrow *et al.* (2005) discovered that when conveying information to older adults it is essential for healthcare professionals to assume a patient-centred approach. This approach has been found to lead to the better understanding of familiar and unfamiliar medications with significantly better recall for the information provided in both verbal and written format. However, there are also many other methods that can help improve recall of information. Some of these are presented in Table 5.3 and the impact of these improvements in Table 5.4.

Table 5.3 Guidelines for improving information recall

Guideline	Example
Keep information simple	Do not over-complicate with medical jargon – use everyday language.
Important information at the start (primacy) or at the end (recency)	Provide the most important information at either the start or the end of the conversation.
Divide the information into chunks	'I am now going to talk about your diagnosis, and now your prognosis, and now your treatment . . .'
Explain and ensure information is meaningful	Relate to the individual patient – make it meaningful for them and ensure that it will fit in with their particular situation.
Ensure understanding	Ask questions to test understanding.
Stress the important message	'This is of central importance . . .'
Repeat information	And repeat, and repeat . . .
Be specific rather than general	'Lose 2lbs in weight' rather than 'Lose some weight'.
Follow up	Phone the patient or discuss at the next consultation to ensure understanding.

Table 5.4 Effectiveness of these techniques for increasing recall

Technique	Control (i.e. without the technique)	With the technique
Primacy	50	86
Stressed importance	50	65
Simplification	27	40
Explicit categorisation	50	64
Repetition: by practitioner	76	90
Repetition: by patient	76	91
Use of specific statements	16	51
Mixture	55	75

Key message

Written information can improve understanding and adherence.

Think about this

How could you improve adherence to treatment in the following:

+ an overweight male on a weight-reducing regime
+ a person with asthma on an exercise regime
+ a male with heart failure requiring considerable medication
+ a person with kidney failure?

5.11 Cognitive models of health behaviour

The cognitive hypothesis model has been useful and indicates some key factors involved in adherence to treatment. However, it does not really address some fundamental concerns about the individual patient – their feelings, concerns and cognitions concerning their health and illness. In order to address this, further models – the social cognition models – have been developed. These models are 'concerned with how individuals make sense of social situations' (Conner and Norman, 1996: 5). These models are the subject of this section. They have been used to explain why people adhere (or don't) to treatment, but also to whether they will engage in health protective behaviour (e.g. going for screening tests or stopping drinking).

Key message

Cognitive models of health behaviour have been a major focus of attention in psychology. They have been used to explain why people engage in health promoting, health protecting or health damaging behaviours.

The earliest models were based on the belief that behaviours were a result of a rational weighting of the potential costs and benefits of that behaviour and that the behaviour is a result of rational information processing of these costs and benefits (spot the potential problem already?). Several models have been proposed as explanations for health behaviour and behaviour change.

The health belief model

The health belief model (HBM) was one of the first and best-known models (Rosenstock, 1974; Becker, 1974) developed in order to predict preventative health behaviours – see Figure 5.10. It has also been used to describe the behavioural response to treatment in patients with both acute and chronic illnesses.

The HBM makes a series of predictions about behaviour and suggests that they are a result of a set of core beliefs. The original core beliefs are the individual's perception of:

✦ susceptibility to illness (e.g. 'My chances of getting cancer are high')

✦ severity of the illness (e.g. 'Cancer is a serious illness')

✦ the costs involved in carrying out the behaviour (e.g. 'Quitting smoking will be stressful')

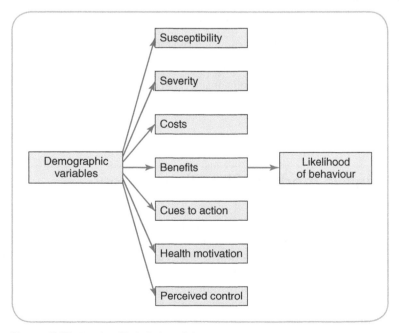

Figure 5.10   The health belief model

+ the benefits involved in carrying out the behaviour (e.g. 'I will be able to run up the stairs')

+ cues to action, which may be internal (e.g. some non-specific symptoms) or external (e.g. health education information/leaflets).

The model suggests that the likelihood of a behaviour occurring is related to these core beliefs. Consequently, the HBM can be used to predict whether a particular behaviour will occur or not. The original HBM has been updated and improved with 'health motivation' added to reflect an individual's readiness to be concerned about health matters (e.g. 'I am concerned that not stopping smoking will seriously damage my health').

Think about this

How can the HBM be used to deal with various health promoting behaviours?

However, there have been criticisms of the HBM such as the absence of a role for emotional factors such as fear and denial. It has also been suggested that alternative factors may predict health behaviour, such as outcome expectancy and self-efficacy. Schwarzer (1992) further criticised the HBM for its static approach to health beliefs and suggests that within the HBM beliefs are described as occurring simultaneously with no room for change, development or process. Also Leventhal *et al.* (1985) have argued that health-related behaviour is due to the perception of symptoms rather than to the individual factors as suggested by the HBM.

As well as this, a recent meta-analysis examined the HBM to determine whether measures of these beliefs could longitudinally predict behaviour, finding suggested weaknesses in some of the predictors and the author concluded that based on this weakness the continued use of the direct version of the HBM is not recommended (Carpenter, 2010). Additionally, earlier research recognised that the HBM had several components that needed to be further developed and some factors needed to be included (Davidhizar, 1983), which prompted researchers to refine this model and in the light of these studies the protection motivation theory (PMT) was developed.

Quick check

What are the components of the health belief model?

Protection motivation theory (PMT)

The PMT was developed by Rogers (1975, 1983) who expanded the HBM to include additional factors (see Figure 5.11).

The PMT suggests that health behaviours can be predicted on the basis of four components:

+ severity (e.g. 'Heart disease is a serious illness')

+ susceptibility (e.g. 'My chances of getting CHD are high')

+ response effectiveness (e.g. 'Doing some exercise would improve my health')

+ self-efficacy (e.g. 'I am confident that I can engage in physical exercise').

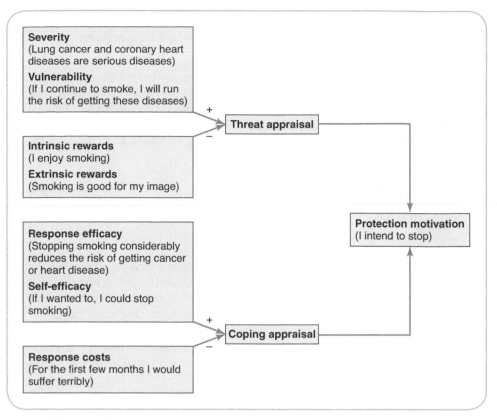

Figure 5.11 Protection motivation theory
Source: Based on Stroebe, 2000.

These components predict behavioural intentions which are related (although somewhat tenuously) to behaviour. The PMT considers that severity, susceptibility and fear are part of the threat appraisal (external factors) and response effectiveness and self-efficacy are related to coping (internal factors). PMT has been successfully utilised in a number of studies, Plotnikoff *et al*. (2010), for example, investigated the utility of the PMT for explaining physical activity in patients with diabetes, suggesting that the PMT was effective in both type 1 and 2 diabetes.

Think about this

How would you use the PMT to increase the chances of a patient attending a breast screening clinic?

Quick check

What are the components of the PMT?

5.12 Social cognition models

The two models described so far have been further developed and revised in order to over-come some of the criticisms levelled against them. In particular, the models have been refined to include a role for the social context of the behaviour and not simply rely on the individual's cognitions or attitudes. Not surprisingly these models have been called 'social cognition mod-els' (as opposed to 'cognition models').

Theory of reasoned action

The theory of reasoned action (TRA) was developed by social psychologists in the 1970s and has been used extensively to examine predictors of behaviours (Fishbein, 1967; Ajzen and Fishbein, 1970; Fishbein and Ajzen, 1975). The TRA was an important model as it was one of the first to place the individual within the social context.

Key message

The theory of reasoned action places the individual within a social context.

The TRA suggests that behavioural intention is a product of an individual's attitude towards performing the behaviour and of subjective norms. Each of these factors has fur-ther elements – see Figure 5.12. So, for example, a person's attitudes towards the behaviour

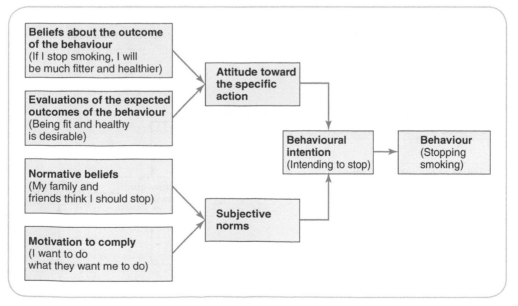

Figure 5.12 Theory of reasoned action

Source: Wolfgang Stroebe, *Social Psychology and Health*, 2nd edn, 2000. Reproduced with the kind permission of Open University Press. All rights reserved.

will be a consequence of the likelihood of that behaviour being associated with a positive outcome. Hence, an individual's attitudes towards starting exercise are a function of the perceived likelihood with which physical exercise is associated with certain consequences, such as being healthier and fitter, and the evaluation of these perceived consequences (i.e. Are they positive? Are they worth the effort?).

The other element to the model is subjective norms and this includes two components:

+ **Normative beliefs** – the beliefs held by us about how people who are important to us expect us to behave.
+ Motivation to comply.

Hence, subjective norms are a product of both normative beliefs and motivation to comply.

Quick check
What are the key components of the TRA?

Theory of planned behaviour (TPB)

The TRA was developed by Ajzen and colleagues into the theory of planned behaviour (TPB) (Ajzen, 1985, 1988) – see Figure 5.13.

The TPB suggests that behavioural intentions (i.e. to engage in a particular practice – to behave in a certain manner) are a consequence of a combination of several beliefs:

+ **Attitudes towards a behaviour:** this comprises a positive or negative evaluation of a particular behaviour and beliefs about the outcome of the behaviour (e.g. 'Exercising is fun and will improve my health').
+ **Subjective norms:** these are composed of the perception of social norms and pressures to perform a behaviour and an evaluation of whether the individual is motivated to comply

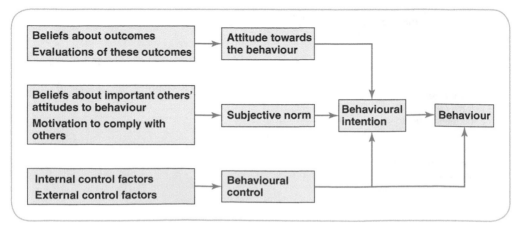

Figure 5.13 Theory of planned behaviour

Source: Jane Ogden, *Health Psychology*, 3rd edn, 2004. Reproduced with the kind permission of Open University Press. All rights reserved.

with this pressure (e.g. 'My husband is important to me and he will approve if I lose weight and I want his approval').

✦ **Perceived behavioural control:** this is an important component and suggests that the individual can carry out the particular behaviour considering both internal (e.g. skills, abilities and information, 'I can play five-a-side football and I know where to join a club') and external (e.g. 'I can make the Friday night when the football sessions are on'). Obviously both of these relate to previous experiences and behaviour.

Think about this

How would you use the TRA and TRB to increase the chances of an individual using a condom when he has sex with his partner? In particular, how would you increase perceived behavioural control?

5.13 Strategies for changing risk behaviour

So far in this chapter the various models that have been devised to predict people's behaviour have been outlined and explored and the value of these to nursing demonstrated. However, of course, one of the important areas for any healthcare professional is in altering an individual's maladaptive behaviour to positive health-promoting behaviour. This will be the focus of the final section of this chapter. In particular, the concept of motivational interviewing will be developed and discussed (Miller and Rollnick, 2002) which was based on the stages of change model (Prochaska and DiClemente, 1982).

One of the most influential psychological models that has been used in behaviour change has been the 'transtheoretical model of change' or 'stages of change' (Prochaska and DiClemente, 1982). The model suggests that change proceeds through six stages summarised in Figure 5.14 and Table 5.5. Importantly, relapse can occur at any stage, and can mean that

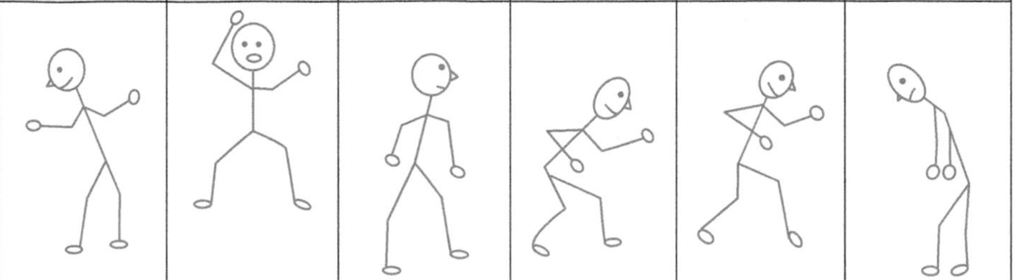

Pre-contemplation	Contemplation	Determination/preparation	Action	Maintenance	Relapse/recycle
	Fence	0–3 Months	3–6 Months	Over 6 months	
No: denial	Maybe: ambivalence	Yes, let's go: motivated	Doing it: go	Living it:	Start over: ugh!!

Figure 5.14 Stages of change model

Table 5.5 Stages of change – definitions and description

Stage	Definition	Description
Pre-contemplation	No intention of change	The person changing the behaviour has not been considered: the person may not realise that change is possible or that it might be of interest to them.
Contemplation	Intention to change	Something happens to prompt the person to start thinking about change – perhaps hearing that someone has made changes or something else has changed, resulting in the need for further change.
Preparation	Intention to change soon and plans of action have been made	The person prepares to undertake the desired change – requires gathering information, finding out how to achieve the change, ascertaining skills necessary, deciding when change should take place. May include talking with others to see how they feel about the likely change, considering the impact change will have and who will be affected.
Action	Making changes	People make changes, acting on previous decisions, experience, information, new skills and motivations for making the change.
Maintenance	Working to maintain behaviour and prevent relapse	Practice required for the new behaviour to be consistently maintained, incorporated into the repertoire of behaviours available to a person at any one time.

the individual goes back to the very first stage. It is not a linear model of simple progression from one stage to another and then relapse means that you simply revert to the previous stage: you can revert to *any* previous stage.

Key message

Always find out where your individual patient is on the stages of change model as this will determine your intervention.

Quick check

What are the stages in the stages of change model?

Think about this

What intervention strategies would you recommend to a smoker in each of the following stages:

pre-contemplation; contemplation; preparation; action; maintenance?

The stages of change model has been used extensively to promote health and assist individuals in smoking cessation (e.g. Aveyard *et al.*, 2009; Prochaska *et al.*, 2007; Anatchkova *et al.*, 2005). This model is important because it allows professionals to identify where individuals are in their behaviour and then develop appropriate interventions (whether these be computer or media based, community or individual based, pharmacologically or psychologically based).

If, for example, an individual smokes and has no intention of giving up (i.e. is in the pre-contemplation stage), the intervention to be developed will be different to that of the individual who is preparing to give up (i.e. is in the contemplation stage) or has started the process (i.e. is in the action stage). In the first case our obligation should be to try to get quitting into the person's thought processes. We want to try to get the individual to consider giving up smoking – we want to shift them from the pre-contemplation stage to the contemplation stage. The most common method in this approach is a simple consciousness-raising exercise: increasing information about the problem and how it can affect the individual concerned. So at this stage it would simply be a case of getting them to realise that smoking is health damaging and that it can affect them individually and then spelling out the individual health problems. This example demonstrates that interventions have to be tailored to the individual's position in the cycle.

Key message

Interventions have to be specific to the individual's stage of change.

Interventions to help people quit smoking, based on the stages of change model, usually incorporate two key elements. First it is necessary to identify accurately an individual's stage of change (or readiness to change), so that an appropriate intervention can be designed and applied. Second, the stage of change needs to be reassessed frequently, and the intervention modified in the light of this assessment. In this way, stage based interventions evolve and adapt in response to the individual's movement through the stages.

The first task that we have to do is identify what stage the individual smoker is at. This is not as difficult as it sounds and can be completed using a simple 'readiness ruler' as indicated in Figure 5.15 along with a confidence ruler (see Figure 5.16) which can assist the practitioner in planning the intervention and the support that will be required. (Note that these rulers can be adapted for any behaviour.)

On a scale of 1 to 10 how certain are you that you want to change your smoking behaviour?

1	2	3	4	5	6	7	8	9	10
Not certain at all								Very certain	
Pre-contemplation			Contemplation			Action			

Figure 5.15 Readiness ruler for assessing stage of change of a smoker

On a scale of 1 to 10 how confident are you that you *want* to change your smoking behaviour?

1	2	3	4	5	6	7	8	9	10
Not confident at all								Very confident	

Figure 5.16 Confidence ruler for assessing an individual smoker

Motivational interviewing

On the basis of the stages of change model a whole series of interventions can be devised, described and implemented. Motivational interviewing has as its goal the simple (some would say!) expectation that increasing an individual's motivation to consider change rather than showing them how to change should be the important step. If a person is not motivated to change then it is irrelevant whether they know how to do it or not. However, if a person is motivated to change then the interventions aimed at changing behaviour can begin.

Motivational interviewing (MI) is a technique based on cognitive behavioural therapy which aims to enhance an individual's motivation to change health behaviour (e.g. Thompson *et al.*, 2011; Russell *et al.*, 2011). The whole process aims to help the patient understand their thought processes and to identify how these help produce the inappropriate behaviour, and how they can be changed to develop alternative, health-promoting behaviours.

Key message

A person must be motivated to change in order to start their change process.

Motivational strategies include components that are designed to increase the level of motivation the person has towards changing a specific behaviour. It is important to note that the motivation is specific to one behaviour – so being motivated to quit smoking does not simply transfer to being motivated to reduce alcohol consumption. Some of the essential skills for motivational interviewing are presented in Table 5.6.

However, before we get to the questions, we need to assess an individual's readiness to change which is usually completed using a 'readiness to change' ruler. This is exactly what it says! Hence, the nurse would ask the patient, 'On a scale of 1 to 10 how ready are you to make the change?' (whether this be change of diet for somebody with diabetes, quitting smoking or

Table 5.6 Key skills for motivational interviewing

Skill	Comment
Use open-ended questions	Encourage the client to do most of the talking: 'What are your concerns about smoking?'
Use reflective listening	Reflect back change talk in a statement: 'I have the shakes in the morning' to 'You are a little concerned about the shakes in the morning . . .'
Use affirmation	Use to build rapport: 'You are right to be concerned about having unprotected sex.'
Summarise	Link together and reinforce what has been discussed: 'You are concerned that your smoking may cause lung cancer.'
Reframe or agree with a twist	Address resistance by reinterpreting: 'My wife nags me to change my diet' to 'It sounds like she really cares about your health.'
Emphasise personal choice	Reinforce that it is the client's choice to change their behaviour.
Evocative questions	
Increasing confidence	Use open questions to evoke confidence: 'How might you go about making this change?'
Confidence ruler	Use the ruler to ask: 'What would it take to score higher?'
Strengths and successes	Review obstacles and how the client has overcome them.
Reframing	'I've tried three times to quit and failed' to 'You have had three good attempts already and are learning new skills'.
Prompt coping strategies	Ask for potential obstacles and putative coping strategies.

reducing alcohol intake). On this basis you could decide whether the patient was in the pre-contemplation stage (probably scoring 3 or below), the contemplation stage (scoring 4-6) or the action stage (7 or above). On this basis you would then tailor your intervention (see Figure 5.17).

Despite the popularity of the stages of change model, there have been several concerns about the validity of its use. One of these concerns was that the stages of change might not reflect real stages, but rather segments of an underlying continuum (Sutton, 2001). In addition, the ordering of the stages, the classification system to define stages and the qualitative differences of the stages have been a subject of debate (West, 2005). The model also focuses on conscious decision-making and planning processes, and assumes that individuals make logical and stable plans, which in fact they do not. Take smoking for example; it has been described as a habitual behaviour which is not a conscious thought process but more of an automatic one.

Think about this

How would you use motivational interviewing to increase an individual's likelihood of quitting smoking?

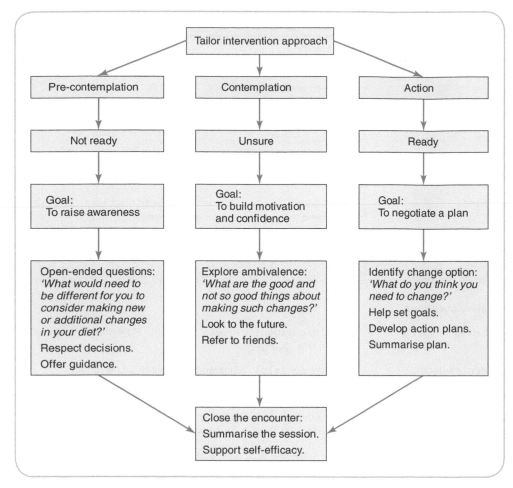

Figure 5.17 Tailoring your intervention strategy according to an individual's readiness to change

Research in Focus

Davis, M.F., Shapiro,D., Windsor, R., Whalen, P., Rhode, R., Miller, H.S., and Sechrest, L. (2011) Motivational interviewing versus prescriptive advice for smokers who are not ready to quit. *Patient Education & Counseling* **83**(1), 129-133.

Background

It is extremely difficult to treat smokers who are not ready to quit. Physicians, nurses and nurse practitioners hold a unique position which enables then to encourage their patients to quit smoking. However, it is unclear as to what would be the best approach in adopting this.

→

Methods

This research was a laboratory-based study adopting a randomised controlled trial of two groups. These groups included 218 pack-a-day pre-contemplative and contemplative smokers recruited from the local community. Each participant was randomised to a 15-minute intervention in order to compare the effectiveness of prescriptive counselling or brief motivational interviewing by a health professional. Intentions to quit and verbal reports were included in 13 outcome variables, which were noted at month 1 and follow-up at 6 months with biological verification.

Results

During the six months in which participants were followed preceding the trial, 33 per cent of the sample reported at least one 24-hour quitting period. It was discovered that neither treatment was superior, however there were subgroup differences. Furthermore, participants within the motivational interviewing condition were more likely to respond to follow-up calls.

Implications

Due to the discovery of both motivational interviewing and prescriptive advice being equally effective for both pre-contemplative and contemplative smokers, practitioners should use the method which appeals to them.

5.14 Conclusion

Perception, attention and memory are all elements in healthcare practice and can impact on your patients' and clients' behaviour. This may help explain adherence to treatment and possible ways of improving this.

5.15 Summary

+ People perceive items and individuals differently.
+ Gestalt principles of grouping including similarity, proximity, continuity, closure and figure/ground and can be used in nursing care practice.
+ Memory is made up of three components: encoding, storing and retrieving information.
+ STM and LTM are different memory stores.
+ Recency and primacy effects are important in conveying and remembering information.
+ Too much information in the environment can lead to distraction and an inability to recall.
+ Chunking and mnemonics can improve recall.

✦ The cognitive hypothesis suggests that understanding, memory and satisfaction influence levels of adherence/compliance.

✦ The HBM is based on susceptibility to illness, severity of illness, costs and benefits of carrying out the behaviour along with cues to action.

✦ The protection motivation theory (PMT) suggests that health behaviours can be predicted on the basis of severity, susceptibility, response effectiveness, self-efficacy and fear.

✦ The theories of reasoned action/planned behaviour are social cognition models which are based on attitudes towards a behaviour, subjective norms and perceived behavioural control.

✦ A particular method for developing behaviour is motivational interviewing which aims to increase an individual's motivation to alter their own behaviour.

Your end point

Answer the following questions to assess your knowledge and understanding of cognition and information provision.

1. Information about how to approach familiar situations such as a day on the ward, organising your studies or ordering in a restaurant is organised into knowledge structures referred to as _____

   (a) sketches
   (b) schemes
   (c) episodes
   (d) schemas
   (e) loops?

2. When some participants read an ambiguous passage about a woman, Sarah, in a nurse's office, which psychological factor reduced the accuracy of their recall of the information from the passage?

   (a) Imagined memories of the event.
   (b) Expectations about recalling the passage at a later time.
   (c) Expectations about Sarah's condition.
   (d) Pre-existing knowledge about people named Sarah.
   (e) The number of times they read the passage.

3. The improved recall of items presented at the end of a consultation compared to the middle of a consultation is referred to as the _____

   (a) last rehearsed effect
   (b) recency effect
   (c) delayed effect
   (d) limited capacity effect
   (e) none of the above?

4. Based on the stages of change model developed by Prochaska and DiClemente (1982), if a woman notices that she has been coughing a lot recently and begins to →

think about stopping smoking over the next six months, she would be at which stage of making behavioural changes:

(a) pre-contemplation
(b) contemplation
(c) preparation
(d) action
(e) maintenance?

5. According to Ajzen's (1985) theory of planned behaviour, behavioural intentions are influenced by:

(a) attitudes towards behaviour
(b) subjective norms
(c) perceived behavioural control
(d) all of the above
(e) none of the above?

Further reading

Atkinson, R.C. and Shiffrin, R.M. (1968) The control of short-term memory. *Scientific American* **225**, 82–90.

Banja, J.D. (2007) My what? *American Journal of Bioethics* **7**(11), 13–15.

Bohner, G., Moskowitz, G.B. and Chaiken, S. (1995) The interplay of heuristic and systematic processing of social information. *European Review of Social Psychology* **6**, 33–68.

Eysenck, W.M., and Keane, T.M. (2010) *Cognitive Psychology: A Student's Handbook.* (6th edn.) Psychological Press: New York.

Floyd, D.L., Prentice-Dunn, S. and Rogers, R.W. (2006) A meta-analysis of research on protection motivation theory. *Journal of Applied Social Psychology* **30**(2), 407–429.

Gillibrand, R. and Stevenson, J. (2006) The extended health belief model applied to the experience of diabetes in young people. *British Journal of Health Psychology* **11**, 155–169.

Levine, J.M., Resnick, L.B. and Higgins, E.T. (1993) Social foundations of cognition. *Annual Review of Psychology* **44**, 585–612.

Navon, D. (1977) Forest before trees: The precedence of global features in visual perception. *Cognitive Psychology* **9**, 353–383.

Watson, P.W.B. and McKinstry, B. (2009) A systematic review of medical advice in healthcare consultation. *Journal of the Royal Society of Medicine* **102**(6), 235–243.

Zimmerman, G.L., Olsen, C.G. and Bosworth, M.F. (2000) A 'stages of change' approach to helping patients change behaviour. *American Family Physician* **61**, 1409–1416.

Weblinks

http://www.memoryarena.com/resources
Memory Resources. This site contains links to the latest memory journal articles.

http://www.umbc.edu/psyc/habits/content/the_model/index.html
Transtheoretical Model of Behaviour Change. This site provides details of how health promotion techniques can be designed using the transtheoretical model.

http://www.mindtools.com/memory.html
Mind Tools. This site contains hints and tips for improving your own memory. Why not have a go!

http://www.patientadherenceroi.com
Patient Adherence. This site contains lots of useful articles on patient adherence to treatment.

Check point

Your starting point		Your end point	
Q1	E	Q1	D
Q2	E	Q2	B
Q3	E	Q3	B
Q4	B	Q4	B
Q5	B	Q5	D

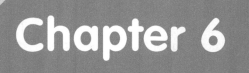

Chapter 6

Stress and stress management

Learning Outcomes

At the end of this chapter you will be able to:

✦ Define, understand and explain stress
✦ Understand and evaluate the various models of stress
✦ Describe the link between stress and ill-health
✦ Review how people cope with stress
✦ Explore and understand how you can employ stress management techniques for your patient.

Your starting point

Answer the following questions to assess your knowledge and understanding of stress and stress management.

1. Being impatient, irritable, always in a hurry, and fixated on deadlines are traits associated with:

   (a) latency stage fixation
   (b) type A personality
   (c) type C personality
   (d) type B personality
   (e) oral stage fixation?

2. As you peek through the door of the ward where you are just about to start, you notice that one of your colleagues is being berated by a drunken youth. Your first stress response is:

   (a) alarm and mobilisation
   (b) plateau
   (c) resistance
   (d) exhaustion
   (e) fixation?

3. On your way to work one morning, you get stuck in traffic and you are 45 minutes late for your shift. This is an example of:

   (a) a background stressor
   (b) a personal stressor
   (c) an uplift
   (d) learned helplessness
   (e) a depressive episode?

4. You tell a patient that he must take a prescribed medicine twice daily to cure his infection. The patient eventually discards the medicine for a 'home remedy' suggested by his grandmother. This demonstrates:

   (a) subjective well-being
   (b) objective well-being
   (c) civil disobedience
   (d) non-adherence
   (e) none of the above?

5. Selye describes the general adaptation syndrome as proceeding in the following order:

   (a) alarm reaction, resistance, exhaustion
   (b) alarm reaction, exhaustion, resistance
   (c) exhaustion, resistance, alarm reaction
   (d) resistance, alarm reaction, exhaustion
   (e) none of the above?

Case Study

Helen is a 40-year-old woman who has worked in the Civil Service for all her adult life. She was committed to her work and, despite having little opportunity to progress, remained loyal and determined to her chosen career. Her father died many years ago, and her elderly mother was her only surviving relative for many years until she died three months ago. Helen married Joe when she was 18 years old and they had twins: Delilah and Joseph Junior (JJ), who are now eight years old. The marriage deteriorated and six months ago the pair split up, and Helen moved into rented accommodation. Helen subsequently filed for divorce and was refused access to her two children because of her drinking habits. Currently, Helen is living alone and sees few people outside her work environment.

At work Helen, although dedicated, has recently been overlooked for promotion and has been told that she is 'next in line for redundancy' by her manager, with whom she does not see eye to eye. Because of this she has been sidelined by her colleagues and has very little interaction with them.

Helen recently consulted her GP after a series of recurrent chest infections, which cleared up with appropriate medication. Other than this, Helen considers herself to be relatively healthy and rarely goes to the doctor. She does tend to overeat and binge drink at the weekends, however, and she took up smoking when her marriage broke up. She takes very little exercise and has few interests, although she enjoys reading historical novels. Helen was recently admitted to the Accident and Emergency Unit after complaining of chest pains that appeared cardiac in nature. She was subsequently admitted to hospital, where it was found that she had suffered a mild heart attack.

Reviewing the case history – why do you think that Helen suffered from a heart attack? Consider all the factors in the case study that you think are relevant to the case – what about her relationships at work? What about the smoking and drinking? What about her chest infections? Obviously she has had some stresses in her life; her marriage has broken up and she has lost contact with her children. Furthermore, she has had trouble at work and is facing redundancy and possible money worries. On top of all this Helen appears to be losing her friends and family. She has lost her parents, and her husband and children no longer have any contact with her. In addition, her work colleagues have deserted her and it appears as if Helen has a particularly joyless existence. It is not surprising, therefore, that Helen has had a heart attack. This is the common view of stress and health: something stressful happens to an individual and, as a result, their health suffers.

Stress probably affects all of us, like Helen, at some time in our lives, and for some it may be a relatively permanent state. There is a popular belief that stress can lead to illness – cancer, heart attacks and so on. A number of studies worldwide have found that heart attack patients report that their health problems were either initiated or compounded by stress. A considerable amount of time, money and effort has gone into investigating stress and how it can affect all areas of our lives, including our health status. Unfortunately, the results of the investigations have not been consistent and there is some debate about the exact impact of stress. This is probably a result of some of the controversies that we will discuss in this chapter.

→

Why is this relevant to nursing practice?

Stress is an everyday phenomenon and can impact on your everyday practice – either because the patients you see will relate their health to their stress levels or may find the healthcare environment stressful, or because your work environment may be extremely stressful. Learning about stress and stress management strategies may be of benefit to both you and your patients. As we have seen with the case study, Helen has been under stress (as most people would define it) and has suffered the consequences (in terms of her heart attack). It is important that we explore the validity of the claim that stress can impact on health, and subsequently what the practising nurse can do about it. Furthermore, we also need to explore the stress in the workplace – how we can recognise it in ourselves and how we can best deal with it.

6.1 Introduction

Stress is a common problem that affects almost all of us at some point in our lives. Take Helen for example; it seems obvious that she would be stressed considering her last few months. But what exactly is stress? The term stress has, in fact, been steadily evolving over a period of several hundred years, if not over centuries. However, there is still some confusion as to how we define stress. Engel (1980) suggests that 'stress is neither a noun, nor a verb, nor an adjective. It is an escape from reality.' Despite this, we all know how and when it affects us, and while everyone may experience stress there are some people who may be susceptible to greater stressors than others. This may be you as a nurse. It may be your patient, or it may even be one of your colleagues. Learning how to identify when you are stressed and recognise the symptoms associated with it, be it the emotional consequences (fear and anxiety) or physiological reactions (increased heart rate and sweating palms), and how to manage these symptoms can greatly improve your mental and physical well-being.

It has long been known that stress can influence health; as Bartlett (1998) postulated, the idea that 'stress' can influence health has had a long history – there are many health consequences that are associated with stress. Considerable amounts of stress may result in heart attacks (Shih-Hsiang *et al.*, 2010), depression (Colman and Ataullahjan, 2010) and cancer (Agallia *et al.*, 2011) to name a few. We are all aware of the reports of top bankers or high-flying business people that suggest they are just heart attacks waiting to happen. Additionally, when under a considerable amount of stress there is the potential threat of suffering with a 'nervous breakdown'. However, we also know that stress can result in milder forms of illness – both physical and psychological. When we are under constant stress we become increasingly susceptible to common illnesses such as a cough or a cold. Thus, the effects of stress and its related factors are evident in relation to the development of both mild and severe illnesses within our everyday lives.

As a nurse you will need to have an understanding of stress and stress management strategies which will benefit both you and your patients. This chapter will draw on relevant theories and explore how stress can lead to both physical and mental health problems and why this is of direct relevance to you and your patients.

Key message

Stress is an everyday phenomenon that affects our lives at all levels.

Think about this

List all the potential stressors of:

✦ working in an acute mental health ward

✦ working on an A&E ward during a multiple road traffic accident (RTA)

✦ working in a hospice for terminally ill children

✦ being a student nurse and coping with university studies and practice

✦ working with a difficult line manager.

6.2 What is stress?

The first thing we have to do is to try and define what stress is. This shouldn't be a difficult thing to do, surely? Probably all of us use the term in our daily lives and we all know what the consequences of it are. However, when you stop and consider this question you begin to appreciate that it may not be as easy as you first thought. Academic research has also had the propensity to meet difficulty when defining stress. The first most generic definition of stress was posited by Selye (1956) who defined stress as 'the non specific response of the body to any demand'. It has also been defined as 'a process in which environmental demands tax or exceed the adaptive capacity of an organism, resulting in psychological and biological changes that may place a person at risk for disease' (Cohen *et al.*, 1997). More simple definitions suggest that it is the 'rate of wear and tear on the body system caused by life' (Stranks, 2005: 7). However, stress can also occur when a person has difficulty dealing with 'life situations, problems and goals' (Videbeck, 2007: 242). Furthermore it has 'physical, emotional and cognitive effects, and although everybody has the capacity to adapt to stress, not everybody responds to similar stressors the same way' (Timby, 2008: 941).

Think about this

Write down all the terms that you associate with stress. Discuss these with your colleagues – have they come up with any different terms?

On completing this exercise you may end up with a number of different terms or phrases. Masse (2000) posed this same question to members of the general public, finding that people identified more than 2,000 terms associated with the concept of stress. This highlights the fact that the term 'stress' has differing meanings to different people. A patient, for example, may define stress in terms of 'strain', being 'tense' or 'worried' – but as a nurse you may define stress as 'having problems at work', 'being distressed' or 'pressure'. Although these are different terms you are both referring to the same concept. Nonetheless, this difficulty is relatively easily overcome – we can usually appreciate when somebody is under stress and we understand what they are really referring to.

Not everybody responds to similar stressors in similar ways due to the individual differences apparent between different people. This is highlighted by the question: what exactly causes stress? If you ask a couple of colleagues what causes stress for them, you will probably come up with a range of different factors.

What causes stress?

Ask a couple of friends to list all of the things that they find stressful on a table similar to the one below.

You	Friend 1	Friend 2

Have you found that there are a couple of things that you all share in common, or are they all completely different? On the one hand, you might have all listed similar activities such as exams, going to the dentist or giving a verbal presentation in front of a large audience. However, there might also be some activities that you cannot agree on. For example, although some of you may consider giving a presentation to an audience stressful, some of you may consider it a 'thrill' or exciting rather than being a negative experience. Similarly, some might consider exams to be useful because they allow us to demonstrate our knowledge and expertise in a subject.

Key message

Stress means different things to different people.

6.3 Models of stress

Stress has been explained in many different ways, although these can essentially be reduced to three different categories:

✦ stress on the outside

✦ stress on the inside

✦ the interaction between the inside and the outside, i.e. between the person and the environment.

Stress on the outside

Stress can be viewed as being on the 'outside' – it is something that happens to us whether this is a big event (e.g. a death in the family) or a minor daily irritant (e.g. not being able to find a parking space at the local supermarket). These 'stressors' can be chronic (e.g. caring for yourself or somebody else with an illness) (Morris *et al.*, 2011), acute (e.g. taking an exam or going for a screening test), a daily hassle (e.g. traffic jams) or life events (e.g. getting married or divorced) (Sparrenberger *et al.*, 2009).

Key message

There are certain life events that are more stressful than others.

Most people can identify with these forms of stressors. Holmes and Rahe (1967) tried to make this approach more systematic and devised a life event scale called the social readjustment rating scale (SRRS). This scale provides respondents with an extensive list of possible life events; each of the stressful life events was awarded a life changing unit, the greater the amount of stress invoked by the stressor then the greater the weighting ascribed to it. The most stressful, as rated by the respondents, was the death of a spouse which scored 100, whilst marriage was rated 50, and Christmas 12 (see Table 6.1).

Think about this

What sort of stresses and strains do you have combining your university work with working in practice? Can you and your friends come up with some items that you think are particularly stressful for you and your colleagues? Rank them in order of stress for each of your friends.

What about patients? What sort of stressors can you imagine them facing when they come into contact with the healthcare system?

Looking back at the information given about Helen and her problems, can you calculate her score using the SRRS?

Many studies have found an association between these stressors, their severity and the onset of some form of illness. For example, Lueboonthavatchi (2009) found that stress severity and stressful life events had the greatest impact on the onset of depressive disorders. But of course, there are problems with the assessment of 'life events'. The relationship between life events and illness is complex due to the understanding that similar events do not necessarily elicit the same response in differing people (Fallon, 2008). The SRRS assumes that each stressor affects people in the same way, and as we saw earlier in the chapter this is not necessary always the case. What you find stressful may not be as stressful to your friends or colleagues (e.g. some people enjoy exams and others don't) (e.g. Matthews and Campbell, 2009; Koolhaas *et al.*, 2010). Furthermore, not every event on the SRRS is

Table 6.1 The SRRS

Event	Weighting	Event	Weighting
Death of a spouse	100	Change in number of arguments with spouse	35
Divorce	73		
Marital separation	65	Mortgage/major loan	31
Jail term	63	Foreclosure of loan	30
Death of family member	63	Change in work	29
Personal injury/illness	53	Child leaving home	29
Marriage	50	Trouble with in-laws	29
Being fired	47	Outstanding personal achievement	28
Marital reconciliation	45	Wife starts/stops work	26
Retirement	45	School starts/ends	26
Change in health of family member	44	Change in living conditions	25
Pregnancy	40	Trouble with boss	23
Sex difficulties	39	School/house move	20
Gain of new family member	39	Minor loan	17
Business readjustment	39	Change in sleeping habits	16
Change in financial state	38	Vacation	13
Death of a close friend	37	Christmas	12
Job change	36	Minor violations of the law	11

Source: Based on Holmes and Rahe (1967)

an everyday event and some people will experience a great many of these life events at certain times in their lives. Kanner *et al.* (1981) tried to overcome this by designing a daily hassles scale which included items that are more common within everyday circumstances. This included losing items, traffic, arguments and physical appearance. Therefore the assessment of life events does not complete the whole picture, suggesting that there must be other elements involved with the process of stress.

Think about this

Close your eyes and try to imagine this scene. You are walking into an Accident and Emergency unit after being told on the phone that your partner is critically ill following a road traffic accident. How do you feel? Can you describe your feelings?

Quick check

What is the most stressful form of life event? What is the relationship between life events and stress?

Stress on the inside

Stress can be defined as being on the 'inside'. The physiological general adaptation syndrome (GAS) was developed by Selye (1956) and describes three stages within the stress process, namely the alarm stage, the resistance stage and the exhaustion stage (see Figure 6.1). It is

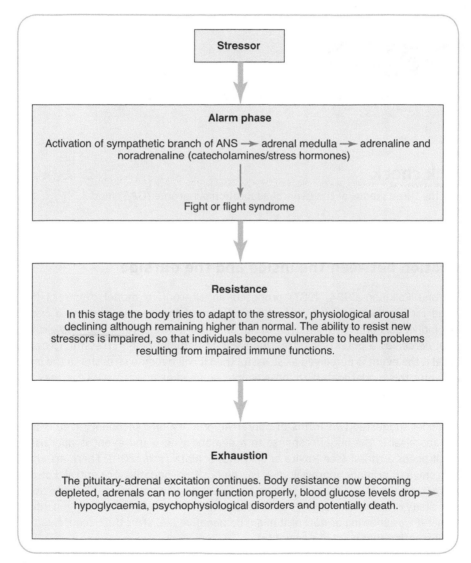

Stressor

Alarm phase

Activation of sympathetic branch of ANS → adrenal medulla → adrenaline and noradrenaline (catecholamines/stress hormones)

Fight or flight syndrome

Resistance

In this stage the body tries to adapt to the stressor, physiological arousal declining although remaining higher than normal. The ability to resist new stressors is impaired, so that individuals become vulnerable to health problems resulting from impaired immune functions.

Exhaustion

The pituitary-adrenal excitation continues. Body resistance now becoming depleted, adrenals can no longer function properly, blood glucose levels drop→ hypoglycaemia, psychophysiological disorders and potentially death.

Figure 6.1 Model of the general adaptation syndrome

one of the earliest models of stress, focusing on the body's continuous reactions to stress (Kemeny, 2003). The type of bodily responses we experience when we are under stress (e.g. increased heart rate, increased blood pressure, increased respiration and so on) are part of the 'fight or flight' syndrome, postulated by Cannon (1932). Cannon suggests that external threats elicit the 'fight or flight' response involving increased activity rate and increased arousal preparing the body for action as mediated through the nervous and endocrine system.

Selye's GAS and Cannon's fight or flight model both regard the individual as automatically responding to an external stressor and describing stress within a straightforward stimulus-response framework. Both have the propensity to ignore the potential roles of individual variability and psychological factors. Despite these criticisms Selye and Cannon laid some important foundations for stress and their model remains influential, and present-day models of stress have attempted to integrate some of the ideas from the GAS.

Key message

Stress can have an adverse effect on the body's physiology.

Quick check

Name the three stages of the general adaptation syndrome (GAS) model.

Interaction between the inside and the outside

Lazarus and Folkman (1984, 1987) proposed an alternative model of stress that also accounted for psychological variables. Lazarus argued that stress involved a *transaction* between individuals and their external world, and that a stress response was elicited if an individual *perceives* a potentially stressful event as actually being stressful. Hence, within this model if the event is perceived as stressful then it will become stressful to the individual. Consequently, this model deals with those people who find exams stressful (i.e. they perceive them as stressful) and those who do not (i.e. they perceive them as fun!), thus accounting for individual differences (see Goh *et al.*, 2010).

This model suggested two forms of **appraisal**; primary and secondary (see Figure 6.2). *Primary appraisal* is the initial response to a demand where the event is appraised as to whether it poses a threat (see Rovira *et al.*, 2010; Schlotz *et al.*, 2011). There are three possible outcomes to primary appraisal: they can be positive, negative or neutral. For example, waking up to a snow storm may be seen as positive (because you will not have to go to work or to university), neutral (because you will be able to carry on with whatever you intended to do whether it was snowing or not) or it might be negative (i.e. stressful because you have an important meeting that you have to get to).

If the situation is perceived to be threatening then *secondary appraisal* occurs. This is when you appraise your perceived ability to cope with the situation and the resources that

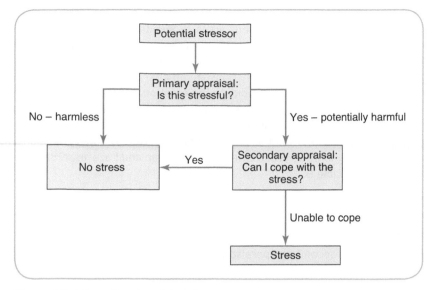

Figure 6.2 Interactional model of stress

you are equipped with to deal with it (see Prati *et al.*, 2010). Within these situations we may ask ourselves: can I cope with this stress, and if so how? The choices available reflect the three dimensions of the locus of control: where an individual can take control of the situation, they can get help from others, or they can do nothing and hope that it goes away. If on the basis of these forms of appraisal the individual considers the situation to be threatening and lacks the resources to cope effectively with it then they will experience some form of stress.

Key message

Stress is an interaction between the person and the environment.

6.4 Coping with stress – how to do it

Coping has been defined as the process of managing stressors that have been appraised as taxing or exceeding a person's resources as the 'efforts to manage environmental and internal demands' (Lazarus and Launier, 1978: 287–327). In the context of stress, coping therefore reflects the ways in which an individual interacts with the stressor in an attempt to return to some sort of normal functioning. The outcome of the appraisal process is referred to as the coping response. Many researchers agree and have identified two contrasting types of coping strategies, and although they are the same concepts they have been named differently. Rosenstiel and Keefe (1983) refer to an active verses passive coping, Roth and Cohen (1986) refer to an approach-focused versus an avoidant-focused coping and Lazarus and Folkman (1984) refer to a problem-focused versus emotion-focused coping. The best recogised of these definitions is that of Lazarus and Folkman (1984). According to Lazarus and Folkman's model coping has two main functions: it can alter the problem causing the stress (i.e. problem-focused coping) or it can regulate the emotional response to the problem (i.e. emotion-focused coping). Research has illustrated that problem-focused strategies are more advantageous for psychological adjustment and health outcomes than emotion-focused strategies (Carver *et al.*, 2010). Nonetheless, a number of different coping mechanisms have been described to lie within these broad categories (Folkman and Lazarus, 1988) and some of these are presented in Table 6.2.

Quick check

What are primary and secondary appraisal?

Table 6.2 Examples of problem- and emotion-focused coping strategies

Problem-focused	Example
Planning: analysing the situation to arrive at solutions to correct the problem	'I knew what had to be done so I doubled my efforts to make things work' or 'I made a plan of action and followed it'.
Confrontative: assertive action taken	'I stood my ground and fought for what I wanted'.
Social support	Gets practical support from friends.

Emotion-focused	Example
Social support	Gets emotional support from friends.
Distancing: detaching from the situation	'I made light of the situation and refused to get too serious about it' or 'I went on as if nothing had happened'.
Escape-avoidance: thinking wishfully about the situation	'I wished that the situation would go away or somehow be over with' or 'I hoped a miracle would happen'.
Self-control: moderating own feelings	'I tried to keep my feelings to myself' or 'I kept others from knowing how bad things were'.
Accepting responsibility: acknowledging own role in the problem while trying to put it right	'I criticised myself' or 'I made a promise to myself that things would be different next time'.
Positive reappraisal: creating a positive meaning from the situation	'I changed or grew as a person in a good way' or 'I came out of the experience better than I went in'.

Think about this

Using the table of coping strategies, how would you advise a person to cope with:

+ an injection
+ their relative being sectioned under the Mental Health Act
+ their child being diagnosed with a life-limiting condition
+ their father dying
+ their colleague failing an exam?

It should also be noted that coping differs in its success ratings for different people – what works for one person may not work for another. Age, type of problem, gender, controllability, personality and available resources have all been said to influence which type of coping strategy works best for a certain individual (Hagger, 2009). In addition to this, Aldwin and Park (2004) illustrate that many individuals adopt more than one form of coping strategy. Tennen *et al.* (2000) examined this by looking at the daily coping strategies in people with rheumatoid arthritis. It was discovered that problem-focused and emotion-focused coping usually occurred together. Moreover, it has also been highlighted that some coping methods (e.g. drinking large amounts of alcohol) may be useful for reducing stress, but increase other problems (see later). For instance, Krueger and Chang (2008) found that high levels of stress led to coping techniques which included higher levels of smoking, drinking or physical inactivity. Each of these has been linked to an increase in particular diseases and in some cases, mortality.

Quick check

List some problem-focused and emotion-focused coping strategies.

What does this mean to me?

The model has three important implications in relation to our clinical practice. First, no event can be characterised as being stressful (or unstressful) *per se*. Any situation can be appraised by one individual as stressful but not by another. It is also important to recognise that something that we may take as an everyday occurrence may be stressful for others. We therefore have to consider this when dealing with patients, clients and members of the general public on a daily basis. Something we view as mundane and routine may be considered stressful and worrying to a patient.

Second, since the model is based on an individual's thought processes (i.e. **cognitive appraisal**) then it is susceptible to changes in mood, health and other mental states. An individual may interpret the same event in different ways depending on the way they are feeling (see Reid *et al.*, 2009).

Third, a stressful response may be experienced irrespective of whether the situation is recalled, experienced or simply imagined. Hence, imagining going to the dentist can be considered by some to be just as stressful as actually going.

Think about this

What daily activities are you involved in that you consider routine and (almost) boring that you think others would consider stressful? How do you think you could best reduce the stress on others?

6.5 The link between stress and health

There are a number of potential indicators of stress and these can be broadly categorised as either psychological or physiological (see Table 6.3). The psychological factors can lead to poor mental health and in chronic cases poor physical health (Yehuda and McEwen, 2004).

A number of illnesses have been linked to stress and continue to be so by both the general public and healthcare professionals (Lundberg, 2006). Surveys have indicated that stress and related conditions form a massive group of work-related ill-health conditions (Jones *et al.*, 2006). About one in seven people say that they find their work either very or extremely stressful (Webster *et al.*, 2007). It is estimated that work-related stress, depression or anxiety affects over half a million people in the UK, with an estimated 13.5 million working days lost due to these work-related conditions between 2007 and 2008 (Kerr *et al.*, 2009). This means that, on average, almost a month per year is lost per affected case and makes stress the largest contributor to the overall estimated annual days lost from work-related ill-health (HSE, 2005).

Table 6.3 Psychological and physiological consequences of stress

Psychological	Physiological
Unease	Persistently elevated BP (leading to clinical hypertension)
Apprehension	
Sadness	Indigestion
Depression	Constipation or diarrhoea
Pessimism	Weight gain or loss
Listlessness	CHD
Lack of self-esteem	Gastric problems
Negative attitudes	Menstrual problems
Short temper	
Fatigue	
Poor sleep	
Increased smoking	
Increased alcohol	

Evidence also suggests that most of those reporting work-related heart disease (some 66,000 people) ascribed its cause to work stress (Chandola *et al.*, 2008). These reports have mainly concerned the mental health effects of stress. However, there are also suggestions, and in some cases evidence, of a link between stress and physical illness (e.g. Cohen, 2005; Lundberg, 2006). This has come from a number of sources and stress has been implicated in a number of different conditions including heart disease (Clark, 2003), cancer (Lillberg *et al.*, 2003), HIV/AIDS (Reif *et al.*, 2011) and other infectious disorders (Langley *et al.*, 2006).

Key message

Stress leads to physical and mental ill-health.

Coronary heart disease (CHD)

Overall, the evidence does suggest that there is a link between stress and coronary heart disease – the greater the stress, the greater the chance of experiencing a heart attack. Coronary heart disease is the physical condition for which there is the most comprehensive evidence of a link with stress (Bunker *et al.*, 2003; SIGN, 2007; Dandana *et al.*, 2011) and one which most members of the general public, including those who have had a heart attack, believe to be linked (Clark, 2003). Research suggests that psychosocial variables may increase the risk of CHD by three or four times, a similar increase to that as a result of biological variables (e.g. hypertension and dyslipaemia).

Breast cancer

Most studies have measured stress and breast cancer in terms of highly threatening or adverse life events. However these have produced conflicting results. On the one hand, studies have reported a relationship between life events and the onset of breast cancer (Kroenke *et al.*, 2004; Nielsen *et al.*, 2005; Schernhammer *et al.*, 2004). Specifically, Lillberg *et al.* (2003) prospectively investigated the relationship between stressful life events and risk of breast cancer. The results indicated that life events, particularly divorce/separation and death of a close relative, were linked to the onset of cancer. Conversely, Michael *et al.* (2009) found no independent association between stressful life events and the breast cancer link. However, some of the research in this area is limited by failure to adjust for confounding factors and small sample sizes. Moreover, a direct cause and effect relationship has not been proven. Nonetheless, some studies have found an indirect relationship between stress and a weakened immune system which in turn may affect the incidence of cancer (Reiche *et al.*, 2004). Despite these criticisms there does appear to be a link between the onset of breast cancer and stressful events (Garsson, 2004).

HIV/AIDS

There is some evidence that stress can lead to a progression of HIV/AIDS (Leserman, 2003). Reif *et al.* (2011) conducted a longitudinal study with 611 HIV-infected individuals, finding that traumatic and stressful experiences were associated with poorer health outcomes. Furthermore, Evans *et al.* (1997) suggested that the more severe the life stress experienced, the greater the risk of early HIV disease progression. For instance, they reported that the risk of disease progression would double for every incident of severe stress within the preceding six-month period.

Infectious diseases

Although stress does not directly cause infectious diseases, it can reduce the body's natural defences against viruses by impairing the immune response. Studies have shown that stress can indirectly influence infectious diseases, including the common cold (Takkouche *et al.*, 2001), pneumonia (Mehr *et al.*, 2001), hepatitis B and C infections (Burns *et al.*, 2002) and recurrent urinary tract infections (Leaver, 2001). Cohen *et al.* (1997) reported that those who had experienced stress of a long duration, primarily as a function of unemployment or family conflict, exhibited a substantially greater risk of developing a cold. They also reported that participants with low numbers of social ties were four times more likely to develop a cold than those with a higher number of ties (Cohen, 2005). Similar findings have been discovered by Park *et al.* (2011) who reported that workers with stress related to high work demands, a lack of job control, and inadequate social support, were at higher risk of developing the common cold.

Other physical conditions

A number of other conditions, for example MS, rheumatoid arthritis, Type I (insulin dependent) diabetes, systemic lupus erythemastosus, bronchial asthma and irritable bowel syndrome, have been reported as being adversely affected by stress. However, for most of these conditions the evidence is equivocal. Although the role of stress in the primary aetiological process is limited, the stronger evidence suggests that the stress process can aggravate the severity of these disorders and is involved in their exacerbation (Schneiderman *et al.*, 2005; Yehuda and McEwen, 2004).

Key message

Stress has been linked to the development and progression of a number of physical disorders.

Think about this

How does this information help you as the nurse? What does it mean for you as a professional?

Stress and mental health

Stress can adversely affect mental health in a number of different ways. It is often reported as a precursor to many mental health problems, but it can also exacerbate any current conditions. Anxiety and depression are the most common mental health problems associated with stress, and often these are a reaction to a difficult life event, for example, moving house, problems at work or bereavement (HSE, 2011). The most common symptoms of anxiety include: palpitations, headache, backache, breathing difficulties, feeling tense, on edge, worrying about things and panic attacks. In contrast the common symptoms of depression include lack of concentration at home and work, impaired sleep, feeling depressed, bouts of crying, poor appetite, sexual difficulties, decreased energy and fatigue.

In practice, it may be difficult to define when 'stress' develops into a 'mental health problem' and when existing mental health problems become exaggerated by other stressors (e.g. stress at work), as many of the symptoms associated with mental health are similar to those people experience when under a considerable amount of pressure. The key difference, however, is the severity and duration of the symptoms and impact they have on someone's everyday life.

Think about this

Next time you talk to someone who has suffered a recent illness – whether it be major (e.g. a heart attack) or minor (e.g. an infection), or a physical health problem (e.g. heart attack) or mental health problem (e.g. a 'breakdown') – discuss with them whether they can link this to any major life events. Use the Holmes and Rahe scale (see Table 6.1, page 192).

They probably can – but what does this mean? Does it mean that the stressful event caused the physical illness, or that people just try to attribute blame? This is one of the problems with retrospective recording of the stressful events; memories differ and there is a tendency to attribute the onset of an illness to a memorable event, even if the two were not related. Consequently, the best type of studies are prospective, where recording of life events is taken before any ill-health onset.

6.6 How does stress affect health?

The research evidence indicates that there does appear to be a relationship between stress and health status. The exploration into how these difficulties come about has led to a number of explanations. Physiological reactions to stress play a role but other routes worthy of further investigation are through the immune system (psychoneuroimmunology) and through changes in one's behaviour.

The three routes from stress to illness are therefore:

✦ direct physiological reactions

✦ psychoneuroimmunology

✦ behavioural change.

Route 1: Physiology

The way stress affects health has been related to three different physiological pathways: the neural pathways, the hormonal pathway and the immune system.

Route 1a: The nervous system

The **nervous system**, which includes the **central nervous system** (CNS) – the brain and spinal cord – as well as the peripheral nervous system (all other neurons), controls the body's reaction to stress. The peripheral nervous system is divided into the somatic nervous system (responsible for movement and senses) and the **autonomic nervous system** (ANS) which serves the involuntary muscles and internal organs. There are two branches to the ANS: the sympathetic division which deals with bodily excitation and the expenditure of energy, and the parasympathetic division concerned with reducing bodily activity and restoring energy.

From this brief description it should be possible to see how the concept of Cannon's fight or flight model can be interpreted in the light of this physiological reaction, especially the sympathetic division of the ANS. Hence, when an individual is under stress the sympathetic division of the ANS innervates the adrenal medulla (part of the adrenal gland) and this results in the release of two chemicals, known as catecholamines: adrenaline (sometimes called epinephrine) and noradrenaline (or norepinephrine). These two neurotransmitters mobilise the body's resources, preparing it for fight or flight. For example, increasing the cardiovascular activity (heart rate, stroke volume and force of contraction), shifting the flow of blood to the muscles rather than digestion or the skin, widening the airways, speeding the rate of breathing and increasing the volume of air intake into the lungs are some of the many reactions. These bodily reactions can be mapped onto the reactions of stress, which are highlighted in Table 6.4.

Table 6.4 Physiological reactions to stress and potential symptoms

Physiological reaction	Potential symptoms
Increase in heart rate	Rapid or irregular heartbeats
Increase in respiration rate	Hyperventilation or some form of asthma
Adrenaline released	Increase in heart rate
Noradrenaline released	Raised blood pressure
Muscle tightening	Tension headache, tense muscles, insomnia, fatigue, loss of concentration
Change in blood flow/circulation	High blood pressure, cold hands, upset stomachs, migraine, pre-ulcerous/ulcerous conditions, increased colitis, constipation and sexual dysfunction
Senses heightened	Emotional irritability, poor impulse control, reduced communication abilities
Increased perspiration	Dehydration
Imbalance in hormone	Frequent infections, auto-immune disease
Saliva consistency change	Dry mouth

The repeated occurrence of these responses is one way in which stress can impact on health. For example, the repeated cardiovascular activation could lead to permanent damage to the arteries and veins and thereby cause elevated blood pressure.

Quick check

List the physiological consequences of stress and how these manifest themselves as symptoms.

Route 1b: The hormonal system

The hormonal (or endocrine) system consists of a number of glands throughout the body which secrete hormones in times of stress. This system is responsible for mobilising your body's resources to deal with threats through acknowledging signals from your brain. Your hypothalamus alerts your pituitary gland, which then releases stress hormones into your blood stream to various parts of the body where they act on target organs (either directly or indirectly). The endocrine or hormonal system acts at a much slower rate than the neuro-transmitters described above but has longer lasting effects. For this reason they are mainly associated with chronic stressors (rather than the acute stressors that influence the nervous system).

One major hormonal pathway through which stress exerts its effects is the adrenocorti-cotrophic hormone (ACTH). The anterior pituitary produces ACTH when it is stimulated by the hypothalamus. ACTH is released into the bloodstream and acts upon the outer area of the adrenal gland causing it to produce a group of hormones – the corticosteroids. These regulate the blood pressure and hence this demonstrates one mechanism whereby hormonal transmitted stress can exert a negative effect. As well as this, when a number of stress hormones are released in large amounts during times of stress, other hormones are decreased to very low levels. The sex hormones for example are inhibited by the stress hormone which leads to a lowered sex drive and to menstrual irregularities in women.

Route 1c: The immune system

Considerable evidence suggests that life stress can weaken immune functioning (Suls and Wallston, 2003; Taylor, 2006). The immune system protects us from infection and illness and consists of a series of coordinated responses to protect the body by defending it against invasion by antigens. When the immune system works well the body is protected and infections and illnesses are absent, however when the immune system overreacts this leads to allergies. The most significant organs involved in the immune system are the lymphoid organs which include bone marrow, lymph nodes, thymus, spleen and vessels. These organs are involved in identifying foreign bodies and disabling them. Immune reactions involve two main types of response. In the first the immunity involves the action of a special white blood cell called the T-cell, which kills invading micro-organisms. In the second, special chemicals known as antibodies or immunoglobulins are released into the bloodstream and attach themselves to the antigen and destroy it. A third type of cell involved in the immune response is known as a phagocyte which envelops and devours foreign substances.

Route 2: Psychoneuroimmunology (PNI)

The term **psychoneuroimmunology** was first coined by Adler (Adler, 1981; Adler *et al.*, 2001) and involves the study of the interactions among psychological factors, the nervous system and the immune system. Early research indicated that there was a link between stress and the immune system and this was first observed in bereaved spouses. The reports suggested that bereaved spouses have a weaker immune system than those in continuing relationships (Bartrop *et al.*, 1977).

Later, Kiecolt-Glaser *et al.* (1987) reported that a sample of women who had recently divorced or separated had a poorer immune system than the control group (Kiecolt-Glaser *et al.*, 2005) and those who had a positive marital environment had a better immune response (Heffer *et al.*, 2004). Thus, those who got divorced had a weaker immune system than those who had not. Women who were more attached to the marriage showed a greater response than those who showed less positive memories of the marriage. Similar findings were reported for men who had been separated or divorced. Similarly, Kiecolt-Glaser and Glaser (1992) found immune suppression in carers of Alzheimer's patients. Those caring for people with a dementing illness had a poorer immune system and hence were more prone to illness – a finding that has been repeated on many occasions (Lovell and Wetherell, 2011).

Workman and La Via (1987) explored the immune system in students taking an exam (an acute stressor) and noted a weakening in the immune system from a baseline prior to the exam, compared to during and after the exam. Studies have also found that the whole immune system appears to be affected, and this appeared to be the case even when behavioural factors such as lack of sleep, diet and drug use were controlled for. Therefore, this study, amongst others, suggests that those students taking exams had a poor immune response – hence they were at a greater risk of developing infectious disorders (Pederson *et al.*, 2010).

Route 3: Changing behaviour

Think about this

Think about the last time you were under exam stress. Did you change your behaviour? Did it become healthier or unhealthier? Did you, for example, smoke more, drink more or eat the wrong things?

It is often the case that when a person is under stress they change their behaviour to try and cope with this stress in a number of different ways. That is, coping strategies are used in order to reduce the stress (as we have seen before with the transactional model of stress). However, some of these coping strategies may be successful in reducing an individual's stress but may, ironically, actually result in an increased health risk (see Table 6.5).

Key message

Coping with stress can lead to more damage if you use inappropriate coping mechanisms.

Table 6.5 How do people cope (badly) with stress?

	What the research suggests	Problems, problems . . .
Smoking	People smoke more when they are stressed, and are more likely to start and restart under episodes of stress. Studies have reported that higher levels of smoking more cigarettes are linked with higher levels of stress (Heslop *et al.*, 2001; Hajek *et al.*, 2010).	Smoking kills you! It leads to a host of health problems including cancer, heart disease and breathing problems.
Alcohol	Research suggests that there is a relationship between stress and drinking alcohol to cope (Rice and Van Arsdale, 2010). The tension-reduction theory suggests that people drink alcohol because of its tension-reducing properties (Cappell and Greeley, 1987). This theory is supported by evidence of a relationship between negative mood and drinking behaviour which suggests that people are more likely to drink when they are depressed or anxious.	Too much alcohol can lead to liver and cardiac problems along with a whole host of other physiological and social consequences.
Eating	There is evidence to support a relationship between eating and stress level. Cartwright *et al.* (2003) found that there was some evidence to support the myth of comfort eating. The report found that those under stress were more likely to eat fatty foods than fruit and vegetables and more likely to snack unhealthily. King *et al.* (2009) also found a significant relationship between high levels of job stress in nurses and disordered eating.	Too much 'comfort food' can lead to increased weight, blood pressure and ultimately cardiac problems.
Exercise	Research has indicated that stress may reduce exercise (e.g. Heslop *et al.*, 2001; Metcalf *et al.*, 2003) whereas stress management that focuses on increasing exercise has been shown to result in some improvements in coronary health.	Lack of exercise can lead to problems with weight, cardiac fitness and lung function.
Safety	Research suggests that individuals who experience high levels of stress show a greater tendency to perform behaviours that increase their chances of becoming injured (HSE, 2011). Furthermore, some research indicates that the greater the stress, the greater the level of accidents at work and in the car.	Try to focus on the task – accidents could cause injuries and even mortality in some cases.

Think about this

?

How did Helen's behaviour alter because of stress? How would you suggest ways in which she could alter her behaviour to cope with the stress?

So, stress can have an influential impact on our health – both physically and mentally. Stress can impact on our physiology, our immune system and the way we behave. Consequently, we need to explore how we can minimise stress in both ourselves and our patients. For this we should explore what variables, or interventions, can be used to try to mediate the stress-illness link.

Quick check

List the three routes that can help explain the link between stress and health. ✓

6.7 We need friends – social support

Social support can be defined as the existence of people on whom we can rely, people who let us know that they care about, value and love us, and the support they provide for us (Sarason *et al.*, 1983). There is a distinction between the existence of social relationships and the functions provided by these. Subsequently the structure would be based on 'how many friends, colleagues, or family relationships' you have and the functional aspect would refer to what these do.

Essentially you can have lots of friends but have no interaction with them which is not useful to us. Social support can come from a variety of different sources and a variety of types of support (Cohen *et al.*, 2000), for instance, spouses, relatives, friends, neighbours, co-workers, or superiors. But it can also come from professional sources (e.g. the nurse) and this can help in reducing stress, thus becoming a useful and advantageous social interaction. The type and amount of social support an individual receives depends upon their social network but also on various demographic factors such as their age, sex, culture, socio-economic status and so on.

Generally social support comes in one of five types (see Figure 6.3).

Social support can play an important part in reducing the effects of stress. Poor social support has been associated with higher mortality rates. Holt-Lunstad *et al.* (2010) reported that people who were less socially integrated had higher mortality rates. Furthermore, an overview of longitudinal studies has shown a continuous increased mortality associated with a lack of social support and weak social ties (Quick *et al.*, 1996). Subsequent studies have confirmed that reliable links exist between social support and better physical health (e.g. Uchino, 2004; Holt-Lunstad *et al.*, 2010). Studies have suggested that those with low levels of social support have higher mortality rates – from cardiovascular disease (e.g. Brummett *et al.*, 2001; Frasure-Smith *et al.*, 2000; Everson-Rose and Lewis, 2005) or

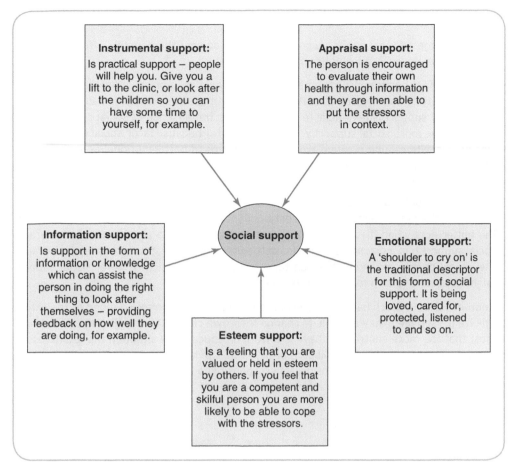

Figure 6.3 Forms of social support

from cancer (e.g. Hibbard and Pope, 1993) and infectious diseases (e.g. Lee and Rotheram-Borus, 2001).

Think about this

How could you use social support in a nursing setting? Think of a number of examples of how healthcare could be less stressful with the presence of some form of support.

Quick check

List the five forms of social support.

How does social support protect health?

It has been suggested that social support can protect against the negative effects of stress. There are two main views on why this may be the case.

✦ **The main effect hypothesis:** states that the more social support an individual has the better the quality of life, regardless of the person's level of stress (Helgeson, 2002). In other words social support is beneficial to health and it is the absence of social support that is stressful. The more social support you have the better because large social networks provide people with regular positive experiences in terms of both emotional as well as physical support. Hence, social support promotes healthier behaviours such as exercise, eating healthily and not smoking, as well as greater adherence to medical regimes.

✦ **The buffer hypothesis:** social support buffers the individual against the stressor. Rather than protect a person all the time against the minor hassles and stresses of everyday life, the buffer acts when it is needed most. For example, when a person with considerable social support has a diagnosis of an illness then they *appraise* it as less stressful because they know people to whom they can turn. In contrast, those with lower social support might be unable to turn to anyone (Cohen *et al.*, 2000).

Another variable which has been investigated thoroughly is **control** – defined as the extent to which a person feels they are able to change their own circumstances. Broadly, the results suggest that the more control you have in a work or educational situation the less stressful it is (e.g. Troup and Dewe, 2002; Gibbons *et al.*, 2011). Obviously, there comes a point where you have more control but also considerable responsibility and this can be stressful as well.

Quick check

What are the models of social support protecting health?

Think about this

How much control do you have over your current working/study life? Are there any areas over which you would like more control? If you had more control, how do you think it would affect your stress levels?

Stress and hardiness

Research has shown that some people are more resistant to stress and are better able to cope with it than others. This is partly due to the fact that some people have particular personality traits that protect them from the effects of stress. This concept was named the hardy personality and was put forward by Kobasa (1979) who identified the three hardy personality traits: commitment, control and challenge.

- *Commitment* is the extent to which a person is engaging in a variety of life domains, and gives us a sense of purpose.

- *Control* represents the extent to which a person believes that they can control events that occur in their lives.
- *Challenge* reflects the extent to which people generally perceive difficult situations as challenging rather than as threats.

A 'hardy' individual copes well with stress and is somebody who has a high sense of personal control, is committed, enjoys challenges and views them positively. Research has shown that people with a hardy personality have increased immune functioning (Dolbier *et al.*, 2001), and therefore are less susceptible to illness which can be caused by stress.

Stress and personality

For some people, personality variables are simply a way of behaving. They represent the way a person reacts to stress – their behavioural response. One personality variable that has received much attention is the so-called Type A personality. The definition of a Type A behaviour pattern (TABP) is 'an overt pattern of behaviour which is elicited from susceptible individuals in an appropriately challenging environment' (Rosenman *et al.*, 1964). TABP was first noted by two US cardiologists (Friedman and Rosenman, 1974) who noted a common type of behaviour in their patients. This behaviour included:

+ job involvement
+ excessive hard-driving behaviour
+ impatience
+ time urgency
+ competitiveness
+ aggressiveness
+ hostility.

There have been attempts at establishing a link between personality types and other illnesses – most particularly cancer – but these have largely met with limited success (e.g. Dean and Surtees, 1989; Greer *et al.*, 1979, 1990; Schapiro *et al.*, 2001).

Stress and hostility

One of the Type A components, hostility, has been researched extensively in recent years. Researchers have suggested that hostility may be the reason why some individuals have more stress than others. Studies have suggested that there is an association between hostility and CHD, where hostility is not only an important risk factor for heart disease but also a trigger for a heart attack (Moller *et al.*, 1999).

Think about this

How would you expect a Type A personality to behave? Think about this in terms of day-to-day activities and when in a healthcare setting.

Key message

Personality variables can influence our physical health.

6.8 How to deal with stress

Given the serious consequences that can arise from stress, we want to try to minimise it as much as possible within our practice. Obviously some would argue that in an ideal world, stress would be removed altogether. However, this is unlikely to happen (ever) and, in reality, we don't want this to occur since a small amount of stress is good for us and can lead to enhanced performance in a number of settings: for instance, when trying to write a challenging assignment, winning a race, an upcoming family event such as a holiday, or a major life event such as moving to university. This positive stress is referred to as eustress.

Think about this

Think about a time when stress was positive. Was there a good amount, and what happens if it tips over into too much stress?

A number of methods or **stress management techniques** have been devised to try to reduce stress or at least teach people how best to cope with it. Stress management can be defined as the application of methods in psychology to reduce the impact of stress. Each of these methods is based upon the models of stress we discussed earlier, so the link should be simple and clear (see Figure 6.4).

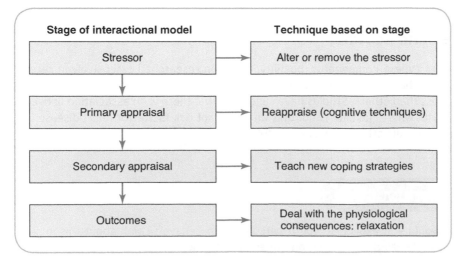

Stage of interactional model	Technique based on stage
Stressor	Alter or remove the stressor
Primary appraisal	Reappraise (cognitive techniques)
Secondary appraisal	Teach new coping strategies
Outcomes	Deal with the physiological consequences: relaxation

Figure 6.4 Stress management techniques based on the interactional model of stress

Quick check

List the elements of the interactional model of stress and how knowledge of this can be used in devising stress management techniques. ✓

Dealing with the stressor

The first method of reducing stress is to remove the stressor, if at all possible! We could take away or modify the demands or exposure to potential stressful conditions. Hence, if the person gets 'stressed out' whenever they ride a horse, don't go near a horse. Obviously, this is easier with certain stressors than others – you can avoid riding a horse, but a person with diabetes may not be able to avoid dealing with needles. If a person gets stressed when going to the dentist and avoids the dentist, then all sorts of problems could follow.

Primary appraisal

If the person cannot avoid the stressor then perhaps attempting to get them to reappraise the situation may prove beneficial. Hence, rather than seeing the dentist as a stressor, get the person to see the visit in a more positive light – this will improve my teeth, my smile, remove my pain and so on. This can take some time and may need professional assistance. This approach underlies many cognitive-behavioural interventions and assertiveness training (e.g. Brown et al., 2010).

Secondary appraisal: improving coping strategies

One of the major psychological approaches to stress management is cognitive-behavioural and this is best developed in the **stress-inoculation-training** (SIT) method (Meichenbaum and Cameron, 1983). This is a self-instructional method for teaching individuals to cope with stress and is basically concerned with developing the individual's competence to adapt to stressful events. SIT enhances one's ability to cope with past, current and future stressors through three phases of treatment. In the first stage individuals learn about the stress response and how to deal with it. Second, they are then taught behavioural and cognitive skills to use emotion-focused and problem-focused coping. Finally, individuals are taught how to generalise their newly acquired skill sets to cope. SIT has been shown to be effective in a number of studies. For instance, Ansari et al. (2010) used SIT with female hypertensive patients, finding that it significantly reduced anxiety, social dysfunction and depression.

Outcomes: dealing with the stress reaction

Stress management can address stress responses directly through relaxation training, biofeedback, visual imagery and meditation techniques (e.g. Ali and Hanson, 2010). The basic premise of relaxation for stress is that it is the opposite of arousal – so relaxing should be a good way to reduce stress. A number of methods have been used to induce relaxation. The most frequently mentioned in psychological terms is **progressive muscle relaxation** (PMR). PMR originated from the work of Jacobson in the 1920s and 1930s. Jacobson (1938) proposed that the main mechanism influencing relaxation lies with the patient's ability to tell the difference between tension and relaxation. PMR involves the successive tensing and relaxing of various muscle groups.

Putting theory into practice: visual imagery

When under stress consider using visual imagery such as that described below. Lie or sit down somewhere quiet, where you are able to relax, and then take yourself through the story, describing it in as much detail as possible to yourself:

Imagine yourself walking along a peaceful old country road . . . The sun is warm on your back. The birds are singing. The air is calm and fragrant. As you walk along your mind naturally wanders to the concerns and worries of the day. Then, you come upon a box by the side of the road and it occurs to you that this box is a perfect place to leave your cares behind while you enjoy this time in the country.

You feel lighter as you progress down the road. Soon, you come across an old gate. The gate creaks as you open it and go through. You find yourself in an overgrown garden. Flowers growing where they have seeded themselves. Vines climbing over a fallen tree. Soft green wild grasses. Shade of trees. Breathe deeply, smelling the flowers . . . Listen to the birds and insects . . . Feel the gentle breeze warm against your skin . . . All of your senses are alive and responding in pleasure to the peaceful time and place . . .

And so on . . .

Putting theory into practice: example of a progressive muscle relaxation script

Do try this at home with a willing volunteer. Ask your guinea pig to lie or sit down in a nice quiet room, allow them to settle comfortably and close their eyes if they wish. Legs, ankles and arms should be uncrossed. Now read aloud to them the following:

Let all your muscles feel heavy. And let your whole body just sink into the surface beneath . . . Good. This exercise will guide you through the major muscle groups from your feet to your head, asking you to first tense and then relax those muscles. If you have pain in a particular part of your body today don't tense that area. Instead, just notice any tension that may already be there and let go of it.

Become aware of the muscles in your feet and calves. Pull your toes back up toward your knees. Hold your feet in this position . . . Notice the sensations. Now relax your feet and release the tension. Observe any changes in sensations as you let go of the tension . . . Good.

Now tighten the large muscles of your thighs and buttocks. Hold the muscles tense and as you do be aware of the sensations. And now release these muscles allowing them to feel soft as if they're melting into the surface beneath you . . . That's it.

Now keep tensing and relaxing muscle groups in your abdomen, chest, hands and fingers, face and head.

Think about this

How could you use some of these stress management programmes in your day-to-day practice?

Think of the ways you could treat Helen on the basis of the stress management techniques outlined.

6.9 Does it work?

Research indicates that stress management programmes can result in reduced stress and generally provide better mental health than having no treatment (Ali and Hanson, 2010). Studies have also indicated that PMR can lead to improvements in the following:

✦ **Hypertension and coronary heart disease:** overall, the evidence (Williams *et al.*, 2003) suggests that: 'structured interventions to reduce stress (stress management, meditation, yoga, cognitive therapies, breathing exercises and biofeedback) have been shown to result in short term reductions in blood pressure'.

✦ **Immune function:** McGregor and colleagues (2004) explored immune function in women with cancer. They found that a psychological intervention to reduce stress resulted in an improved immune function. This improvement was noted both immediately after the programme and three months later when the group was followed up.

✦ **Mental health:** the role of stress in the development of mental health issues is considerable. Lolak *et al.* (2008) used PMR training on anxiety and depression in patients. They found that PMR was effective in improving both anxiety and depression. There are also suggestions that PMR is useful for reducing substance misuse problems.

Quick check

List the main methods of stress management – how do they relate back to the interactional model of stress?

6.10 Stress and nursing practice

Chronic workplace stress and the related concept of 'burnout' is a widely recognised phenomenon in healthcare workers. There is a considerable literature base on stress and burnout in both qualified and student nurses (Wallbank and Hatton, 2011; Bragard *et al.*, 2010). There are three major symptoms of burnout: emotional exhaustion, depersonalisation and trivialisation of personal accomplishments. The Nursing Stress Scale (Gray-Toft and Anderson, 1981) has been used extensively to investigate stress and its relationship to clinical areas, job satisfaction and well-being. Nursing provides a series of potential stressors and French *et al.* (2000) have identified nine workplace stressors that might impact on nurses:

✦ conflict with physicians
✦ inadequate preparation
✦ problems with peers
✦ problems with supervisor
✦ discrimination
✦ workload
✦ uncertainty concerning treatment
✦ dealing with death, and dying patients
✦ dealing with patients and their families.

The outcomes of stress may be severe. Ultimately, it may lead to psychological and physiological distress, low job satisfaction and burnout. Obviously, some of these sources of stress need to address the working and structural conditions in order to ameliorate any problems.

Key message

You need to care for yourself, just as much as you care for your patients.

6.11 Conclusion

Stress is a major part of all our lives. Its impact can be significant and can harm physical and psychological health through a number of pathways. Medical, and more importantly, psychological interventions can help ameliorate and extinguish stress. This can be of benefit to both the patient/client and the healthcare professional.

Think about this

What do you do when you are under stress? How can you deal with the stress of working clinically? Are there any elements in your workplace over which you can exert additional control? Or have you developed your own coping style?

Research in Focus

Simpson, E.E.A. and Thompson W. (2009) Stressful life events, psychological appraisal and coping styles in postmenopausal women. *Maturitas*, **63**(4), 357-364.

Background

Stress associated with menopause can be a result of psychosocial factors which coincide with midlife. These stressors have been shown to be associated with greater severity of symptoms reporting anxiety and depression in peri- and postmenopausal women. It is important to consider the coping styles in these women as stress may be prolonged and lead to risks of coronary heart disease, stroke and some form of cancers at midlife. Therefore this study aimed to gain a better understanding of what events postmenopausal women report as stressful, their psychological appraisal of such events and how this predicts coping styles employed. This study used the transactional theory of stress as is useful when examining appraisal, prolonged physical changes, coping strategies and mediators of stress.

Methods

Participants: One hundred and seventy-nine postmenopausal women attending a menopause clinic for the first time were recruited. Inclusion criteria included: being recently diagnosed as postmenopausal, which was determined by the World Health Organization (WHO) definition, no major physical or psychiatric problems, not taking hormone replacement therapy, and FSH levels >30 u/L.

Measures: Data was collected by self-reported questionnaires. Menopausal symptoms were assessed by the Green Climacteric scale. Stress was measured by the Perceived Stress Scale (PSS) and stressful life events, cognitive appraisal of events and coping were assessed by the Daily Coping Inventory.

Results

Stressful life events were categorised into family problems, menopause symptoms, work problems, daily hassles and other health problems. The most commonly reported coping styles were: catharsis (68%), direct action (66%) and seeking social support (63%).

Socio-demographic variables, menopausal symptoms and general stress levels were not predictive of coping styles. Specific aspects of psychological appraisal were predictive of distraction, direct action, catharsis and seeking social support.

Implications

This study gives support for the transactional theory of stress to gain a better understanding of stress and coping in post menopause. Coping styles most commonly implemented were also the ones predicted by psychological appraisal of the stressful event and tended to be used by older women. The findings should be used to inform practice and to develop appropriate interventions for this group, such as encourage specific →

coping styles within interventions and stress management techniques, to promote a better quality of life, general health and well-being. The use of social support groups could also provide valuable opportunities to give and receive support to others going through similar experiences.

Think about this

Returning to Helen, what type of stress was she suffering from? What could have mediated the impact of the stress? What sort of risk is Helen putting herself at?

6.12 Summary

+ Stress is a difficult concept to define, even though it is a feature of our everyday lives.

+ Stress can be defined as coming from the inside (GAS), from the outside (life events) and as an interaction between the two (transactional model).

+ Coping with stress can take one of two broad forms: problem-focused or emotion-focused.

+ Stress has been implicated in mental health and in certain physical illnesses such as coronary heart disease, cancer and some infectious disorders.

+ Stress can influence health through a number of routes: through physiology, psychoneuroimmunology, and because of changes in behaviour.

+ There are several mediators of the stress–health link. For example, social support, control, hardiness, personality types and hostility have all been suggested as impacting on the stress–health link.

+ Social support can prove effective in promoting health and reducing the consequences of stress.

+ Stress management techniques include teaching improved coping techniques, increasing social support and promoting relaxation techniques.

+ Workplace stress can lead to considerable problems for both individuals and organisations.

Your end point

Answer the following questions to assess your knowledge and understanding.

1. Which of the following *is not* true of stress?
    (a) The external environment is a potential stressor.
    (b) The response to the stressor is stress or distress.
    (c) The concept of stress involves biochemical, physiological, behavioural and psychological changes.

→

(d) All stress is harmful and damaging.

(e) All of the above.

2. Alarm, resistance and exhaustion describe three stages represented in which model of stress:

(a) life events theory

(b) self-regulatory model

(c) Selye's GAS

(d) health belief model

(e) protection motivation theory?

3. Social support from others is undoubtedly important for human beings, but it *cannot*:

(a) buffer the impact of high stress

(b) stave off loneliness

(c) compensate for the loss of a marriage partner

(d) promote better health and longevity

(e) be treated simply as a number.

4. Which of the following is *not* a good method for dealing with stress:

(a) regular exercise

(b) increasing alcohol consumption

(c) eating less fatty foods

(d) cutting back on sweets

(e) seeking out support from friends?

5. When would you expect that your immune system would be weakest:

(a) during summer holidays

(b) just after receiving good news

(c) during exam week

(d) immune activity would remain the same during all of the above

(e) at coffee break?

Further reading

Ader, R. and Cohen, N. (1975) Behaviourally conditioned immunosuppression. *Psychosomatic Medicine* **37**(4) 333–340.

Gibbons, C. (2010) Stress, coping and burn-out in nursing students. *International Journal of Nursing Studies* **47**(10), 1299–1309.

Grossman, P., Niemann, L., Schmidt, S. and Walach, H. (2004) Mindfulness-based stress reduction and health benefits: A meta-analysis. *Journal of Psychosomatic Research* **57**, 35–43.

Lazarus, R.S. and Folkman, S. (1984) *Stress, Appraisal and Coping.* New York: Springer.

Sapolsky, R.M. (1994) *Why Zebras Don't Get Ulcers.* New York: Freeman.

Schwarzer, R. and Knoll, N. (2007) Functional roles of social support within the stress and coping process: A theoretical and empirical overview. *International Journal of Psychology* **42**(4), 243–252.

Uchino, B.N., Cacioppo, J.T. and Kiecolt-Glaser, J.K. (1996) The relationship between social support and physiological processes: A review with emphasis on underlying mechanisms and implications for health. *Psychological Bulletin* **119**, 488–533.

Weblinks

http://www.stress.org.uk
Stress Management Society. A resource for individuals wishing to de-stress their lives. The website contains useful tips for stress reduction.

http://www.stress-anxiety-depression.org
Stress, Anxiety and Depression Resource Centre. This site provides information on stress, including the causes of stress and how you can manage the stress in your life. The site also details how stress can lead to anxiety and depression.

http://www.guidetopsychology.com/pmr.htm
Progressive muscle relaxation technique. This site contains a comprehensive explanation of the progressive muscle relaxation technique for stress reduction.

http://www.mbsr.co.uk
Mindfulness based stress reduction technique. The site provides detailed information on the mindfulness stress reduction technique.

https://www.pnirs.org
Psychoneuroimmunology Research Society. This site contains details of the latest research and developments in the field of PNI.

http://www.hse.gov.uk/
Health and Safety Executive (HSE). This site gives information about work-related stress, including statistics and psychosocial factors involved in work-related stress.

Check point

Your starting point		Your end point	
Q1	B	Q1	D
Q2	A	Q2	C
Q3	B	Q3	E
Q4	D	Q4	B
Q5	A	Q5	C

Chapter 7

The psychology of pain

Learning Outcomes

At the end of this chapter you will be able to:

✦ Understand the definition of pain
✦ Appreciate the biopsychosocial nature of pain
✦ Be able to distinguish between chronic and acute pain
✦ Be able to identify how to assess pain and what to consider during assessment
✦ Appreciate the various methods through which pain is managed (medical, behavioural, cognitive and multi-modal methods)
✦ Be aware of the role of psychology in pain.

Your starting point

Answer the following questions to assess your knowledge and understanding of pain and pain management.

1. Which of the following is a measure for pain assessment:

   (a) Spielberger's
   (b) HAD
   (c) Melzack and Wall
   (d) 16-PF
   (e) all of the above?

2. Which factors are the most important in pain perception:

   (a) biological variables
   (b) psychological variables
   (c) social variables
   (d) cultural variables
   (e) all of the above?

3. Pain behaviours are:

   (a) behaviours that result from acute pain, but not chronic pain
   (b) obvious when reported by the patient
   (c) behaviours that are a manifestation of pain
   (d) helpful in understanding the physiology of pain
   (e) all of the above?

4. The perception of pain can be influenced by:

   (a) anxiety
   (b) learning
   (c) the meaning of the pain
   (d) all the above
   (e) none of the above?

5. According to the gate controlled theory of pain, which factors close the pain gate:

   (a) depression
   (b) boredom
   (c) low activity levels
   (d) focusing on the pain
   (e) none of the above?

Case Study

Andrea is a 45-year-old woman who is married with two teenage children. She used to be a senior administrative officer with the local council. However, 18 months ago she was involved in a minor car accident, which has resulted in her suffering from lower back pain (LBP) ever since. This bad back pain has continued despite all other symptoms now being resolved. Andrea was signed off sick from her employment initially, but was eventually forced to resign. She is now receiving benefits in order to support her period without employment. A recent medical assessment has not revealed any significant anatomical or physiological abnormality but has revealed significant anxiety and depression. Andrea maintains that both these psychological ailments are a consequence of the bad back and her inability to work any more. At the medical assessment, various additional home support was provided: she now has a wheelchair, a stair lift and a bath hoist. Andrea's husband, Emile, took time off work in order to look after her and subsequently lost his job. The only relief that Emile gets is two nights a week when the two teenage children 'sit' with their mother while he plays five-a-side soccer with his local pub team. However, he is considering giving this up (at Andrea's request) so that he can remain at home at all times to support her.

Andrea reports that she is in considerable pain, and she is on an increased dose of painkillers. The dose has been increased steadily over the last 18 months and the medical staff caring for her consider that there is a danger that she may become dependent on the painkillers. However, Andrea states that she is unable to sleep and survive throughout the day without these painkillers. As a consequence, the drugs remain at a high level. During the day, Andrea spends most of her time in the wheelchair watching TV, but now and again she attempts to work in her garden – although after a few steps Emile usually has to support her and help back to the chair, where she takes a considerable time to recover.

Andrea was asked to attend a pain clinic, which she did because she has 'tried everything else'. She only lasted a day and felt that the therapists did not understand the pain and suffering that she was experiencing. She feels that she needs effective drugs and possibly surgery.

Looking at Andrea's case, she is clearly reporting pain and is confined to a wheelchair, but there is no medical evidence of any damage of underlying structure. What does this mean – is she in pain or not? Do you think that there could be a psychological component to her experiences of pain? If so, what methods could be introduced to help Andrea reduce her pain? Similarly, what about Emile and the two children – are they helping Andrea deal with her pain or are they hindering her recovery?

Why is this relevant to nursing practice?

Pain will happen to all of us. Although this is an unpleasant thought it is a reality that at some stage of our life we will be in considerable pain. It may be related to an injury – an acute pain – or it may be more long-term such as a chronic illness. Despite being unpleasant, it must be remembered that pain has a vital survival value as it serves to warn us that we are in danger and should escape the situation and is consequently vital to our continued existence. Those animals or humans that are born without the ability to experience pain do not live for very long.

Pain is one of the most common reasons for people to seek healthcare assistance. For example, over 80 per cent of the population will experience disturbing lower back pain problems at some time during their life. Similarly, some 30-40 per cent of the population will have experienced a tension headache in the previous year. Not only does this have serious consequences for the individual but it also has an impact on society – the costs in terms of lost employment time, benefits and visits to healthcare practitioners are considerable. Furthermore, many people will experience pain when they enter the healthcare system and the treatment they receive may actually cause more pain in the short term. Obviously, for the nurse there is the requirement to minimise and reduce pain throughout treatment using a range of methods.

How can pain be described and how does it occur? What about the different forms of pain, for example the difference between acute and chronic pain? If we can answer these questions we should gain some insight into how pain can be treated and managed. What role does psychology have in ameliorating pain, and how can this be used in practice? These questions will be addressed in this chapter.

7.1 Introduction

As a keen and conscientious student you are probably reading this book over your morning hot coffee. Being fully engrossed in the text, you reach for your mug and sip your black coffee – it burns your tongue and you don't attempt to sip it again (unless you're a bit odd) until you believe the risk of this pain returning has decreased. This is one example of pain – it is something that is an everyday experience and happens to us all. Of course, many will experience more severe instances of **acute pain** in their lifetime, from tripping and falling or burning your tongue on hot coffee, to more long-term pain that may accompany **chronic disorders** such as back pain, arthritis and so on.

It is clear from this example that, although extremely unpleasant, pain can serve as a useful survival function, assisting us in identifying and avoiding potentially damaging activities (such as drinking boiling liquids). Similarly, from this we would expect that those who do not have this tool and therefore continue to drink the boiling hot coffee, walk on broken glass and iron their thumbs would not last long, as they would soon fall victim to nasty injuries and infections.

It is not just a matter of acute pain as a consequence of injury; pain also occurs chronically. For instance, over 80 per cent of the population will experience disturbing lower back pain problems at some time during their life, and some 30-40 per cent of the population will have experienced a tension headache in the previous year. Together these figures help explain why pain is one of the most common reasons for people to seek healthcare assistance. Not only does this pain have serious consequences for the individual but it also has an impact on society – the costs in terms of lost employment time, sick pay and benefits, visits to healthcare practitioners and medication are considerable (see daCosta *et al.*, 2011; Leider *et al.*, 2011).

With pain being a by-product of many problems leading to hospital attendance and treatment, the minimising of this pain becomes an important role for all healthcare staff, particularly nurses. As a consequence the role of psychology in pain and how nurses can use this knowledge is of central importance. We will begin this chapter by looking at what pain is and how to categorise it. Following this, methods of assessing pain will be explored and then how this information has been used to select interventions to manage differing types of pain.

Key message

Pain is a useful evolutionary tool that can protect us from harm.

7.2 What is pain?

The term pain encompasses a broad range of experiences, from a bang on the knee as you walk into a piece of furniture, to a paper cut, to the sharp internal pressure of a broken collar bone or a chronic dull ache. Pain can be described as a private and internal sensation that cannot be directly observed or measured. The International Association for the Study of Pain (IASP) defines pain as 'An unpleasant sensory and emotional experience associated with actual or potential tissue damage, or described in terms of such damage' (IASP, 1992). The literature on pain distinguishes between a number of different forms which are worth outlining here. The distinction most commonly referred to relating to pain is between acute and chronic pain.

Quick check

Define pain.

Acute pain is characterised as a short-term pain with an easily identifiable cause. It is often fast and sharp followed by aching pain which is usually centralised to one area. It has an adaptive function, in that it makes us move away quickly from the pain-inducing stimulus, and teaches us to avoid pain and associated dangers in the future. It generally results from tissue damage or disease. This pain usually improves throughout the tissue healing process. Acute pain may be mild and last just a few seconds, or it may be more severe and last for a few weeks. In most cases acute pain does not last longer than three months; however, if the pain is unrelieved and becomes persistent then it can become chronic pain.

Chronic pain is a long-term pain, outliving any original tissue damage. Definitions have the propensity to differ in relation to how long pain has to be present for it to become chronic. However it is generally accepted that for pain to be characterised as chronic it needs to have persisted for approximately three months. The IASP (1992) defines chronic pain as 'pain that persists beyond normal tissue healing time, which is assumed to be three months'; similar to this is Elliot *et al.* (1999) who define chronic pain as 'pain or discomfort, that persists continuously or intermittently for longer than three months'. Chronic pains can include arthritis (Neva *et al.*, 2011), lower back pain (Crowe *et al.*, 2010) and pain associated with cancer (Chapman, 2011). In chronic pain the link between injury and pain is less clear, suggesting there is more to this particular pain than mere biology – leaving room for the impact of the person's psychology in pain perception. Although psychology has played its primary role in the treatment of chronic pain, it does have some role in treatment of acute pain.

The distinction between acute and chronic pain is a general and simplistic division but can be further sub-divided into:

✦ **Recurrent acute pain** caused by benign conditions that are sometimes intense and sometimes disappear (e.g. migraines).

✦ **Intractable-benign pain** is pain that is persistent and never really goes away (e.g. lower back pain).

✦ **Progressive pain** is that which is both continuous and worsens over time (e.g. arthritis or cancer).

Quick check

What are the various forms of pain? Can you define what pain Andrea is suffering from?

Another distinction that can be made is between the various known or assumed biological causes of pain. There are two groups of pain and these are identified in the following box.

Types of pain, defined by cause (or assumed causes)

Nociceptive **(pain resulting from the stimulation of specific pain receptors)**

✦ **Somatic:** pain occurring from stimulation of receptors within tissues such as skin, muscle, joints, bones, and ligaments; often known as musculo-skeletal pain.

✦ **Visceral:** pain occurring from stimulation of receptors within internal organs of the main body cavities. This pain originates from ongoing injury to the internal organs or the tissues that support them.

Non-nociceptive **(pain arising from within the peripheral and central nervous system – assumed to be independent of any initial injury/damage)**

✦ **Neuropathic:** pain occurring from within the nervous system itself – also known as pinched nerve or trapped nerve. The pain may originate from the peripheral nervous system or from the central nervous system. It can result from diseases that affect nerves (such as diabetes), from trauma or because chemotherapy drugs can affect nerves as a consequence of cancer treatment.

✦ **Sympathetic:** pain that occurs due to possible over-activity of the **sympathetic nervous system** and central/peripheral nervous system mechanisms.

By distinguishing between types of pain the nurse can identify its likely duration and the patient's response to possible pain treatments.

The biopsychosocial model of pain

The **biopsychosocial** model of pain is offered as an alternative to the predominant biomedical model (Gatchel *et al.*, 2007). As pain is complex and multidimensional, a single explanation is rarely enough to give a full explanation. The biopsychosocial model focuses on multiple factors in which the experience of pain could be affected by:

✦ **Biological factors** – intensity of stimulation; the biological component seeks to understand how the causes of pain stem from the functioning of one's own body.

✦ **Psychological factors** – emotions, cognition and intentions; the psychological component looks for potential psychological causes for the pain such as lack of self-control, emotional turmoil and negative thinking.

✦ **Social factors** – experiences; the social component investigates how different social factors such as socio-economic status, culture, poverty, technology and religion can influence pain.

With these distinctions in mind it is important to realise that a biological cause for pain is not always present and that psychological factors also have an important role in relation to all aspects of pain (Gatchel *et al.*, 2007). As pain is not experienced independently from our culture, social situation, or our upbringing (e.g. what we have learnt about injury, how our friends see us, whether the expression of pain is appropriate), then we have to appreciate that:

Psychological factors are always present, whether or not they are acknowledged by patients or therapists. They can be ignored, although their effect on pain may be powerful, or they can be systematically managed in such a way as to maximise pain relief.
(IASP, 1992)

Key message

Pain is a biopsychosocial concept.

7.3 Concepts of pain

Attempts at understanding pain have a long history, with one of the first explanations being provided by Descartes in 1644 (Joyce, 2006) who 'conceived of the pain system as a straight through channel from the skin to the brain' (Melzack and Wall, 1973: 126).

In other words, when you hit your thumb with a hammer the hurt and damage from this area is sent up to the brain via one channel that tells you that you are experiencing pain.

A development of this theory was the **specificity theory** developed by Von Frey in 1894 who assumed that there were specific sensory receptors responsible for the transmission of sensations, such as touch, temperature and pain. Therefore pain would be caused by painful stimuli exciting specific nerve endings via specific pathways to the pain centre. In a similar discussion, Goldschneider (1920) developed the **pattern theory** of pain which suggested that the pattern of nerve impulses determined the degree of pain and that messages from the damaged area were sent to the brain via these nerve impulses.

These are rather simple ways of viewing the pain process, all of which have the same series of underlying principles:

✦ Damage to the body causes the sensation of pain.

✦ Psychological reactions are a consequence of the pain.

✦ No psychological variables are associated with modifying the pain.

✦ Pain is an automatic response.

✦ Pain has a single cause.

✦ There are only two forms of pain – organic ('real' pain when an injury is visible) or psychogenic ('all in the patient's mind').

If we were to visualise this process it might look something like this:

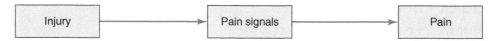

If these models were correct then it should be relatively easy to treat pain by interfering with activity in pain pathways:

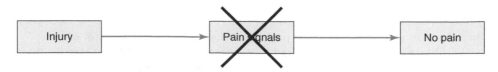

This model of pain (known as the **linear-biomedical model**) is still around today (e.g. McLean and Clauw, 2005) and underlies surgical treatments discussed later in this chapter.

Think about this ?

What evidence are you aware of that might bring a simple link between injury and pain into question? What do you do when you experience pain in an attempt to reduce it? Why do these activities/behaviours work?

Quick check ✓

What is the linear-biomedical model of pain?

Problems with earlier models

This earlier view of pain as a simple linear concept was very popular until the twentieth century when evidence to suggest that pain was not as simple as a mere linear relationship between injury and perceived pain started to mount up (Joyce, 2006). So what evidence do we have against this view of pain?

First, it was noted that when attempts were made to interfere with these pain signals through biological interventions such as medication or surgery, the treatment was not as useful for more persistent or chronic pain.

Second, it was observed that two people reporting the same level of injury in the same location did not necessarily report the same level of pain and often required differing levels of pain relief. This suggested that pain was not simply a direct response to a given stimulus (Quintner et al., 2008). A classic study which reported on this phenomenon is that of Beecher (1959). Beecher reported on the pain experiences of civilians compared to soldiers returning from the battlefield. He found that similar levels of tissue damage needed greater levels of pain medication in the civilian group compared to soldiers. Only one in three soldiers required painkillers, whereas in the civilian group it was four out of five. Beecher suggested that it was the meaning of the situation that was affecting the pain experience. The soldiers' pain was offset by the fact that they had escaped death on the battlefield and could now spend weeks or months in safety and relative comfort while they recovered. The civilians had been removed from their home environment and now faced an extended period of illness and the fear of possible complications. This suggests that pain in itself is not simply a consequence of excited nerve impulses, but that psychological and social factors play a part (Quintner et al., 2008).

Another form of evidence is that of **phantom limb pain** where there are no nerve transmissions but there is pain (e.g. Bosmans et al., 2010; Fieldsen and Wood, 2011): in other words the part of the body where the pain is reported isn't there so cannot be responsible for the pain. People who have lost limbs through amputation often have severe pain in the missing limbs. Phantom limb pain has no physical basis but the pain can feel excruciating and feel as if it is spreading. Not only is the pain not related to actual tissue damage but not all people who have had a limb amputated experience this pain, or the level of pain may vary from individual to individual (Bosmans et al., 2010).

These pieces of evidence – the variation in medication's success at reducing pain, the variation in individuals' perception of pain relating to the same tissue damage and pain without injury – indicate the pain process is more complex than the linear-biomedical model, and that pain does not equate to injury.

7.4 The gate control theory of pain

In order to overcome some of these identified problems, Melzack (a psychologist) and Wall (an anatomist) published a new theory of pain: the **gate control theory** (Melzack and Wall, 1965). It described a role for both physiological and psychological causes and interventions. The simple description of the gate control theory is that pain is a consequence of pain messages. However, importantly, these pain messages travel through a gate – if the gate is open then more pain messages get through and consequently more pain is experienced (see Figure 7.1). On the other hand, if the gate is closed then fewer pain messages get through and therefore less pain is experienced.

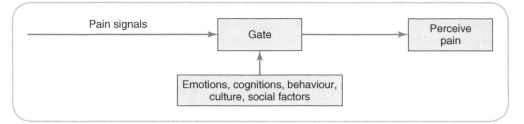

Figure 7.1 The gate control theory of pain

The central idea of the gate control theory is the presence of neural mechanisms in the spinal cord which can somehow close or open a gate, and therefore alter the amount of pain messages travelling to the brain (Deardorff, 2003). The theory proposes that the gating mechanism is in the **substantia gelatinosa** of the **dorsal horns**, which are part of the **grey matter** of the spinal cord.

Quick check

What is the gate control theory of pain?

In this model you can see that signals from the injury enter the gating mechanism (substantia gelatinosa) of the spinal cord from pain fibres (**A-delta** and **C fibres**). These pain fibres are responsible for different sensations. C fibres are slow, small and unmyelinated and are responsible for pain, whereas A-delta fibres are large, fast and myelinated and are responsible for things such as touch (Deardorff, 2003). After these signals pass through the gating mechanism they activate transmission cells which send impulses to the brain. When the signals reach a critical level the person perceives pain: the greater the output beyond this level, the greater the pain intensity. When the pain signals enter the spinal cord and the gate

Think about this

How could you use these ideas to develop an intervention for managing pain without medical treatment?

What could you suggest to Andrea to help relieve her pain?

Key message

The gate control theory suggests that a variety of physiological, psychological or social factors can open the gate (i.e. make pain worse) or close the gate (i.e. relieve pain) and hence alter the perception of pain.

is open the transmission cells send impulses freely. But if the gate is closed then the output of the transmission cells is inhibited. There are differing factors influencing whether the gate is open or closed, and these are:

✦ **The amount of activity in the pain fibres:** the greater the injury the more active the pain fibres, the more open the gate, meaning larger injuries often cause more pain than smaller ones.

✦ **The amount of activity in other peripheral fibres:** some small fibres and A-beta fibres carry information about harmless stimuli (e.g. touching or rubbing of the skin) and tend to close the gate. This is why you can rub a cut better.

✦ **Messages that descend from the brain:** impulses from **neurons** in the brainstem and **cortex** can open or close the gate. The effects of some of these (e.g. anxiety or excitement) may open or close the gate, so what would normally bring a child to tears goes unnoticed when they are having fun with their friends at their birthday party.

Other factors in the negotiation of pain signals are presented in Table 7.1. Many of these factors may be visible in your own and others' natural responses to pain (e.g. rubbing it better).

Table 7.1 Factors influencing pain

	Opens the gate	Closes the gate
Emotional factors	✦ Anxiety	✦ Happiness
	✦ Worry	✦ Optimism
	✦ Tension	✦ Relaxation
	✦ Depression	
Cognitive and behavioural factors	✦ Focusing on the pain	✦ More involvement and interest in life activities
	✦ Boredom	✦ Distractions or focus on other activities
	✦ Other reactions	✦ Other reactions
Physical factors	✦ Extent and type of injury	✦ Medication
	✦ Low activity level	✦ Counter-stimulation (e.g. rubbing)

Quick check

What can open and close the gate?

Problems with the gate control theory

Obviously the gate control theory considers a number of aspects not addressed by a more linear biological model and consequently has advanced our understanding of pain (Melzack, 1993; Novy *et al.*, 1995; Findley, 2004). The model has also stimulated a wealth of additional pain research. Most, although not all, of these studies have offered support for these proposals (Greener, 2009). Nevertheless there are still several problems with the model that have been highlighted (see Price *et al.*, 2009):

✦ Although a great deal of investigation has centred on the search for the neural mechanism of the gate, there has been little advance in locating this mechanism.

✦ The model still focuses on physiological rather than psychological input: an organic basis for the factors impacting on pain is still assumed (it is not the emotion but the chemical basis of the emotion that is relevant).

✦ Although the gate control theory attempts to integrate mind and body it still sees them as separate processes.

However, this being said, the gate control theory has moved the concept forward considerably from the original linear-biomedical approach.

7.5 Psychological factors influencing pain

On the back of the development of the gate control theory considerable research has explored the psychosocial factors of pain. This research has indicated that there are many factors that can influence pain. For example, **self-efficacy** – the extent to which somebody believes they are able to cope with pain – can influence their pain perception (Rahman *et al.*, 2008; Walker and Watts, 2009). Similarly, the way in which a person copes with challenges (e.g. an **emotion-focused coping** vs. **problem-focused approach**) can influence their success in managing pain experiences (Elfant *et al.*, 2008). Research has also shown that **anxiety** can lead to increased self-reported pain intensity (Jones *et al.*, 2002), reduced pain tolerance (Carter *et al.*, 2002), and decreased pressure pain thresholds (Michelotti *et al.*, 2000).

Key message

If a person believes they have control over their own pain they will experience less of it.

This research supports the need to look at pain in terms of individual experience and consider the factors important in each person's case. As you can see from what has been discussed so far, attempting to measure pain objectively will be difficult. Nevertheless, it is essential in the treatment of pain to understand the nature of the pain experienced; this can help practitioners distinguish between the types of pain and focus on the evidence base relating to the management of this type of pain (Al-Shaer *et al.*, 2011). We will now consider some of the methods used to assess the total pain experience.

7.6 The assessment of pain

In order to assess pain it is important to understand the way the *individual* patient experiences it and to ensure that all of the components of the pain experience are assessed. Consequently, most measures of pain include at least three dimensions:

+ **sensory:** the nature, location and intensity of pain
+ **affective:** the emotional component and response to the pain
+ **impact:** functioning, level of activity and participation in daily life.

On this basis we can evaluate the individual's readiness for treatment and develop an appropriate intervention which focuses on the specific pain experience of each patient. We can also monitor the effectiveness of any intervention applied to the pain and modify treatment based on these findings.

There are a number of issues that will influence how a nurse should measure pain; why, who and for how long you want to review the individual will all influence this selection process.

Quick check

What are the elements of pain measurement?

Think about this

When you are in pain, what sorts of components does this have? How would you assess the pain (e.g. location, duration and so on)?

Self-report measures

The most obvious thing to do when you want to know about somebody else's experience is to ask them about it (e.g. Huguet *et al.*, 2010). Self-report measures rely on the individual's own subjective view of their pain level. There are a number of methods for approaching this: from the **unstructured interview** to the more formally structured rating scale. Interview discussions can focus on such items as the history of the pain, where the pain is, what it feels like, when it tends to occur, how strong it is, what treatments have been tried, what has or has not worked, emotional adjustment and the social context of the pain (e.g. Souze and Frank, 2000). In any format, the gathering of a detailed pain history is vital in understanding the patient's pain experience and the possible causes or factors involved in this experience.

There are four categories of pain assessment tool which are reported that provide a useful guiding framework:

✦ uni-dimensional

✦ numerical

✦ categorical

✦ multidimensional.

Uni-dimensional measures

Uni-dimensional tools record a single aspect of the pain (e.g. the degree of pain relief or pain intensity). This is then compared throughout the treatment processes. The advantage of the pain relief scale is that comparisons can be made between interventions, as all participants start with a baseline of zero (e.g. Farrar *et al.*, 2010). However, this type of measurement does not take into account the complexity of the pain experience and as such will not give a full picture of the impact of treatments on the pain experience.

Numerical measures

Numerical assessments such as the **visual analogue scale** (VAS) involve patients rating their pain on a scale of 0–10; 0 indicating no pain and 10 the most extreme pain (see Figure 7.2). This may be represented as a list of numbers or as a 10-cm. line on which patients mark their current position (e.g. Hjermstad *et al.*, 2011).

The VAS is quick and simple to administer and easy to score; however it does require the ability to transform a pain experience into a visual display, which involves continuous judgement and accuracy. This may not be possible in certain populations such as elderly

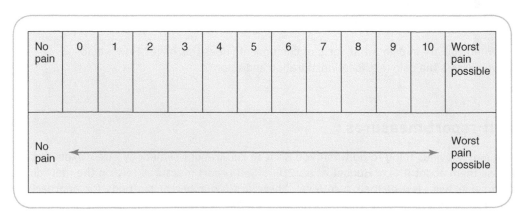

Figure 7.2 Example of a numerical measure of pain

No pain	Some pain	Considerable pain	Worst pain possible

Figure 7.3 Example of a verbal rating scale

individuals with organic brain disorders. In fact it has been found that the VAS could not be used in around 7 per cent of the population (Kremer *et al.*, 1981). As well, factors that may influence reliability and validity are learning, memory and perceptual judgement (Coll *et al.*, 2004). Furthermore, the VAS can assess only one aspect of the pain experience (Hjermstad *et al.*, 2011).

Categorical measures

A variation on the VAS is the **verbal rating scale** (VRS) where people are asked to describe their pain by choosing a word or phrase from several that are given (see, for example, Figure 7.3). These scales can be used to measure how someone estimates their pain in general and how this changes over time, either with or without treatment (Williamson and Hoggart, 2005). Again this approach is quick and easy to administer, and it has been reported as the most appropriate for use with older adults (Closs *et al.*, 2004). However, improvements in the pain experience are more difficult to identify when comparing these responses than numerical scores (Williamson and Hoggart, 2005). Adjustment from one category to another may require a greater degree of improvement than does a 5-mm. shift along a line. Additionally, the score depends on the individual's ability to translate their pain experience into words, which may not be easy. As well as this words can be ambiguous and the same word does not necessarily mean the same thing to each patient. Also the VRS can assess only one aspect of the pain experience (Williamson and Hoggart, 2005).

Multidimensional measures

The self-report measures discussed so far only inform us of one element of an overall experience. Healthcare professionals are now recognising the multidimensional nature of pain, which suggests that these scales may be too simplistic to cover the full nature of the pain process. Melzack (1975) developed the **McGill pain questionnaire** (MPQ), one of the first widely used multidimensional pain assessment measures developed based on observations and some intensive research.

The McGill pain questionnaire focuses on location, quality, intensity and sensory dimensions of pain. The measurement tool first uses a verbal descriptive scale consisting of 102 pain descriptors which are sorted into groups describing different aspects of pain. These are classified into three major groups of words. The classes are: first, words that describe the sensory qualities of the experience (e.g. quivering, pulsing, pressure); second, words that describe affective qualities (e.g. tension, fear, punishing); and third, words that are evaluative to describe the subjective overall intensity of the pain experience (e.g. annoying or troublesome). People in acute pain tend to score higher on the sensory descriptors while those in chronic pain score more highly on the emotional words. It has also been noted that people suffering from the same sort of conditions choose the same pattern of words (Wilson *et al.*,

2009). The questionnaire also investigates the pain location, medication, previous pain and changes in pain over time (e.g. what things may have increased or relieved it). The question-naire also includes a verbal rating scale of present pain intensity (PPI), which is based on an intensity scale of 1–5 where 1 is labelled mild and 5 as excruciating. A short form of this ques-tionnaire has also been developed; the short form McGill pain questionnaire (SF-MPQ) which includes 15 descriptive words that are rated on an intensity scale of 0–3, where 0 is none and 3 is severe. The questionnaire also includes the PPI and the VAS. This questionnaire takes less time to administer than the long form.

The main limitation of the questionnaire is that it requires a fairly strong vocabulary (e.g. 'lancinating'), which was reported by a number of researchers (Graham *et al.*, 1980; Deschamps *et al.*, 1988; Fernandez and Towery, 1996) who all found that a number of descrip-tors are actually incomprehensible to many participants. Also individuals are required to make fine distinctions between groups of words (e.g. 'beating' and 'pounding'). As well as this, specific descriptors may be classified into more than one domain, for example, 'fear-ful' has been categorised as both a threat (Dehghani *et al.*, 2003) and affective word in the MPQ (Melzack and Katz, 2001). This would be particularly limiting for those reporting their experience in a second language. However, the instrument has been translated into a variety of languages including German, French, Dutch, Hindi, Kannada, Malayalam, Marathi, Urdu, Spanish and Chinese. An alternative is to use a scale with pictures rather than words (e.g. the Wong-Baker facial grimace scale – see Figure 7.4).

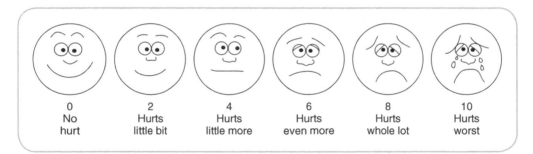

0	2	4	6	8	10
No hurt	Hurts little bit	Hurts little more	Hurts even more	Hurts whole lot	Hurts worst

Figure 7.4 The Wong-Baker FACES Pain Rating Scale

Source: From Hockenberry MJ, Wilson, D: *Wong's essentials of pediatric nursing* ed. 8, St Louis, 2009, Mosby. Used with permission. Copyright Mosby.

Physiological measures

Although there are no objective measures of pain, physiological measures may be used to assess associated factors such as heart rate, respiratory rate and blood pressure. These measures include **electromyography (EMG)** – see Figure 7.5 – which can be used to measure muscle tension in patients with headaches and lower back pain (e.g. Binderup *et al.*, 2010). This psychological approach not only investigates a possible cause of pain but also indicates a possible method of intervention (see progressive muscle relaxation later in the chapter). However, most research using these measures has failed to demonstrate a consistent rela-tionship between these physiological measures and the experience of pain as a number of other factors can affect these results (Solowiej *et al.*, 2010). For example, Hatch *et al.* (1991) recorded EMG activity of 12 individuals who had tension type headaches and nine individuals who rarely or never suffered from headaches, finding that the EMG activity in the headache

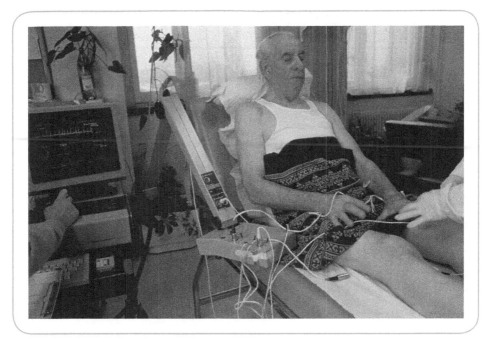

Figure 7.5 Attempting to measure pain with an EMG
Source: Science Photo Library/BSIP Laurent

or control groups did not significantly differ and EMG activity did not vary with pain, stress or negative affect.

Quick check

With what population would you use the Wong-Baker facial grimace scale?

Key message

There are many questionnaire methods for assessing pain.

Behavioural measures

Another factor influenced by pain is outward behaviour. These are behavioural measures which assess the behaviours associated with pain, either by counting them or observing how they change over time (e.g. Chen *et al.*, 2011): for example, physical symptoms (e.g. limping or rubbing), verbal expressions (e.g. groaning or sighing) or facial expressions (e.g. grimacing or frowning). These measures are generally useful and can be used either in everyday situations or in structured clinical sessions. They are also particularly useful for patients who are unable to communicate, for example, those with severe cognitive deficits or newly born infants (Boyle, 2011). These observations may be used in addition to information gained from self-reports. One

Table 7.2 Checklist of non-verbal pain indicators (CNPI)

Behaviour	With movement	At rest
1. Vocal complaints: non-verbal (sighs, gasps, moans, groans, cries)		
2. Facial grimaces/winces (furrowed brow, narrowed eyes, clenched teeth, tightened lips, jaw drop, distorted expressions)		
3. Bracing (clutching or holding onto furniture, equipment or affected area during movement)		
4. Restlessness (constant or intermittent shifting of position, rocking, intermittent or constant hand motions, inability to keep still)		
5. Rubbing (massaging affected area)		
6. Vocal complaints: verbal (words expressing discomfort or pain – 'ouch', 'that hurts'; cursing during movement; exclamations of protest – 'stop', 'that's enough')		

limitation of this approach is that it may be more difficult to apply to the assessment of chronic or recurrent pain because the overt behavioural signs usually associated with pain tend to become habit as time passes, making them difficult to observe reliably. These behaviours are also easily faked or modified based on what patients perceive is expected of them.

A non-verbal measure of pain is the checklist of nonverbal pain indicators (CNPI) developed by Feldt (2000) which can be used in a range of different settings – see Table 7.2.

Scoring

Score a 0 if the behaviour was not observed. Score a 1 if the behaviour occurred even briefly during activity or at rest. The total number of indicators is summed for the behaviours observed at rest, with movement, and overall. There are no clear cutoff scores to indicate severity of pain; instead, the presence of any of the behaviours may be indicative of pain, warranting further investigation, treatment and monitoring by the practitioner.

Think about this

In what types of situation and with which types of patient would you use the CNPI?

Quick check

What sort of behaviours are associated with pain? How can you assess these?

Assessing children's pain

As you can see, some of these measures rely heavily on verbal communication (with the exception of the CNPI), so obviously assessing the pain of an articulate adult would involve different measures to those we would expect to be applied to a child (Boyle, 2011). Therefore these methods need to be adapted to the individual patient; for example, pre-verbal children have to be assessed through observational methods (e.g. facial expressions, crying (Boyle, 2011)) while older children can be assessed through picture-based pain scales (e.g. the picture scale (Frank *et al.*, 1982)).

Assessing the pain of older adults

Similarly, assessing older patients introduces other issues. Older adults are often reluctant to acknowledge or report pain and the increases in problems such as sensory impairment and memory loss at this age can make communicating effectively with this group equally difficult (Royal College of Physicians *et al.*, 2007). Nonetheless, evidence suggests that verbal descriptors or the numerical rating scales are both appropriate for use with older adults and can also be used with individuals with mild or moderate dementia (Schofield, 2010). However, when communication difficulties exist such as post-stroke or severe dementia, observational assessments may be more appropriate.

When using self-reports or interviewing patients from these groups it may also be beneficial to consult with others close to the patient, such as family members or carers, in order to expand the level and breadth of information available to you.

The FLACC scale

The Faces, Legs, Activity, Cry, Consolability (FLACC) scale relies on behavioural indicators to assess pain. This multidimensional tool is a checklist that guides the healthcare professional in examining the child's behaviour in response to pain. This checklist was developed for children aged two to seven years for use after surgery or when experiencing sharp, acute pain during a procedure.

Face

0	1	2
No particular expression or smile	Occasional grimace or frown, withdrawn, disinterested	Frequent to constant frown, clenched jaw, quivering chin

Legs

0	1	2
Normal position or relaxed	Uneasy, restless, tense	Kicking or legs drawn up

Activity

0	1	2
Lying quietly, normal position, moves easily	Squirming, shifting back/forth, tense	Arched, rigid or jerking

→

Cry

0	1	2
No cry, awake or asleep	Moans or whimpers, occasional complaint	Crying steadily, screams or sobs, frequent complaints

Consolability

0	1	2
Content, relaxed	Reassured by occasional touching, hugging, or 'talking to', distractible	Difficult to console or comfort

How to use the FLACC scale:

✦ Rate the patient on each of the five categories (i.e. Face, Legs, Arms, Cry, Consolability). Each category is scored on the 0–2 scale.

✦ Add the scores together (for a total possible score of 0–10).

✦ Document the total pain score.

Interpreting the score:

0 = Relaxed and comfortable

1–3 = Mild discomfort

4–6 = Moderate pain

7–10 = Severe pain or discomfort or both

Think about this

How would you assess pain in these cases:

✦ a 6-month-old child undergoing orthopaedic treatment

✦ a 27-year-old man with paranoid schizophrenia with a cut forehead

✦ Joe, a 35-year-old man with chronic lower back pain

✦ an 18-year-old woman undergoing dental treatment

✦ an 88-year-old adult with dementia following a fall

✦ a 16-year-old boy with learning disabilities complaining of stomach pain?

Key message

There are different forms of pain assessment, dependent on the population, the nature of the pain and the injury.

7.7 The management of pain

It is very often the case that the elimination of pain is not a realistic goal, therefore it is more common to refer to the management of pain, in which interventions are aimed at improving the situation of the patient without the intention of removing pain altogether (Cox, 2010). This terminology also affects the way in which patients perceive, and what they expect from the treatment. Expecting pain to be eliminated altogether may be an unrealistic goal which could lead to negative impacts on the individual's quality of life and overall mental health.

The management of different types of pain, particularly acute pain and chronic pain, are very different. You are unlikely to give someone with a severe leg injury a single aspirin and expect it to relieve their pain, although this may be sufficient for a mild headache. Nevertheless, there are common elements in the form of approaches that may be useful for different types of pain: for example someone who has a severe leg injury is likely to be offered some form of **medical intervention**. It may also be that those with chronic pain benefit from some form of psychological support and intervention as the management of pain should be diverse enough to take into account the various dimensions of the pain experience (e.g. Jacobson *et al.*, 2010).

In this section each of these types of approaches will be explored and their application to both acute and chronic pain will be discussed. The benefits and problems for the nurse and patient for each of these approaches will also be outlined. However, with all of these approaches it is important to remember that there is no single answer to pain; **multi-modal methods** are often required.

Key message

Pain management should be diverse enough to take into account the various dimensions of the pain experience.

Methods of pain management

The most obvious method of pain management is by medication intervention which temporarily reduces/relieves pain but does not eliminate its cause (Swann, 2010). This is most useful in reducing acute pain and can be extremely effective. There are many forms of drugs that can be taken to reduce acute pain and three of the most common are listed in Table 7.3.

Although effective drug treatments are available, not all patients receive appropriate pain relief 'resulting in the needless suffering of countless millions of patients' (IASP, 1992: 3). This is in part the result of pain medication being administered based on what health professionals expect to be the problem as opposed to resulting from a consultation with the patient about the nature of their pain experience. This may result in many patients remaining in pain. A survey of over 3,000 individuals discharged from hospital showed that some 87 per cent reported moderate or severe pain on leaving hospital (Bruster *et al.*, 1994). In children the picture is the same: Karling *et al.* (2002) reported that almost three-quarters of those children discharged were in pain and that a quarter of these were experiencing moderate or severe pain. This, coupled with the length of hospital stays reducing, means that the need for effective pain management at home is essential (Swann, 2010).

Table 7.3 Methods of drug pain management

Pain-analgesic	How it works
Aspirin and ibuprofen	Reduces fever and inflammation by interfering with the transmission of pain signals.
Narcotics (e.g. codeine and morphine)	Inhibits the transmission of pain signals and can be very effective at reducing severe pain.
Local anaesthetics (e.g. for tooth pain or for an epidural)	Blocks the nerve cells in a small region from generating impulses.

As indicated in the Beecher (1959) study, people often respond differently to pain and this can affect the treatment offered and requested. A difference in response to pain by different ethnic groups has been identified, with different groups expressing the quality and intensity or frequency of pain differently and using varying amounts of analgesics in an attempt to control their pain, which illustrates the influence of culture on pain perception (Cleland *et al.*, 2005). The impact on medication prescribing can be affected by the patient's ideas, concerns and expectations. For instance, Matthys *et al.* (2009) found an association between the presence of concerns and/or expectations and less medication prescribing. As well as this the researchers concluded that exploring the patient's ideas, concerns and expectations may lead to fewer new medications prescribed. The prescribing of pain medication may also be influenced by the healthcare professional's expectations of the patient (Swann, 2010). For example, it is suggested that men are viewed as 'tough' or 'macho' and hence are often prescribed less medication than a woman irrespective of the individual's rating of pain.

Key message

Drug management of pain must be optimal.

Placebos

A **placebo** is an assumed inactive substance or dummy treatment which is traditionally administered to a control group within **randomised control trials**. It serves as a baseline when trying to determine some comparison of the effects of an active drug or treatment. Placebos have been shown to have an effect in pain relief, especially in patients with chronic pain. For instance, Dimond *et al.* (1960) carried out several sham operations to examine the placebo effect on pain relief. Patients were given a general anaesthetic, cut open and sewed back up again without actually having anything operated on. The patients believed that they had the operation and their pain was reduced. More recently, Kaptchuk *et al.* (2010) found that a group of patients with irritable bowel syndrome (IBS) reported significant symptom relief even when they were told in advance that their medication was fake. This explains that placebos may be useful in pain management and should be incorporated within care, which may explain the success of complementary therapies. However, given that placebos are not an active drug, prescribing them to patients and deceiving them cause ethical issues.

Quick check

Highlight three methods of medical pain management. What types of pain can they be used for?

Surgical methods

Another intervention resulting from the **medical model** of treatment is the surgical approach. Obviously mild headaches would not be best tackled through surgery; on the other hand, this intervention may be considered if the pain becomes severe or persistent.

As mentioned when looking at concepts of pain, the thinking behind surgical approaches to pain management/reduction is relatively simple: if the pain pathway to the brain is broken then the pain message cannot get through. Hence surgery involves the division of nerve pathways, either by severing or destroying them, thus reducing the perception of pain (e.g. Bolivor, 2009). This technique is most commonly used in those with chronic lower back pain (mainly in the USA).

However, as predicted from evidence refuting this simple linear link, the technique is not particularly successful and there may be limited benefits. Indeed, there may be some negative consequences resulting from the removal of these pathways: numbness, pins and needles and even paralysis in the region involved in the surgery. Additionally, since pain messages can travel to the brain via different routes the pain may return a month or two after the surgery.

Hence, surgery may have little to offer most people with chronic pain. However, in patients with pain from arthritis, joint replacement surgery can offer a great pain relief (Gullaspie, 2010). As well as this, surgery can help relieve pain caused by cancer in some patients if other treatments have failed (Chakraborty *et al.*, 2011).

Think about this

Looking back at the case study, would it be appropriate to give Joe surgical treatment?

Transcutaneous electrical nerve stimulation (TENS)

A further method of interfering with the pain signals is through the use of **transcutaneous electrical nerve stimulation** (TENS). TENS is based on the principle of counter-stimulation. It works on the premise of replacing pain signals with a tingling sensation through the stimulation of the skin area over the site of the pain, using an electrical stimulator. This is similar to when you rub your knee after banging it: stimulation of the receptors around the pain site can reduce the overall perception of pain. It consists of a battery operated device that delivers small variable electrical current to the region of pain via adhesive pads. The patient can operate this device, which also allows for personal control. This form of pain management is reported to be effective for some individuals in some forms of chronic conditions: phantom limb pain, labour pain and pain following surgery (e.g. Planton *et al.*, 2010). However, despite being extensively used there is conflicting evidence about whether TENS is beneficial (Khadilkar *et al.*, 2008). Reviews of its effect on other chronic pains, including back pain, have been inconclusive (Carrol *et al.*, 2006). The major methodological problem has been the lack of sufficient numbers of placebo-control groups in the studies, a trend you will see throughout research on the value of pain management techniques.

Key message

TENS machines can be useful as a pain management tool, particularly in labour.

Biofeedback

Another approach used to manage pain through the modifying of biological processes is **biofeedback**. This technique involves the monitoring of physiological data (e.g. heart rate, muscle activity, brain wave patterns and skin response) which is then presented to the patient who attempts to control and change these originally involuntary biological variables. For example, a patient's muscle group is wired to an electromyography (EMG) machine and the results of the muscle tension presented to the patient. The patient is then shown how the muscle tension can be increased or decreased – by either tensing their muscles or relaxing. By providing feedback on how the biological variables respond, the patient over time learns how to control their physiological responses by changing thoughts or behaviour.

Biofeedback has been used in cases such as tension headaches, migraines, lower back pain and with traumatised refugees. Vasudeva *et al*. (2003) reported that using biofeedback techniques in those with migraine headaches reduced their reports of pain, depression and anxiety. The biofeedback treatment involved the patients learning to control their cerebral blood flow velocity which was measured in the middle **cerebral artery** with a **transcranial doppler**. Furthermore, Muller *et al*. (2009) discovered that when used with traumatised refugees who were experiencing chronic pain, pain management increased significantly, although the authors did note that it is far more advantageous to the patient when combined with other forms of management. However, biofeedback can be time consuming and expensive, especially as it is often considered nothing more than relaxation.

Relaxation

Relaxation is most commonly used as a treatment for tension headaches or migraines (see also Chapter 6); it has also been found to be one of the most effective treatments for tension headaches (Bendtsen and Jensen, 2011). The thinking behind these relaxation approaches to tension headaches, for example, is relatively straightforward: tension headaches are assumed to result from persistent muscle contractions around the head, neck and shoulders and if this occurs then relaxing these muscles should have the opposite effect: the person becomes relaxed and pain free (there are, of course, other theories of headache development).

Since there appears to be a link between the tension and the pain then a suitable intervention would be **progressive muscle relaxation** (PMR). In essence the PMR approach involves the tensing and relaxing of muscles to demonstrate to the patient the difference between the two. The patient is then taught how best to relax. They will also be taught to identify the signs of an onset of a pain episode so they can start to relax early to prevent the pain from increasing. It is not only the PMR method that can be used to relax and reduce the tension and hence the pain; there are a number of other forms of relaxation techniques.

Research into the issue of whether relaxation works for a range of pains has produced mixed results (e.g. Sarafino and Goehring, 2000), with most research reviewed in the literature displaying weaknesses in methodology, which limits the ability to draw conclusions about this intervention. Furthermore, comparisons between relaxation and attention-training techniques have indicated that relaxation is inferior in relation to managing pain (Sharpe *et al.*, 2010). Relaxation appears to benefit some but not others and as it has little if any negative impact on patients, it is generally agreed that it should be integrated into approaches to reduce pain as part of a multimodal intervention (Chan *et al.*, 2011). Whether relaxation is effective as a stand-alone intervention is debatable (Persson *et al.*, 2008).

With this in mind it must be noted that the encouragement to 'take it easy' and to avoid social, leisure and work activities is not classed as a relaxation technique, as avoiding these may lead to negative impacts on someone's quality of life (see Dysvik *et al.*, 2011). Furthermore, reductions in these activities can lead to patients becoming more and more inactive over and beyond the recommended rest period. Ultimately, they may avoid more activities and this can cause an increased focus on the pain since they no longer have any other outlets on which to focus. Thus, the individual's life will tend to revolve around the pain and its treatment, which in turn may lead to the patient **catastrophising**. Also a loss of rewards from environmental stimulus may cause the patient to become depressed. This depression can lead to a greater increase in pain and a vicious downward spiral can develop.

Think about this

In what situations would relaxation be useful as a method of pain management? Would it be appropriate in Joe's case?

Quick check

Using the material throughout this book, think of a relaxation strategy for pain management.

Acupuncture

Acupuncture is aimed at channelling the body's motivational energy in an effort to stimulate the body's natural healing response and to restore balance. Fine needles are used that pierce the skin at points on the body where it is believed to stimulate the release of endorphins. Developed in the Far East, this method is now being used more and more as a complementary therapy to tackle pain. Reviews suggest that there is evidence both for and against the effectiveness of this treatment (Furlan *et al.*, 2005). Some evidence has been noted in relation to the effectiveness of acupuncture in the treatment of musculoskeletal pain (Ezzo *et al.*, 2000) and cancer pain (Lee *et al.*, 2005). Moreover, Gamus *et al.* (2008) examined acupuncture in relation to the perception of pain. They posited that acupuncture may be efficient in changing a patient's pain perception from chronic to acute. Also, it was able to enhance their sense of personal and treatment control over their experience of pain.

There are a range of approaches to acupuncture and a variety of **control methods** have been used to evaluate its effectiveness: these variations make an examination of acupuncture's value as a pain intervention difficult to assess. Therefore, clinical research into the use of acupuncture as an effective treatment is currently difficult to interpret (Birch *et al.*, 2004).

Hypnotism

Hypnosis refers to an altered state of consciousness brought about by a trained therapist. There are anecdotal reports of hypnotised patients undergoing cardiac surgery, caesarean sections and appendectomies with no medication. Hypnosis is an intervention that has been shown to be effective for reducing a variety of forms of pain (e.g. Patterson and Jensen, 2003; Barber, 1998). Controlled clinical trials have continuously provided consistent support for the efficacy of hypnosis in reducing the average daily pain intensity in individuals with various chronic conditions (Dillworth and Jensen, 2010; Jensen and Patterson, 2006). Hypnosis has also been demonstrated as working merely as a placebo or as a relaxation technique (e.g. Spanos and Katsanis, 1989). Overall, however, the evidence is not substantial enough to be used in place of psychological or medical methods in the treatment of pain (Landolt and Milling, 2011).

Recent developments with the use of hypnosis in children have explored the role of virtual reality in this process and introduced a range of new possibilities (Patterson *et al.*, 2006). Furthermore, it has been postulated that the virtual reality hypnosis is more advantageous to an individual as a treatment in offering hope to those whom might otherwise be unable to experience hypnotic analgesia (Milling, 2008). Research also supports the conclusion that adding hypnosis to cognitive behavioural therapy (CBT) treatments enhances the overall treatment efficacy, suggesting that combining hypnosis with CBT may improve clinical outcome (Jensen *et al.*, 2011).

Mindfulness meditation

Mindfulness meditation training (MMT) teaches patients to increase awareness of their immediate experiences through intensive meditative practice. Specifically the goal is acceptance of one's experience without judgment (Jensen, 2011). Mindfulness has been found to be a potentially effective intervention in pain with research supporting the efficacy of treatment that includes MMT for pain management (Grossman *et al.*, 2007). However, despite the support for this intervention, there is a lack of specific, reliable and validated mindfulness measures.

Think about this ?

How would you manage pain in these cases (using both medical and psychological approaches):

+ a 6-month-old child undergoing orthopaedic treatment
+ a 27-year-old man with paranoid schizophrenia with a cut forehead
+ Joe, a 35-year-old man with chronic lower back pain
+ an 18-year-old woman undergoing dental treatment
+ an 88-year-old adult with dementia following a fall
+ a 16-year-old boy with learning disabilities complaining of stomach pain?

7.8 Behavioural approaches to pain and pain management

Behavioural approaches (see Chapter 2 for more details) to the treatment of pain argue that pain is a series of pain behaviours (or **operants**) and that pain can either be increased by reinforcing these pain behaviours (i.e. **positive reinforcement**) or decreased by individuals avoiding an unpleasant or aversive situation (i.e. **negative reinforcement**). For instance, it is posited that an individual experiencing pain may often receive certain benefits which may act as a reinforcer for their behaviour: if an individual loses their stressful job but receives compensation they will avoid the stress and burden associated with a stressful job as well as benefiting from the compensation. There might be other benefits as well – others within the family may fulfil the domestic chores and so these pressures will be removed (negative reinforcement). In addition, they may receive the sympathy and attention of friends and family and have more spare time to engage in other activities (positive reinforcement).

Key message

Pain behaviours can be rewarded by well-meaning family and friends of the patient.

Think about this

Looking back at the case study, how does this relate to Andrea?

This approach was first applied to pain research by Fordyce et al. (1984). In a behavioural approach the pain behaviours are noted: for example, how often the patient makes an audible remark (e.g. moaning), expression (e.g. grimacing teeth), distorted posture or movement (e.g. limping), negative affect (e.g. depression) or avoidance of activity (e.g. not walking). Initially the patient is asked to do something small (e.g. walk a few paces) and this is reinforced by the healthcare practitioners and the family. This is in contrast to negative reinforcement, where the pain behaviours are left unrewarded. Hence, the grimaces and other pain behaviours are ignored and not reinforced by healthcare professionals. At the same time the pain medication is reduced and given on a time-based schedule rather than on need as expressed by the patient. Over time this period is lengthened and/or the dosage reduced. This environment allows for more positive behaviours to be reinforced and pain behaviours to be extinguished. Important to the behavioural approach is the patient's family. It has been found that those with chronic pain are more likely to have 'caring' and 'over-supportive' families (Bebbington and Delemos, 1996). Hence the patient's family are trained to avoid reinforcement of pain behaviours by not providing sympathy and not taking on more of the domestic work.

These interventions have been shown to be successful in reducing patients' target pain
behaviours, resulting in a reduced use of pain medication and an increase in activity levels
(Roelofs *et al.*, 2002), thus this is more so when family and friends are supporting adoption
of this approach. Therefore the behavioural functioning of patients can be improved through
these techniques. Nevertheless, as these activities are not a direct objective measure of pain,
their reduction cannot automatically be assumed to be associated with reduced pain.

Indeed, Roelofs *et al.* (2002) also suggest that there is evidence that there is no reduction in
subjective measures of pain. Consequently, patients may still report the same amount of pain,
but not show it. Furthermore, detractors of the behavioural approach argue that as soon as
the intervention ends the old pattern of inactivity and pain behaviour reappears. It should also
be evident that this type of programme may not be suitable for all – certainly those with progressive chronic pain (e.g. cancer sufferers) would not benefit in the long term. In addition to
this, although these types of approaches can be effective in the long term they can be hard for
the patient to complete and there is a large drop-out rate from programmes with this form of
intervention. In certain cases this drop-out rate can be as much as one-third of all participants.

Finally, reviews suggest that many of the behavioural trials in the current literature should
perhaps use a combination of behavioural and medication treatments, or behavioural treatment following non-optimal medication treatment, as few studies have systematically isolated behavioural treatments alone (Andrasik, 2007).

7.9 Cognitive approaches

Instead of the focus on outward pain behaviour, cognitive therapists, as the name would suggest, focus on the way that people think and the importance of this regarding their experience of pain. It is these thoughts that are the target for change in any cognitive programme.

If we take the example of someone who is waiting in the reception area for a dentist appointment, a number of thoughts may be going through this person's head: 'this is going to hurt', 'I don't want them to use those drills', 'I am really anxious'. These thoughts are likely to increase the pain experienced. Research by Klages *et al.* (2006) lends support for the idea that those with high anxiety amplify pain anticipation which influences their evaluation of treatment-related pain. Similarly research into pain perceived to be intentional and that which is non-intentional lends further support to the role of cognitions in pain perception, with those believing the behaviour leading to pain to have been intentional experiencing a higher level of pain than those who believed it to be an accident (Lavoie, 2008).

If we return to the dentist situation and reverse these **cognitions**, someone may be waiting and thinking 'I am going to be brave . . . there are experiences a lot more painful than this . . . it won't take long'; this is more likely to reduce tension and the experience of pain. This is known as **reconceptualisation**, viewing the same experience in a more positive light to elicit different beliefs about the event (e.g. Meeus *et al.*, 2010).

You can use three elements of cognitive therapy with your patients:

✦ Patients are taught to reconceptualise their pain by emphasising how it can be controlled by thoughts, feelings and beliefs.

✦ Imagery and diversion techniques are important.

✦ The practice and consolidation of these techniques in general situations are assessed.

Key message

The way a patient thinks about the pain will affect the extent and nature of their pain.

Quick check

What are cognitions and how do they contribute to pain?

Think about this

How can we use cognitions and cognitive behavioural therapy to improve pain management? Talk to a person in pain and see what sort of thought processes they are going through.

Pain redefinition

The situation in a dentist's reception area outlined above is a good example of this technique. The patient is asked to redefine their pain in more positive terms, for example rather than something being painful they may find it easier to refer to it as unpleasant but necessary, or less unpleasant than . . . . Similarly, they may wish to redefine the sensation as a scratching or vibration, or hot/cold, rather than a feeling of pain.

Distraction

This is a technique where the focus of attention is away from the painful experience. For instance, a nurse may encourage a child to look away from the needle while having an injection, or may distract them by asking them about a game or television programme they enjoy. This technique has been significantly supported by recent research into the effects of an animation distraction on reported pain by children during venipuncture (Hana *et al.*, 2011).

Strengths of the distraction technique are that it is simple to do, it requires no special training or equipment, requires minimal effort and can be used in multiple settings. As may be predicted, this approach (like relaxation) can influence the success of a number of techniques and has been used to explain some and even all of the success of other pain-reducing interventions, e.g. acupuncture.

Quick check

Where would you use the distraction technique and with what type of patient?

Imagery

Similar to the distraction technique is **imagery**. With this technique a patient is asked to focus on an imagined activity that makes them feel happy, pleasant or safe, as opposed to focusing on the situation around them. Images may include lying on a beach, walking through a meadow or sitting in their sister's living room on a noisy Christmas morning. The therapist may guide them through the process, asking them to pay attention to various sensations, smells, sounds, tastes; this can then be applied outside the therapy session. This technique has been supported by recent research by Gonzales *et al.* (2010) who found imagery to be effective in reducing pain when using it in an ambulatory surgery setting.

Group interventions

So far all of these techniques have been discussed on the basis of their application to individuals; however, a number of benefits have been identified in the administration of group therapy for those with chronic pain. The use of group interventions, particularly CBT group therapy, is becoming commonplace (Thorn and Kuhajda, 2006). It is suggested that these benefits may result from a number of factors:

✦ Putting an individual's pain up against others' helps them to realise the extent of their pain experience.

✦ Social support gained from this approach may improve opportunities for distractions and interest in other activities, thus reducing boredom and a focus on the pain experience alone.

✦ The group may provide positive reinforcement for reductions in negative pain behaviours such as avoidance and for an increase in positive behaviours such as returning to work or increased physical activity.

Key message

Using a range of methods to manage pain can be extremely beneficial.

7.10 Conclusion

Pain is one of the most common occurrences in healthcare and as such it is vital that nurses and all other healthcare professionals are aware of the factors influencing this experience. Previously pain was viewed merely from a medical perspective, but psychological factors are now recognised as having an important role to play in its experience. Consequently there are now numerous psychological approaches to the management of pain which can easily be incorporated, where necessary, into nursing care.

Research in Focus

Bair, M.J., Matthias, M.S., Nyland, K.A., Huffman, M.A., Stubbs, D.L., Kroenke, K. and Damush, T.M. (2009) Barriers and facilitators to chronic pain self-management: a qualitative study of primary care patients with comorbid musculoskeletal pain and depression. *Pain Medicine* **10**(7), 1280–1290.

Background

Self-management can be defined as 'the ability to manage the symptoms, treatment, physical and psychosocial consequences and life style changes inherent in living with a chronic condition' (Barlow *et al.*, 2002). Self-management programmes have been suggested to be effective in improving chronic pain conditions, they also differ from self-help in that self-management emphasis is on patient skill development which serves to increase confidence or self-efficacy to manage symptoms. As well as this depression, a comorbid condition, is present in 30% to 50% of patients with chronic pain. Therefore the aim of this study was to identify barriers and facilitators to self-management of chronic musculoskeletal pain among patients with comorbid pain and depression.

Method

Participants: 18 participants from Roudenbush Veterans Affairs (VA) Medical Center and Indiana University (IU) primary care clinics in Indianapolis, Indiana, were recruited after their participation in a randomised clinical trial called 'Stepped-Care for Affective Disorders and Musculoskeletal Pain' (SCAMP) study.

Design: The study was a qualitative study using four focus groups.

Protocol: 3–6 patients were in each focus group. Open-ended questions were asked, combined with a series of probing questions, which were designed to elicit perceived barriers and facilitators to the use of pain and self-management strategies.

Results

Barriers: The most common complaint was physical effects of pain and how these limitations interfered with self-management. Patients also expressed fear that engaging in activities would exacerbate their pain. Another barrier was not receiving instruction on pain self-management strategies from primary care physicians and instead patients reported that their primary care physicians exclusively relied on analgesics to treat the pain. Depression was also a barrier. Some patients had a negative view of the self-management programme and they were not interested in it; they also thought that it was not effective in relieving pain. Other barriers included not having support from those around them, either at home or at work; not having enough time to engage in self-management practices; a lack of self-discipline; and a lack of financial resources for transportation to and from appointments.

Facilitators: Effective treatment of patient's depression was the most frequently cited facilitator to pain self-management as this improved mental focus and a greater desire or motivation to do things with a more positive outlook. Another facilitator was the support from friends, family and nurses; as well as this encouragement from nurse care managers was a facilitator. Being able to compare themselves to others helped put their pain into perspective and helped facilitate the pain.

Implications

This study has several implications. First, identifying barriers and needs is helpful in the development and implementation of successful self-management programmes for patients with chronic illnesses. Second, using self-management programmes is believed to promote physical and emotional health; they also may be able to help both providers and patients be aware of barriers and facilitators in chronic pain. Third, interventions should be designed that capitalise on the facilitators identified while at the same time addressing the barriers to pain self-management. Finally, effective treatment for comorbidities may help to reduce pain by optimising outcomes for self-management.

Think about this

Looking back at Andrea and Emile in the case study, devise a programme for Andrea. What role would Emile and their children have in the programme? What role would the nurse have?

7.11 Summary

✦ The nature of pain is individual, varying in nature, pattern, severity and so on.

✦ There are many categories of pain representing some of these variations in the pain experience: chronic, acute, recurrent, progressive, intractable, benign.

✦ Early theories of pain proposed a direct link between injury and pain.

+ Three groups of evidence bring early theories into question: (1) biological interventions successful at managing acute pain are sometimes ineffective with persistent pain; (2) the same injury in two individuals may produce different levels of pain; (3) phantom limb pain, pain without injury.

+ Melzack and Wall proposed the gate control theory of pain which suggests there is a gate between injury and pain perception that moderates the level of perceived pain and is influenced by psychosocial as well as biological factors.

+ Frequently researched psychological factors of pain in current literature include coping styles, self-efficacy and anxiety.

+ There is no universally agreed objective measure of pain, but different measures for different patient groups with different forms of pain.

+ Three dimensions of pain that most assessments consider are sensory, affective and impact.

+ When designing an assessment this must be tailored to the individual.

+ The most common form of assessment is verbal rating scales and these can be uni-dimensional (measuring one aspect of pain) or multidimensional (e.g. the McGill pain questionnaire).

+ Interventions are designed to manage pain and are not considered a cure for this pain.

+ The treatment of pain will vary depending on the type of pain presented.

+ The most common intervention for pain is pharmacological. Although successful in the short term, there are associated problems such as tolerance and dependence.

+ Behavioural interventions focus on reducing behaviours associated with pain, and the involvement of family and friends is key to the success of this approach.

+ Cognitive approaches to pain reduction focus on replacing or modifying thoughts around pain, e.g. through imagery, pain redefinition and distraction.

+ Group interventions, particularly group CBT, are growing in popularity.

+ Interventions are most often multi-modal in nature.

Your end point

Answer the following questions to assess your knowledge and understanding of pain and pain management.

1. Which of the following tools is most appropriate for pain assessment:

    (a) uni-dimensional
    (b) numerical
    (c) multidimensional
    (d) categorical
    (e) all of the above?

2. Which of the following pieces of evidence have been used to support the presence of psychological factors in the experience of pain:

    (a) people with amputated limbs can experience phantom limb pain
    (b) people can experience pain without injury
    (c) people differ in their perceptions of pain
    (d) people vary in the medication needed to relieve their pain
    (e) all of the above?

→

3. The linear-biomedical model of pain suggests that:

   (a) injury leads to pain signals
   (b) pain signals lead to the experience of pain
   (c) pain signals can be blocked
   (d) pain is an automatic response
   (e) all of the above?

4. Cognitive behavioural therapy can relieve pain through:

   (a) electrically stimulating muscle tissue around the source of the pain
   (b) changing the way a patient thinks about pain
   (c) slowly tensing and relaxing the muscles surrounding the painful area
   (d) negatively reinforcing pain behaviours
   (e) none of the above?

5. According to the gate controlled theory of pain, which factors open the pain gate:

   (a) depression
   (b) boredom
   (c) low activity levels
   (d) focusing on the pain
   (e) all of the above?

Further reading

Brodie, E., Whyte, A. and Niven, C. (2007) Analgesia through the looking-glass? A randomized controlled trial investigating the effect of viewing a 'virtual' limb upon phantom limb pain, sensation and movement. *European Journal of Pain* **11**(4), 428–436.

Brodner, G., Mertes, N., Buerkle, H., Marcus, H.A.E. and Aken, H.V. (2000) Acute pain management: Analysis, implications and consequences after prospective experience with 6349 surgical patients. *European Journal of Anaesthesiology* **17**(9), 566–575.

Jensen, M.P. (2011). Psychosocial approaches to pain management: An organizational framework. *Pain* **152**(4), 717–725.

Melzack, R. and Wall, P.D. (1996) *The Challenge of Pain*. London: Penguin.

Morley, S., Eccleston, C. and Williams, A. (1999) Systematic review and meta-analysis of randomized controlled trials of cognitive behaviour therapy and behaviour therapy for chronic pain in adults, excluding headache. *Pain* **80**, 1–13.

Morris, D.B. (1999) Sociocultural and religious meanings of pain. In R.J. Gatchel and D.C. Turk (eds), *Psychosocial Factors in Pain*. New York: Guilford Press.

Zhou, X. and Gao, D.G. (2008) Social support and money as pain management mechanisms. *Psychological Inquiry* **19**(3), 127–144.

Weblinks

http://www.iasp-pain.org
International Association for the Study of Pain. This site provides detailed information on the study of pain and how this can be used to improve relief from pain.

http://www.britishpainsociety.org
British Pain Society. This site involves all aspects of pain and its management.

http://pediatric-pain.ca
Paediatric Pain. This site provides information on pain experienced by children. It includes links to paediatric pain research and self-help materials for families.

http://www.ampainsoc.org
American Pain Society. This site contains links to the latest pain research and news.

http://www.painsupport.co.uk/ps_home.html
Pain Support. This site provides detailed descriptions of a range of techniques that can be used to manage pain, including conventional medicine and alternative therapies.

http://www.biofeedbacktherapy.net
Biofeedback. This site contains detailed information on the biofeedback pain management technique.

Check point

Your starting point		Your end point	
Q1	C	Q1	C
Q2	E	Q2	E
Q3	C	Q3	E
Q4	D	Q4	B
Q5	E	Q5	E

Chapter 8

Psychology of mental health

Learning Outcomes

At the end of this chapter you will be able to:

✦ Define mental health

✦ Evaluate the classification of mental health and abnormality

✦ Understand the nature of schizophrenia, including the subtypes, symptoms, aetiology and treatment

✦ Appreciate the nature of anxiety disorders including their nature, aetiology and treatment

✦ Interpret specific knowledge about the diagnosis, aetiology and treatment for both major depression and bipolar disorder

✦ Understand the differing concepts for personality disorder (clusters A, B and C), particularly the diagnosis, aetiology and treatment for antisocial and borderline personality disorder

✦ Understand the nature of anorexia and bulimia nervosa, the various aetiological explanations and effectiveness of treatments

✦ Appreciate the range of substance misuse disorders and their diagnosis, aetiology and treatment

✦ Understand what is meant by the Mental Health Act.

Your starting point

Answer the following questions to assess your knowledge and understanding of the psychology of mental health.

1. What is schizophrenia?

    (a) Another term for multiple personalities.

    (b) A major psychiatric disorder which is characterised by psychotic symptoms that alter a person's perception, thoughts, affect and behaviour.

    (c) A term used for people who hear internal voices only.

    (d) An untreatable disorder in which individuals can't lead a productive life and have to be hospitalised.

    (e) None of these.

2. Which of the following are the symptoms of panic disorder:

    (a) hyperventilating

    (b) nausea and stomach problems

    (c) dizziness and palpitations

    (d) sweating and trembling

    (e) all of the above?

3. What term describes individuals who predominately suffer from depressive episodes, but may also have periods of hypomania:

    (a) major depression

    (b) bipolar i

    (c) a personality disorder

    (d) bipolar ii

    (e) none of these?

4. What are defined under cluster B personality disorders?

    (a) Paranoid, antisocial, obsessive compulsive and dependent.

    (b) Schizoid, avoidant and narcissistic.

    (c) Schizotypal, borderline and histrionic.

    (d) Antisocial, histrionic, narcissistic and borderline.

    (e) Antisocial, paranoid and avoidant.

5. What are considered acceptable forms of treatment for anorexia nervosa?

    (a) Individual cognitive behavioural therapy, family therapy and weight restoration.

    (b) Weight restoration and eye movement desensitisation and reprocessing.

    (c) Exposure therapy and antidepressants.

    (d) Mindfulness and acceptance and commitment therapy.

    (e) All of the above.

Case Study

Jennie is a 40-year-old mother of four, who, with her husband Bob, struggles to pay the bills each month. Jennie owned a clothing business but unfortunately due to the economic downturn this went into liquidation. At the same time as this happened, her husband returned from his army tour of duty in Afghanistan with some minor physical injuries. Due to this, her current unemployment and some difficulties with her daughter she has recently reported that she has been under a lot of stress. She is continuously worrying about any little thing which may be wrong. This has left her feeling extremely low to the point where she often stays in bed throughout the day as she does not feel any need, or point, in getting up. Additionally, Jennie has recently been experiencing disturbing, repetitive thoughts centred on her children's well-being. After supposedly hearing that something was wrong with one of her children she rushed to their school in a panic to find that nothing had happened.

Jennie's daughter Lisa, 15, has recently lost a large amount of weight resulting in her becoming seriously underweight. In addition to this, Lisa's behaviour has also become unusual, and she is continually washing her hands due to believing that they are always dirty. Jennie feels excessive guilt for Lisa's current problems as she believes that these are due to deterioration in the financial situation along with the marriage problems. Jennie decides to speak with Lisa regarding her size to see if they can work out how to make it better. Unfortunately, Lisa becomes extremely defensive saying that she is normal weight, showing her mother a magazine to illustrate her point. Lisa continues by saying that all her friends are thinner than she is and that she needs to be the same. Ultimately the 'chat' deteriorates into a slanging match and Lisa storms off shouting at her mother: 'Stop trying to control me – it is my life.'

Jennie's husband, Bob, returned home after being away for six months on active service as an infantryman in the army. Since being home, Bob has been complaining of constantly being tired and has been having difficulty sleeping due to experiencing vicious nightmares. Bob has also decided he can't go back as he is afraid of experiencing more trauma. Jennie has become concerned about Bob's behaviour; since he has returned home, he refuses to take any form of transport but walks everywhere. This has put a strain on the family as they are now unable to partake in any activities together as a family. Bob has started spending a considerable amount of time down the local pub which he visits both at lunchtime and in the evening. Jennie has estimated that Bob spends at least eight hours at the pub where he is currently consuming over 15 pints a day, along with the whiskey he consumes on his return home in the evening.

As well as this Jamie, Jennie and Bob's eldest son, has not been returning home at night. Recently, his school informed them that he has been missing a lot of school lately. They are also concerned as when he does attend he refuses to take part in lessons and is continuously aggressive towards the teachers. When confronted by Bob, Jamie argues that he has been going to school. However he does become extremely aggressive to both of his parents and siblings. He has already been warned by the police on several occasions for his bad behaviour, and underage drinking.

Think about this

Considering the case study can you think of any mental health issues that Jennie, Bob, Lisa or Jamie may be confronting?

8.1 Introduction

Defining mental health is not an easy task and by a similar token, defining abnormal mental health is also difficult. You may have recently encountered an individual with mental health issues and you may have struggled to understand why a patient did or felt something that was out of the ordinary and did not behave in the way that you and your colleagues do. However, can you say that this behaviour was abnormal and if so, to what extent? How do you draw the line between normal and abnormal behaviour? You could define abnormality as behaviour that is infrequent, unusual or rare, or a deviation from the norm, meaning that the behaviour is undesirable. You could also define abnormality as behaviour that is socially or culturally unacceptable, or if a behaviour adversely affects them – either physically, psychologically or both. But are any of these acceptable? Are any of these suitable definitions for Jennie's or Bob's behaviour?

Think about this

Think about how you would define abnormality. Is Bob's drinking habit unusual in his particular culture (the army)? Does he drink abnormally? If so, where would you make the cutoff on a daily basis and over what period?

This chapter will also look at a variety of disorders including schizophrenia, anxiety disorders (including specific phobias, social phobias, panic disorders, general anxiety disorder, obsessive compulsive disorder and post-traumatic stress disorder), mood disorders (including major depression and bipolar disorder), personality disorders (clusters A, B and C), eating disorders (anorexia and bulimia nervosa) along with substance misuse. The nature, diagnosis, aetiologies and treatments of these disorders will also be considered.

8.2 What is mental health?

Mental health is an integral and essential component of health. The World Health Organization (WHO) defines mental health as:

a state of well-being in which the individual realises his or her own abilities, can cope with the normal stresses of life, can work productively and fruitfully, and is able to make a contribution to his or her community. In this positive sense, mental health is the foundation for well-being and effective functioning for an individual and for a community.
(WHO, 2007).

In the evolving global definitions of health, the World Health Organization emphasised the importance of mental health to overall health, claiming that there can be 'no health without mental health'. Mental health problems can range from the worries we experience as part of our everyday life to those that are more serious and cause more long-term conditions. People with mental health problems can experience problems in the way that they think, feel or behave, which can affect their relationships, work and quality of life. It has been estimated that one in four British adults experience at least one diagnosable health problem in any one year.

Key message

Mental health is an integral and essential component of health.

8.3 Classification of mental health

The historical roots of the classification system lie in the work of Emil Kraepelin in the early twentieth century. He grouped together numbers of existing diagnoses that all appeared to have certain signs and symptoms that when present together warrant designation as a 'disease' or '**syndrome**'. This went on to form the basis of the classification systems seen today.

There are two diagnostic classifications used to diagnose mental illness; the American Psychiatric Association's DSM-IV-TR: *Diagnostic and Statistical Manual of Mental Health Disorders* (APA, 2000), and the World Health Organization's ICD-10: *International Classification of Disease* (WHO, 1992). Both these diagnosis classifications of symptoms are based upon the clustering of symptoms resulting in a diagnosis such as schizophrenia, personality disorders or anxiety disorders.

ICD-10

The ICD-10 consists of 22 chapters, with chapter 5 concerning mental and behavioural disorders, which are shown in Table 8.1.

DSM-IV-TR

The DSM-IV-TR is probably the most widely consulted classification system for psychiatric disorders. It uses a multi-axial design allowing an individual's mental state to be evaluated on five different axes. Axes I and II cover the classification of psychopathology; axes III, IV and V are not required to make a psychopathological diagnosis, but to appreciate the individual's life situations. The axes of the DSM-IV-TR are shown in Table 8.2.

Key message

There are two diagnostic classifications used to diagnose mental illness: the DSM and ICD.

Table 8.1 ICD-10 Mental and behavioural disorders

Code Block	Type of disorder
F00-F09	Organic, including symptomatic, mental disorders
F10-F19	Mental and behavioural disorders due to psychoactive substance use
F20-F29	Schizophrenia, schizotypal and delusional disorders
F30-F39	Mood (affective) disorders
F40-F49	Neurotic, stress-related and somatoform disorders
F50-F59	Behavioural syndromes associated with physiological disturbances and physical factors
F60-F69	Disorders of adult personality and behaviour
F70-79	Mental retardation
F80-89	Disorders of psychological development
F90-98	Behavioural and emotional disorders with onset usually occurring in childhood and adolescents
F99	Unspecified mental disorder

Table 8.2 The five axes of psychiatric diagnosis in the DSM-IV-TR

Axis	Included
Axis I: Clinical disorders, including major mental disorders, and learning disorders	Depression, anxiety disorders, bipolar disorder, ADHD, autism spectrum disorders, anorexia nervosa, bulimia nervosa, and schizophrenia.
Axis II: Underlying personality disorders and mental retardation	Paranoid personality disorder, borderline personality disorder, antisocial personality disorder, narcissistic personality disorder.
Axis III: Acute medical conditions and physical disorders	Brain injuries and other medical/physical disorders which may aggravate existing diseases or present symptoms similar to other disorders.
Axis IV: Psychosocial and environmental factors contributing to the disorder	Family, educational, financial, housing or social problems which may contribute to the disorder.
Axis V: Global Assessment of Functioning	Global Assessment of Functioning (GAF). This is a 100-point scale that the mental health professional uses to describe the patient's overall level of performance in usual daily activities and social, occupational, academic and interpersonal functioning.

Think about this

(?)

Consider these classification systems; are they useful? Can you think of any problems with them or their use? What about comparing them – is one better than another?

8.4 Evaluation of the classification system

These classification systems provide a standard for classifying mental disorders, with a common language, explaining that anyone presenting with a set of problems will receive the same diagnosis across the world and will therefore receive the same treatment wherever they are (Bennett, 2011).

However, there are some major criticisms to consider when using these classification systems. First, although the diagnostic criteria for the DSM and ICD systems are similar, they are not identical. Research has suggested that concordance rates between some disorders have noticeable differences; compared to the DSM-IV-TR the ICD-10 criteria yield higher prevalence rates for social phobia and post-traumatic stress disorder (Andrews *et al.*, 2001) and lower rates for personality disorders (First and Pincus, 1999).

Second, both the ICD and DSM exemplify the medical model of psychological disorders. Therefore they largely ignore both the social and psychological aspects of the individual's experience, although the DSM does try to include psychosocial factors in axes IV and V. The medical model implies that biological factors are the main cause of the development of the disorder, and therefore biological treatments are the first line of treatment. This explains that the individual's diagnosis is treated and not the individual.

A third criticism is that using criteria to label an individual with a diagnosis can be stigmatising and harmful. Indeed, this can give the individual more difficulties than they may already have. For instance, symptoms may be exacerbated by diagnostic labels and may actually encourage an individual to adopt a 'sick' role, which can result in patients adopting a long-term role as someone with what they perceive to be a debilitating mental disorder (Scheff, 1975). As well as this, **stigma** within mental health problems assumes that all individuals with the same disorder have homogeneity, which does not take into consideration the fact that two people with the same diagnosis can present with entirely different patterns of symptoms (Trossman, 2011). Also research has suggested that many people choose not to attend mental health services because they do not want to be labelled as a 'mental patient' or suffer the prejudice and discrimination that the label entails (Kessler *et al.*, 2001; Aromaa *et al.*, 2011), thus delaying treatment.

Another criticism is that both the DSM and ICD have distinct categories of disorders; however it is more than likely that an individual with a mental disorder will be given more than one diagnosis. This is often referred to as a **comorbidity**. This may suggest that the diagnostic classification systems do not have independent categories as they claim, and instead represent symptoms of either hybrid disorders or more broad ranging syndromes or a disorder spectrum that represents a higher-order categorical class of symptoms (Krueger *et al.*, 2005; Widiger and Samuel, 2005).

In the case study, what were the comorbidities? What sort of issues could this raise in treatment?

Finally, the DSM has been criticised for its growing number of diagnoses, which has increased from 106 in 1952 in the DSM-I to 297 in the newest DSM-IV. This is set to grow even more in the DSM-V, with additional disorders such as a sexual interest/arousal disorders (Flaskerud, 2010).

Quick check

What are the criticisms of the classification systems?

Specific issues

In this next section, some of the disorders shown in the classification systems will be discussed; these will include schizophrenia, anxiety disorders, mood disorders, personality disorders and eating disorders. The DSM-IV-TR criteria, prevalence and common comorbidities will be discussed, along with the causes and main treatments.

8.5 Schizophrenia

Schizophrenia is a major psychiatric disorder, or cluster of disorders, characterised by psychotic symptoms that alter a person's perception, thoughts, affect and behaviour (NICE, 2009c). It affects around 1 per cent of the population and has been ranked as one of the most disabling condition in the general population (Ustun *et al.*, 1999; Novick *et al.*, 2009). For a diagnosis of schizophrenia to be made, the DSM-IV-TR states that two or more of the following criteria A symptoms are present for a significant proportion of time during a one-month period:

✦ delusions
✦ hallucinations
✦ disorganised speech (e.g. frequent derailment or incoherence)
✦ grossly disorganised or **catatonic** behaviour
✦ negative symptoms (e.g. affective flattening, **alogia** or **avolition**).

Only one of these is required if delusions are bizarre, or hallucinations consist of a voice keeping up a running commentary on the person's behaviour or thoughts, or two or more voices conversing with each other.

Other criteria for a diagnosis of schizophrenia include:

✦ Social and occupational dysfunction for a significant amount of time and declined since onset.
✦ Signs of disturbance persist for at least six months. This six-month duration must include at least one month of symptoms that meet criteria A.

✦ Where schizoaffective disorder and mood disorder with psychotic features have been ruled out.

✦ The disturbance is not due to the direct physiological effects of a substance.

✦ If there is a history of Autistic Disorder or another pervasive developmental disorder, then a diagnosis of schizophrenia is only made if hallucinations are also present for at least a month.

Key message

Schizophrenia is one of the most disabling mental health disorders.

Think about this

Looking back at the case study, can you describe Jennie as having any of these criteria?

The DSM-IV-TR divides schizophrenia further into five subtypes (Table 8.3). Paranoid, disorganised and catatonic schizophrenia all have specific symptoms that differentiate them from one another; the other two types, undifferentiated and residual type, are characterised not by specific differentiating symptoms but rather by mixed symptoms.

Symptoms

Schizophrenia is often characterised in terms of **positive symptoms** and **negative symptoms**. Positive symptoms are noted by an excess or distortion of normal behaviour or cognition; they include hallucinations, disorganised thought, speech, catatonic behaviour and delusions, and are usually a distressing experience for the client (Lakhan and Vieira, 2009). Negative symptoms are distinguished by the absence of some normal capabilities, which include

Table 8.3 Types of schizophrenia in the DSM-IV-TR

Type	Features
Paranoid schizophrenia	Delusions and hallucinations with themes of persecution and grandiosity.
Disorganised schizophrenia	Incoherent speech, with behaviour which has an inappropriate affect.
Catatonic schizophrenia	Motor abnormalities (immobility) and a lack of responsiveness.
Undifferentiated schizophrenia	Where an individual has psychotic symptoms but the criteria for paranoid, disorganised or catatonic types have not been met.
Residual schizophrenia	Where positive symptoms have been present but have not been present for some time.

blunted affect, alogia and avolition. These symptoms may go unnoticed by the patient but be apparent to others who are in contact with them (Rollins *et al.*, 2010). Negative symptoms are typically more stable and enduring having a rapid onset and remission and have a more profound effect on everyday life such as social functioning and quality of life (Lysaker and Davis, 2004).

Quick check

What are positive and negative symptoms of schizophrenia?

Aetiology

The causes of schizophrenia are difficult to identify, and it is generally said that schizophrenia may be caused by a combination of factors, such as genetics, brain abnormalities, neurotransmitters and psychosocial factors.

Genetics

Based on twin, family and adoption studies there is clearly a strong genetic component to the risk of schizophrenia (Gottesman and Reilly, 2003). Studies have found that the closer you are related to someone with schizophrenia the more likely you are to develop the disorder. For example, Gottesman (1991) suggested that children with both parents with schizophrenia have a 46 per cent risk of developing schizophrenia, whereas when only one parent has schizophrenia the risk drops to 13 per cent. He also suggested that if your monozygotic (identical) twin has been affected by schizophrenia you have an elevated risk of 46 per cent, whereas if your dizygotic (non-identical) twin has been affected then your risk drops to around 14 per cent for developing schizophrenia.

Brain abnormalities

The most common findings of brain scans of people diagnosed with schizophrenia include enlarged ventricles (Lawrie *et al.*, 2008). Individuals with large ventricles tend to show social, emotional, and behavioural deficits, they also tend to have more severe symptoms and are less responsive to treatment than individuals diagnosed with schizophrenia without enlarged ventricles (Andreassen *et al.*, 1987; Nolen-Hoeksema, 2011). Studies have also shown that individuals with schizophrenia have abnormalities in the prefrontal cortex, which seems to be smaller and to have less blood flow compared to controls. The hippocampus is another brain area seen to be affected by schizophrenia (Barch, 2005). The hippocampus plays an important role in the formation of long-term memories, which seems to be affected in individuals with schizophrenia when encoding and recalling information (Schachter *et al.*, 2003).

Neurotransmitters

The neurotransmitter dopamine has been shown to play a role in schizophrenia, suggesting that schizophrenia is the result of excess levels of dopamine. Neuroimaging studies suggest that individuals diagnosed with schizophrenia have more dopamine receptors and higher levels of dopamine in some areas of the brain (Conklin and Iacono, 2002; Kendler and Schaffner, 2011). Evidence has also suggested that amphetamine use increases dopamine levels that are similar to the positive symptoms seen in schizophrenia (Lieberman *et al.*, 1990). However, some evidence is less supportive showing some antipsychotic medication appearing to work by its impact on the serotonin levels and not the dopamine system, suggesting that other neurotransmitters may be involved in schizophrenia (Duncan *et al.*, 1999).

Psychosocial

Although not a cause of schizophrenia, psychosocial factors can be a trigger for developing schizophrenia. It has been found that individuals from a lower socio-economic group are more likely to develop schizophrenia (Werner *et al.*, 2007). This could be due to higher amounts of stress being associated with lower socio-economic groups. Furthermore, evidence has also suggested that stressful life events such as losing your job, divorce or losing someone close to you may trigger psychotic episodes (Docherty *et al.*, 2009; Phillips *et al.*, 2007). Family interactions have also been associated with schizophrenia, suggesting that individuals with a diagnosis of schizophrenia who have families with a high expressed emotion are more likely to relapse than those with families with a lower expressed emotion (Bebbington *et al.*, 1995).

Quick check

What are the main causes of schizophrenia?

Treatments

Antipsychotic medication

Most people diagnosed with schizophrenia will receive some form of medication, which works by blocking the effect of dopamine in the brain. Antipsychotics have been very useful in decreasing the amount of time spent in hospital for individuals with schizophrenia (Lavretsky, 2008). However, there are many side effects related to antipsychotic use, such as Parkinsonism symptoms and tardive dyskinesia (Guo *et al.*, 2011). Fortunately, newer drugs called atypical antipsychotics have been developed to treat schizophrenia, which have been more effective than the typical antipsychotics and have fewer side effects (Dossenbach *et al.*, 2004; Guo *et al.*, 2011). However despite this, serious side effects have still been evident when using atypical antipsychotics.

Psychological approaches

Cognitive behavioural therapy (CBT) is recommended by the National Institute for Clinical Excellence (NICE, 2009c) to treat schizophrenia. The main aim of CBT for schizophrenia is to help identify the thinking patterns that are causing the unwanted feelings and behaviour and learn to replace these with more realistic, useful thoughts. CBT can help individuals adjust to the realities of the outside world, help medication compliance, assist training for memory and attention and facilitate individuals to cope successfully (Perivoliotis *et al.*, 2010). Studies have found that CBT is more useful for reducing the positive symptoms of schizophrenia than standard psychiatric care or no treatment (Tarrier and Wykes, 2004; Zimmerman *et al.*, 2005). Evidence has also shown that CBT effects for schizophrenia are long lasting (Zimmerman *et al.*, 2005), and reduce future symptoms in individuals at risk of developing psychotic symptoms (Morrison *et al.*, 2002).

Family therapy has also been recommended for use for schizophrenia by the National Institute for Health and Clinical Excellence (NICE, 2009c). As discussed earlier on, high negative expressed emotion contributes to relapses, therefore much research has been devoted to family interventions to reduce relapse rates. Family interventions have a well established evidence base, and have efficacy in reducing relapse rates in schizophrenia (NICE, 2009c). Pharoah *et al.* (2000) suggested that family interventions reduce risk of relapse by about half in comparison to standard medical care. Therefore family interventions may be particularly useful for families of people who have recently relapsed or are at risk of relapsing or have persisting symptoms.

Quick check

What are the main treatments for schizophrenia?

8.6 Anxiety disorders

An **anxiety disorder** is an excessive or aroused state characterised by feelings of apprehension, uncertainty and fear. Anxiety disorders are relatively common affecting an estimated 28.8 per cent of individuals over the course of their lives (Kessler *et al.*, 2005a). They encompass a range of different disorders, including specific phobias, social phobias, panic disorders, general anxiety disorders, obsessive compulsive disorder and post-traumatic stress disorder.

Key message

An anxiety disorder is an excessive or aroused state characterised by feelings of apprehension, uncertainty and fear.

Specific phobia

Specific phobias are defined as an excessive, unreasonable persistent fear triggered by a specific object or situation. The main DSM-IV-TR diagnostic criteria for social phobia are:

+ Marked, persistent fear triggered by objects or situations.
+ Exposure to the trigger leads to intense anxiety.
+ Individual recognises the fear is excessive and unreasonable.
+ Object or situation is avoided and interferes with daily functioning.

Specific phobias are extremely common, with a lifetime prevalence of between 7 and 11 per cent. Phobic responses can occur in variety of types: blood-injection-injuries (e.g. seeing blood or injuries (Sarlo *et al.*, 2011), situation fears (e.g. enclosed spaces, flying or public transport), animals (e.g. snake, spiders or dogs), and natural environment (heights, storms or water).

Attempts to explain the aetiology of specific phobias come from a psychoanalytical approach devised by Freud (see Chapter 2). Freud suggested that phobias act as a defence against the anxiety experienced by repressed id impulses, which results in displacement of the repressed feelings onto an object or situation. This object or situation becomes the phobic stimuli which are then avoided by the individual. The most famous case of this type of phobia is 'Little Hans' who developed a phobia of horses, and would avoid leaving the house because of a fear of being bitten by one. Freud explained this by the fact that he was avoiding confrontation with the real underlying issue, which in this case was a repressed childhood conflict.

Key message

Freud suggested that phobias act as a defence against the anxiety experienced by repressed id impulses.

Another explanation for the aetiology of specific phobias is a behavioural approach, which explains phobias as the result of conditional experiences (see Chapter 2). This is when an inappropriately feared object or situation is associated with the experience from some time in the past. This can be seen in another classical case of 'Little Albert' who was conditioned with a fear of a white rat, which was then generalised to all furry animals and similar looking stimuli, such as cotton wool and white fur. However, despite its popularity (Davey, 2008) the classical conditioning model cannot explain the range of features possessed by specific phobias, such as the fact that many individuals who have a phobia cannot recall a traumatic event.

A further explanation is an evolutionary model, whereby phobias tend to have a biologically preparedness (Seligman, 1971) or a non-associative fear response (Poulton and Menzies, 2002). This would explain why phobias are centred around snakes, spiders and heights as these are life threatening. However, there does not need to be one single explanation for a phobia to occur, in fact different types of phobias may be acquired from many different factors, and it is now generally agreed that different sub-types of phobias (e.g. situational, animals) may have many different aetiologies and be acquired through quite different psychological mechanisms (Davey, 2007).

Key message

Seligman argued that the potential to develop some phobias may be hardwired into our brains – preparedness theory.

The treatment of phobias focuses on **exposure therapy**, which puts individuals in a situation where they can experience evidence that is contrasting to their dysfunctional beliefs (Price *et al.*, 2011). Exposure therapy has been empirically demonstrated and is currently recognised as the treatment of choice for specific phobias (Emmelkamp *et al.*, 1995; Price *et al.*, 2011). In particular, in vivo exposure is generally more effective than other forms of exposure (Emmelkamp, 1982).

Social phobia

Social phobia is the severe and persistent fear of social or performance situations. The main DSM-IV-TR diagnostic criteria are:

✦ Persistent fear triggered by social or performance situations.

✦ Exposure to the trigger leads to intense anxiety.

✦ Individual recognises the fear is excessive.

✦ Trigger situations are avoided which interferes with daily functioning.

Key message

Social phobia is the severe and persistent fear of social or performance situations.

Kessler *et al.* (2008) suggested that social phobia is a common, under-treated disorder which leads to significant functional impairment. Social anxiety disorder has lifetime and 12-month prevalence rates of 12.1 per cent and 7.1 per cent, respectively (Ruscio *et al.*, 2008). The psychological distress associated with social phobia results in clearly diminished involvement in normal activities of daily living and reduced behavioural flexibility across contexts (e.g. education, employment, relationships). The consequences of this pattern of responding are a dissatisfaction with life (Quilty *et al.*, 2003; Stein and Kean, 2000).

Family and twin studies have explored genetic factors to explain the aetiology of social phobias, suggesting that there is a heritable contribution (Tillfors, 2004). For example, Lieb and colleagues (2000) found an association between parental social phobia and social phobia among their children. There also seems to be genetic inherited evidence for related constructs such as shyness, social avoidance and behaviour inhibition (Gladstone, 2004; Buss *et al.*, 1973). However, evidence has suggested that social phobias appear at a very early age, which may explain that there may be other causes of social phobias, such as from a developmental perspective or from early childhood experiences (Neal and Edelmann, 2003; Altman *et al.*, 2009).

Another possible cause for social phobias comes from a cognitive perspective. This is where individuals with social phobias tend to rate their social performance higher than individuals without a social phobia (Gilboa-Schechtman *et al.*, 2000; Turk *et al.*, 2001). An individual with social phobia also tends to focus on more negative aspects, evaluating themselves more harshly and finding it hard to process positive feedback, which maintains their avoidance of social situations (Alden *et al.*, 2004).

The treatment of social phobia has mostly focused on CBT in the form of social skills training and exposure therapy (see Price *et al.*, 2011). Social skills training consists of behavioural rehearsal, modelling, corrective feedback and positive reinforcement and has also been shown to be effective in treating social phobias (Bogels and Voncken, 2008; Scharfstein *et al.*, 2011). As well as this, exposure therapy (which involves helping the individual to become gradually more comfortable with the social situations that they once avoided) has been shown to be very effective in treating social phobia.

Panic disorder

Panic disorder is the experience of repeated and uncontrollable panic attacks. The main DSM-IV-TR diagnostic criteria are:

+ Recurrent unexpected panic attacks.
+ At least one month of persistent concern about the consequences of an attack, or behavioural changes because of an attack.
+ Not accounted for by the physical effects of a substance or general medical condition.

Although most of us will experience a panic attack in our lifetime the number of people who actually have a diagnosis is about 2 per cent (Batelaan *et al.*, 2006). Common features of a panic attack include hyperventilating, nausea, sweating, trembling, palpitations and dizziness. Other symptoms may include depersonalisation (a feeling of being outside one's body), and derealisation (a feeling of the world being unreal).

The current explanations for the causes of panic disorders can be defined as being either biological or psychological. Biological explanations are popular because of the intense nature of the physical symptoms that are included in panic disorder (e.g. hyperventilation). It has been proposed that individuals who have panic disorder can induce a panic attack by hyperventilating (Ley, 1987). This suggests that people who have panic attacks may suffer from a poor regulation of several neurotransmitters (e.g. norepinephrine and serotonin (Charney *et al.* (2000)).

Psychological explanations suggest that individuals who have panic attacks may have a 'fear of fear'. This is where individuals may detect what they may think is an internal sign of a panic attack and immediately become fearful of the consequences, which can be closely linked to a classical conditioning perspective. Also cognitive theorists would argue that individuals suffering from panic attacks may have a catastrophic misinterpretation of bodily sensations where an individual pays close attention to their bodily sensations and misinterprets these in a negative way and then exaggerates their symptoms which then leads to a panic attack (Teachman *et al.*, 2010).

Medication such as tricyclin antidepressants can reduce panic attacks in the majority of patients (Katon, 2006). However, CBT has been shown to be extremely effective when it focuses on changing negative interpretations of bodily sensations and helping individuals get used to changes in autonomic sensations (Craske and Barlow, 2007; Gould *et al.*, 1995; Koszycki *et al.*, 2011). CBT has been found to reduce anxiety in response to biological challenges that evoke panic sensations and also to reduce self-report measures of catastrophic misinterpretation and related cognitions (Wenzel *et al.*, 2006).

General anxiety disorder

General anxiety disorder (GAD) is a continual apprehension and anxiety about future events, leading to chronic and pathological worry. The main DSM-IV-TR diagnostic criteria are:

+ Worry occurring more days than not, over a period of six months.
+ Associated with three or more physical symptoms (irritability, sleep disturbances, on edge).
+ The anxiety causes significant distress in daily functioning.

People with GAD worry about minor, everyday issues, but find it difficult to control the extent to which they worry. Prevalence rates are among 5 per cent for women and 3 per cent for men (Kessler *et al.*, 2005a). GAD has high levels of comorbidity; over 50 per cent of individuals with GAD also develop another anxiety disorder, 70 per cent have a mood disorder and 33 per cent have a substance use disorder (Conway *et al.*, 2006; Craske and Waters, 2005).

GAD appears to be associated with an over-activation in part of the brain system, which Gray (1983) called the behavioural inhibition system. This results in GAD sufferers consistently responding to perceived threats which the system would ordinary deal with; however the system fails to achieve this and becomes chronically activated leading to consistent worry.

As well as the biological explanation, a cognitive explanation has been proposed which recognises that individuals with GAD have an information processing bias which appears to maintain their hyper-vigilance for threat which creates further sources for worry and anxiety (Wilson *et al.*, 2006).

A psychoanalytical explanation can also help to explain the aetiology of GAD. Freud explained that general anxiety in adulthood could arise from excess punishment or protection during childhood. This may lead to distorted id impulses or inadequate defence mechanisms.

Key message

Freud explained that general anxiety could arise from excess punishment or protection during childhood.

CBT has been shown to be an effective treatment for GAD, especially when self-monitoring, relaxation, cognitive restructuring and behavioural rehearsal are included (Hunot *et al.*, 2007; Taylor and Clark, 2009). Self-monitoring involves making the individual aware of their behaviour and triggers that lead to worry. Relaxation involves learning to physically relax and to control breathing. Cognitive reconstruction involves identifying the cognitions leading to anxiety and challenging any inappropriate assumptions. Finally, behavioural rehearsal involves either the actual or imagined rehearsal of adaptive coping responses that need to be deployed when a worry or trigger is encountered. As well as this, **mindfulness** and acceptance and commitment therapy (ACT) techniques have proved to be effective in the treatment of GAD (Roemer *et al.*, 2008; Wetherell *et al.*, 2011); however, more randomised control trials are needed in this area to show its reliability in treating GAD.

Obsessive compulsive disorder

Obsessive compulsive disorder (OCD) is defined as recurrent obsessions or compulsions which are severe enough to be time consuming or cause distress. The main DSM-IV-TR diagnostic criteria are:

+ Recurrent and persistent thoughts, impulses or images which are intrusive and inappropriate.
+ Repetitive behaviours or mental acts that a person feels driven to perform.
+ Recognition that these obsessions or compulsions are excessive and cause marked distress.

OCD has been cited as one of the most common and debilitating psychological disorders. It is the fourth most common psychological disorder following phobias, substance abuse and depression (Twohig *et al.*, 2006). It affects around 1-3 per cent of individuals at some point in their life (Kessler *et al.*, 2005a).

OCD may be caused by a memory deficit which causes a 'doubting' that things have been done properly. Damage to brain systems may also lead an individual to over-respond to environmental stimuli, and therefore be unable to prevent their cognitive and behavioural responses to them.

Key message

OCD can be caused by anxiety triggers that the individual cannot avoid.

A psychoanalytical explanation could also be considered. Freud thought that OCD was a result of an individual's fear of their id impulses and their use of ego defence mechanisms to reduce this anxiety. According to Freud this conflict was not played out in the unconscious, but instead involves explicit and dramatic thoughts and actions.

Another cause of OCD is described as inflated responsibility (Salkovskis, 1985), which will motivate the individual to persist with rituals and compulsions until they are fully confident they have avoided the negative outcomes, for example, avoiding contamination by compulsively washing.

The most common and effective treatment for OCD is **exposure and response prevention** (ERP: Foa *et al.*, 1998; Simpson *et al.*, 2011), which is recommended by the National Institute for Health and Clinical Excellence as the best form of treatment for OCD (NICE, 2005a). EPR involves individuals being repeatedly exposed to the situation and thoughts that trigger distress. Individuals also practise competing behaviours, such as habit reversal or modification of compulsive rituals.

Post-traumatic stress disorder

Post-traumatic stress disorder (PTSD) is a set of persistent anxiety-related symptoms that occur after experiencing or witnessing an extremely traumatic event. The main DSM-IV-TR diagnostic criteria are:

+ Exposure to a traumatic event that caused extreme fear, helplessness or horror.
+ The event is re-experienced, such as by nightmares or recurrent distressing thoughts of the event.
+ The individual avoids stimuli associated with the trauma.
+ Increased arousal which may cause sleep disturbances, irritability and hyper-vigilance.
+ Duration of disturbances is more than one month.

Post-traumatic stress disorder (PTSD) is a highly prevalent, often chronic and disabling psychiatric disorder that can occur after experiencing or witnessing a major traumatic event, such as a major accident, torture, rape, terror actions, natural disasters and war experiences (Bisson and Andrew, 2009; Lennmarken and Sydsjo, 2007). Lifetime prevalence rates are estimated to affect approximately 7.8 per cent of individuals (Nelson, 2011). Prevalence rates among groups that regularly encounter traumatic events are much higher, for example, emergency personnel

(Bennett *et al.*, 2005). PTSD is also frequently comorbid with other psychiatric disorders such as other anxiety disorders, depression and substance abuse (Kessler *et al.*, 2005a).

Individuals who have a vulnerability factor seem to be more susceptible to developing PTSD after experiencing a major traumatic event. For example, individuals who are already experiencing increased anxiety or depression have an increased vulnerability for developing PTSD (Cardozo *et al.*, 2003). Lack of social support (King *et al.*, 1999) and avoidant or self-destructive coping strategies increase an individual's vulnerability to develop PTSD following a traumatic event. Neuroimaging findings have also found that individuals who develop PTSD seem to have an amygdala which responds more actively to emotional stimuli (Francati *et al.*, 2007).

Key message

Individuals who have a vulnerability factor seem to be more susceptible to developing PTSD after experiencing a major traumatic event.

Prolonged exposure (PE) is an exposure-based treatment for PTSD; it helps individuals confront and experience events and stimuli relevant to their trauma and symptoms. PE has been shown to be very effective in the treatment of PTSD (Nemeroff *et al.*, 2006; Nacasch *et al.*, 2010), and has proved to have lasting benefits (Powers *et al.*, 2010). Another treatment for PTSD is **eye movement desensitisation and reprocessing** (EMDR), where individuals are required to focus their attention on the traumatic memory while simultaneously visually following the therapist's finger moving backwards and forwards. EMDR is currently one of the most recent, most extensively researched and controversial treatments for PTSD (Boschen, 2008). And increasingly a growing number of guidelines recommend EMDR for their preferred treatment for PTSD (NICE, 2005b; ACPMH, 2007).

Think about this

Looking back at the case study, do you think Bob has post-traumatic stress disorder? And if so, how do you know? And how would you treat it?

Quick check

List the causes and treatments for the following:

+ specific phobias
+ social phobias
+ panic disorder
+ general anxiety disorder
+ obsessive compulsive disorder
+ post-traumatic stress disorder.

8.7 Mood disorders

Everybody may feel down at some point and at other times feel a sense of excitement or emotional pleasure, but for someone to be diagnosed with a **mood disorder** the feelings need to be extreme. A mood disorder is defined as a significant disturbance in mood, and the lifetime prevalence rate of mood disorders is estimated at 20.8 per cent (Kessler *et al.*, 2005a). This section will discuss **major depression** and **bipolar disorder**, the diagnostic criteria, prevalence rates, aetiology and treatment.

Major depression

Major depression is a condition where the individual experiences a significant degree of impairment as a result of depression. For major depression to be diagnosed the DSM-IV-TR criteria specifies the presence of at least five of the following for at least two weeks:

+ depressed mood
+ a markedly diminished interest or pleasure in almost all activities
+ weight loss or gain that is significant
+ physical agitation
+ fatigue or loss of energy
+ distress or impairment that is significant
+ feelings of worthlessness or excessive guilt
+ reduced ability to think or concentrate, or indecisiveness.

The DSM-IV-TR also states that at least one of these symptoms should be either depressed mood or loss of interest in pleasure. Symptoms must also cause significant distress or daily impairment and not be accounted for by other significant losses, such as bereavement. These symptoms must also last longer than two months.

Over 70 per cent of individuals with major depression have other comorbidities, such as an eating disorder, substance abuse disorder, or an anxiety disorders (Kessler *et al.*, 2003). It is estimated that about 5 per cent of the European population is clinically depressed at any one time (Paykel *et al.*, 2005). The DSM-IV-TR also suggests that it is more common in women than in men, with lifetime prevalence rates of between 10–25 per cent for women and 5–12 per cent for men.

The causes of major depression can be explained by biological and psychological factors. First, biological factors can explain that two neurotransmitters, norepinephrine and serotonin, seem to be implicated in the aetiology of major depression. It is suggested that mood is the result of an interaction between these two neurotransmitters (Rampello *et al.*, 2000).

Second, psychological factors provide the behavioural, cognitive and socio-cultural perspectives that can help explain the aetiology of major depression. Behavioural explanations assert that major depression is the result of a low rate of positive social reinforcement, which leads to low mood and reductions in behaviour to gain rewards (Lewinsohn *et al.*, 1979). The theory of learned helplessness can also help to explain the causes of major depression (Bougarel *et al.*, 2011). This suggests that the type of stressful event most likely to lead to depression is an uncontrollable negative event (Seligman, 1975).

These events, especially if they are frequent or chronic, can lead an individual to believe that they are helpless to control important outcomes in their environment. This theory was reformulated to help explain the cognitive factors that may influence whether a person becomes helpless and depressed following a negative event (Peterson and Seligman, 1984). This theory focuses on an individual's casual attributions for an event. Casual attributions explain that individuals tend to blame themselves for the negative events and expect to experience more negative events in many areas of their life. This in turn leads to long-term learned helplessness deficits as well as a loss of self-esteem in many areas of an individual's life. Socio-cultural factors may also help to explain the aetiology of major depression, which can be shown from the high prevalence rates of major depression in poor, ethnic minorities, and those who have poor social or marital support (Plant and Sachs-Ericsson, 2004).

Quick check

What are the biological and psychological causes of major depression?

Antidepressant medication is generally considered the primary treatment for major depression (Hougaard, 2010). This works by increasing the levels of serotonin and norepinephrine in the brain. There are also selective serotonin reuptake inhibitors (SSRIs), another drug which works by preventing serotonin re-uptake by the pre-synaptic neuron. However, a recent meta-analysis found that although drugs seem to be better at treating major depression there has been an increased improvement for placebo groups in randomised control trials (Papakosta and Fava, 2010), explaining that there must be other psychological processes involved.

Electroconvulsive therapy (ECT) is another form of treatment for depression, which involves passing an electrical current of around 70 to 130 volts through the head of the patient for around half a second. ECT is usually given when the individual has severe depression and is not responding well to other treatments (Cohen *et al.*, 2000). It seems that ECT works by affecting the levels of serotonin and norepinephrine. However, the effects of ECT are only short-lived (Breggin, 1997) and produce a number of severe side effects, such as an inability to learn new material and recall new material.

Cognitive therapy (CT) can help treat major depression by helping depressed individuals identify their negative beliefs and negative thoughts and challenging these in the hope of disproving them. Studies have shown that CT is more effective than no treatment or a placebo (Dobson *et al.*, 2008; Gloaguen *et al.*, 1998; Wampold *et al.*, 2002), and it is as effective as interpersonal psychotherapy (IPT), which is a short-term therapy that has proved to be effective for the treatment of depression, and is supported by the National Institute for Health and Clinical Excellence (NICE, 2009d).

Mindfulness-based cognitive therapies (MBCT) have also shown effectiveness in treating major depression, particularly in reducing relapse rates (Piet and Hougaard, 2011). Ma and Teasdale (2004) found that MBCT reduces relapse rates by as much as 36-78 per cent, showing that MBCT should be used to help combat relapses in depressed patients.

Bipolar disorder

Bipolar disorder (BD) is a condition in which individuals fluctuate between periods of profound depression and manic behaviour. According to the DSM-IV-TR manic episodes include at least three of the following:

+ inflated self-esteem or grandiosity
+ decreased need to sleep
+ more talkative, or a pressure to keep talking
+ racing of thoughts and/or a flight of ideas
+ distractibility
+ increased activity or psychomotor agitation
+ excessive engagement in high-risk activity.

There are two types of BD, namely bipolar I and bipolar II disorder. Bipolar I is where individuals typically experience alternating episodes of depression and mania, lasting weeks or months. Bipolar II describes individuals who predominately suffer from depressive episodes, but may also have periods of hypomania, which is defined as an increase in activity more than normal; but not excessive enough to be labelled mania. BD has a lifetime prevalence rate of between 1 and 5 per cent; bipolar II disorder appears to be less prevalent and it has been suggested that the lifetime prevalence rate for bipolar II disorder ranges from 0.5-3 per cent (Muller-Oerlinghausen *et al.*, 2002; Weissman *et al.*, 1996).

Quick check

What are the two types of bipolar disorder? And how are they defined?

BD appears to have some important biological determinants. First it seems that there is an inherited component to the disorder. Kelsoe (2003) suggested that first-degree relatives of individuals with BD are seven times more likely to develop BD than the general population. Evidence also suggests that like major depression there is an imbalance of neurotransmitters. High levels of norepinephrine have been found to be associated with elevated mood and mania and low levels in a depressed mood (Schildkraut *et al.*, 1985). Some researchers have suggested that the rapid alternating between depression and mania in BD may be related to how the brain controls levels of different neurotransmitters (Hirschfeld and Goodwin, 1988) and thyroid functioning (Chakraborti, 2011). Freud's psychoanalytical approach (see Chapter 2) attempts to define the aetiology for BD, with the view that mania is a defence mechanism to counteract unpleasant emotional states, explaining why individuals with BD can rapidly alternate between periods of depression and mania.

Antidepressants such as lithium carbonate are used to treat BD as standard antidepressants have been shown to provoke severe mood swings (Keck *et al.*, 2007). The National Institute for Health and Clinical Excellence (NICE, 2006) has recommended lithium as a first-line treatment for BD. It has also been shown to have long-term effectiveness and long recognised benefits in terms of preventing suicidal behaviours (Smith *et al.*, 2007). ECT as described earlier for major depression can also be used to treat BD patients. CT, another treatment used to treat major depression, can also be used to treat BD. CT is used in conjunction with appropriate medication in individuals with BD, and has been shown to reduce symptoms, enhance social adjustment and functioning and reduce relapses and hospitalisations in patients with BD (Jones, 2006).

8.8 Personality disorders

A **personality disorder (PD)** is categorised by pervasive, inflexible and enduring patterns of cognition, affect, interpersonal behaviour or impulse control that deviate markedly from culturally shared expectations and lead to significant distress or impairment in social, occupational or other important areas of functioning.

The DSM-IV-TR identifies ten personality disorders which can be divided into three clusters; these are shown in Table 8.4. This section will briefly explore each of these clusters.

Table 8.4 The three clusters of personality disorder

Cluster A: Odd/Eccentric disorder	Paranoid, schizoid, schizotypal
Cluster B: Dramatic/Emotional	Antisocial, histrionic, narcissistic, borderline
Cluster C: Anxious/Fearful	Avoidant, dependent, obsessive-compulsive

Odd-Eccentric personality disorders (cluster A)

According to the DSM-IV-TR, people with a cluster A personality disorder have symptoms similar to those individuals with schizophrenia, including inappropriate flat affect, odd thought and speech patterns, and paranoia. However, unlike schizophrenia, cluster A personality-disordered individuals do not seem to lose touch with reality or experience sensory hallucinations.

Key message

Cluster A diagnoses are also known as the schizophrenia spectrum disorders, and include paranoid, schizoid and schizotypal disorders.

Dramatic-Emotional personality disorders (cluster B)

Cluster B personality disorders are defined by the DSM-IV-TR as individuals who are maladaptive, volatile and uncaring in social relationships. They are prone to impulsiveness and violent behaviours, and also show little regard for their own safety or the safety of others.

One particularly severe form of personality disorder is the antisocial personality disorder, characterised as a perceived pattern of disregard for, and violation of, the rights of others occurring from the age of 15. It includes:

+ failure to conform social norms
+ repeatedly lying, use of aliases, or conning others for personal benefit
+ impulsivity or failure to plan ahead
+ lack of remorse
+ reckless disregard for the safety of themselves or others.

Antisocial personality disorder has a prevalence rate in the general population of between 0.7 and 3.6 per cent. The prevalence rate of the disorder is even higher in selected populations, such as people in prisons. For example, a survey of prison populations in 12 western countries found that 47 per cent of male inmates and 21 per cent of female inmates met the diagnostic criteria for antisocial personality disorder (Fazel and Danesh, 2002).

As antisocial personality disorder is closely linked to criminal behaviour there has been much interest in identifying the aetiology for antisocial personality disorder (Walters and Knight, 2010). It has been recognised that conduct disorder diagnosed in children may be one of the best predictors of antisocial personality disorder (Abramowitz et al., 2004; Moffitt et al., 2001). Using meta-analytic techniques to combine results of five retrospective and prospective studies, Loeber et al. (2003) revealed that those with conduct disorder are 17 times more likely to develop antisocial personality disorder than those without conduct disorder. However, it is unclear how antisocial behaviour may develop in childhood. It has been suggested that problems such as smoking, alcohol use, illicit drug use, police trouble and sexual intercourse all before the age of 15 significantly predicted antisocial behaviour later on in life. McGue and Iacono (2005) suggested that those who exhibited four or more of these problem behaviours prior to the age of 15 were 90 per cent more likely to develop an antisocial personality disorder in males and 35 per cent more in females. There are also suggestions that ineffective parenting styles, poor peer relationships, an impoverished neighbourhood and educational failure can lead to antisocial personality disorder later on in life (Hill, 2003; Eamon and Mulder, 2005). Some research has suggested that individuals with antisocial personality disorders have developed a **dysfunctional schema**, which causes responses to various situations to be extreme, impulsive and changeable. These dysfunctional schemas have been suggested to develop as a result of abuse or neglect as a child (Horwitz et al., 2001).

Think about this

Looking back at the case study, some suggested that Jamie had an antisocial personality disorder. Is there any evidence for this?

Key message

Antisocial behaviour seems primarily to be the result of adverse social circumstances.

Lithium and atypical antipsychotic drugs have been effective for the treatment of antisocial personality disorder to control impulsive and aggressive behaviours (Markovitz, 2004). The psychological intervention recommended for antisocial personality by the National Institute of Health and Clinical Excellence (NICE, 2009b) is group-based cognitive and behavioural therapy which is intense and over a long period. This focuses on teaching social and problem-solving skills and exploring dysfunctional schemas that might be underlying the problematic behaviour.

Quick check

What are the main causes and treatment for antisocial personality disorder?

Borderline personality disorder

The DSM-IV-TR defines borderline personality disorder as a pervasive pattern of instability of interpersonal relationships, self-image and affect and marked impulsivity. The main diagnostic criteria according to the DSM-IV-TR include:

+ frantic efforts to avoid real or imagined abandonment
+ unstable or intense interpersonal relationships
+ unstable self-image
+ impulsivity
+ recurrent suicidal behaviours or threats
+ difficulty controlling anger and feeling empty.

The prevalence of borderline personality disorder ranges from 0.7 to 1.8 per cent (Swartz *et al.*, 1990; Torgersen *et al.*, 2001); findings from these studies also suggest that the disorder is more common in women than in men. There is also a high suicide rate, where 75 per cent of individuals with a borderline personality disorder attempt suicide and 10 per cent die by suicide, a rate almost 50 times higher than in the general population (Kraus and Reynolds, 2001). Borderline personality disorder is often comorbid with depression, anxiety, eating disorders, post-traumatic stress disorder, alcohol and drug misuse, and bipolar disorder (NICE, 2009a).

There are various aetiologies for borderline personality disorder. First, developmental factors such as events during childhood, including ongoing experiences of neglect and abuse, are reported by many individuals with borderline personality disorder (Zanarini *et al.*, 1997). The most frequent of these is childhood sexual abuse, which is reported by 40–71 per cent of inpatients (Westen *et al.*, 1990). A psychodynamic theory can explain this through the object relations theory, which can explain that a lack of support and love from important others (such as parents) results in an insecure ego which is likely to lead to lack of self-esteem and fear of rejection. As well as this the theory of object relations suggests that individuals with insecure egos engage in a defence mechanism called splitting where they evaluate people, events or things as either black or white, often judging people as either good or bad.

Key message

Borderline personality disorder seems to be largely linked to the experiences of childhood rejections and trauma.

Dialectical behaviour therapy (DBT) is currently the most frequently investigated psychosocial intervention for borderline personality disorder (Kliem *et al.*, 2010). Although more research needs to be completed in this area, studies to date have shown it to be an effective treatment

(McMain *et al.*, 2009; Robins and Chapman, 2004). DBT has been shown to be effective in reducing depression, anxiety, hopelessness, self-destructive and impulsive episodes, suicidal ideation and hospitalisation (McQuillan *et al.*, 2005; Van den Bosch *et al.*, 2005). DBT focuses on helping individuals with borderline personality disorder gain a more realistic and positive sense of self, learn adaptive skills for solving problems and regulating emotions, and correcting dichotomous thinking. DBT helps individuals to challenge the thoughts of their black-and-white judgements and help control their impulsive behaviour by learning alternatives.

Anxious-Fearful personality disorder (cluster C)

Cluster C personality disorders have been described by the DSM-IV-TR as individuals who are extremely concerned about being criticised or abandoned by others and therefore have dysfunctional relationships with others.

Key message

A personality disorder can be identified in three clusters: A – odd or eccentric; B – dramatic or emotional; and C – fearful and anxious.

8.9 Eating disorders

Many of us may feel we would like to lose some weight and go on a diet at some point in our lives; however, this cannot be considered an **eating disorder** unless it becomes extreme and beyond the norm. Aside from obesity there are two forms of significant eating disorder: anorexia and bulimia nervosa.

Anorexia nervosa

Anorexia nervosa can be defined as when an individual maintains a low weight as a result of a preoccupation with body weight, which is constructed either as a fear of fatness or pursuit of thinness. In anorexia nervosa weight is maintained at 15 per cent below what is expected, or a body mass index (BMI) below 17.5 (NICE, 2004). The main DSM-IV-TR diagnostic criteria for anorexia nervosa are:

✦ a refusal to maintain body weight above minimally normal weight for age and height

✦ intense fear of gaining weight, even though underweight

✦ disturbances in the way individuals perceive their body shape

✦ cessation of menstruation if this has already begun.

The DSM-IV-TR also defines two differing types of anorexia nervosa. These are the restricting type of anorexia nervosa, where an individual starves themselves in order prevent weight gain, therefore not associated with purging; and the binge eating/purging type of anorexia nervosa, where an individual regularly engages in purging activities to help control weight gain. Anorexia nervosa is more common in females, who are said to account for about

90 per cent of all cases (Hudson *et al.*, 2007), and the lifetime prevalence rate is between 0.5 and 2 per cent (Preti *et al.*, 2009). Major depression is a common comorbid diagnosis, with rates up to 63 per cent reported in some studies (Herzog *et al.*, 1996); around 35 per cent of individuals also have a diagnosis of OCD (Rastam, 1992) and around 8 per cent have a substance abuse problem (Salbach-Andrae *et al.*, 2008).

Key message

There are two types of anorexia nervosa: the restricting type and the binge eating/purging type.

Bulimia nervosa

Bulimia nervosa is characterised by recurrent episodes of binge eating, and secondly by compensatory behaviour, such as vomiting, purging, fasting, exercising, or a combination of these in order to prevent weight gain. The main DSM-IV-TR criteria are defined as:

✦ recurrent episodes of binge eating

✦ recurrent inappropriate compensatory behaviour

✦ compensatory behaviour occurs, on average, at least twice a week for three months

✦ undue influence of weight or shape on self-evaluation.

Like anorexia nervosa, bulimia nervosa is more common in females, affecting around 90 per cent of all cases with lifetime prevalence rates of between 1 and 3 per cent (Keel *et al.*, 2006; Preti *et al.*, 2009; Wade *et al.*, 2006). There are also two types of bulimia nervosa: the purging type, where the individual regularly engages in self-induced vomiting or the misuse of laxatives; and the non-purging type, where the individual attempts to compensate for binge eating by indulging in excessive fasting or exercise. Bulimic episodes are usually planned, with food purchased or prepared in order to be consumed without interruption. The amount of food consumed in binges can be vast, perhaps up to and beyond 5,000 calories; the food is not eaten for pleasure, and is usually eaten in secret and quickly. Bulimia nervosa is usually associated with guilt, shame and high levels of self-disgust, low levels of self-esteem and feelings of inadequacy.

Aetiology for anorexia and bulimia nervosa

Biological factors can help to explain the aetiology of anorexia and bulimia nervosa, albeit to a minor degree. First there has been clear evidence that it runs in families (Young, 2010). Twin studies have found that anorexia nervosa has a 56 per cent heritability factor (Bulik *et al.*, 2006), whereas bulimia has a heritability of between 50 and 83 per cent (Striegel-Moore and Bulik, 2007). Second, individuals with anorexia and bulimia seem to have hypothalamus deficits. The hypothalamus is in charge of such things as regulating appetite. The hypothalamus is largely mediated by two neurotransmitters: dopamine and serotonin, which initiate, maintain and then inhibit eating.

The fact that individuals with anorexia and bulimia place importance on shape and weight suggest that socio-cultural factors could also be important in its aetiology. It is argued that societal pressure to be thin promotes an internalisation of the thin ideal and body dissatisfaction, which in turn leads to dieting behaviour and creates a risk of developing an eating disorder (Stice, 2002).

Just like the societal pressure, peer pressure can affect the occurrence of an eating disorder. For instance, Eisenberg *et al.* (2005) found that the use of unhealthy weight control behaviours was significantly influenced by the dieting behaviour of close friends.

Cognitive models, such as Fairburn's (1997) weight-related schema, suggest that the over-evaluation of appearance is of prime importance in the development of eating disorders. This theory suggests that people who consider their body shape to be one of the most important aspects of their self-evaluation and who believe that achieving thinness will bring about social and psychological benefits will engage in behaviours to reduce their weight (Robles, 2011). Another cognitive model involves a distorted body image, where individuals think they are overweight even when their weight is clinically subnormal (Robles, 2011). Gupta and Johnson (2000) suggested that many people with anorexia considerably overestimate their body proportions, have a low opinion of their body shape, and consider themselves to be unattractive.

A family systems theory can account for the fact that individuals with eating disorders are embedded within a dysfunctional family structure that actively promotes the development of eating disorders (Minuchin *et al.*, 1978). According to Minuchin, families of individuals with eating disorders show enmeshment, overprotection, rigidity or lack of conflict resolution.

Severe life stresses have been implicated in the aetiology of both anorexia nervosa and bulimia nervosa, with approximately 70 per cent of cases being triggered by severe life events or difficulties (NICE, 2004). One form of adverse life experience that has been implicated as a risk factor in eating disorders is childhood sexual abuse. There is consistent evidence for higher levels of childhood sexual abuse in bulimics (Steiger *et al.*, 2000) and in anorexics (Brown *et al.*, 1997) compared to controls.

Individuals who develop eating disorders also appear to have particular personality and dispositional characteristics. Perfectionism has been implicated as a risk factor for eating disorders as well as impulsivity, low self-esteem, neuroticism and a negative or depressed mood (Robles, 2011).

Treatment for anorexia nervosa

As neurotransmitters such as dopamine and serotonin play a role in anorexia, pharmacological interventions can be used; however, there has been a limited evidence base for their use and no evidence has been found that they change core anorexic symptoms. Results of studies with SSRIs for weight restoration in patients with anorexia have revealed no benefit (Barbarich *et al.*, 2004). However, SSRIs have been shown to improve relapse rates in patients whose weight was restored prior to SSRI therapy (Kaye *et al.*, 2001). As well as this atypical antipsychotics, particularly olanzapine, risperidone and quetiapine, have been evaluated for the treatment of anorexia nervosa and have been shown to induce weight gain and improve symptoms of depression and obsessive thoughts (Powers *et al.*, 2002; Yasuhara *et al.*, 2007). All this evidence suggests that medication should not be used as the sole or primary treatment in anorexia.

For inpatients with anorexia nervosa, a structured symptom-focused treatment regimen with the expectation of weight gain should be provided in order to achieve weight restoration. It is also very important to carefully monitor the patient's physical status during refeeding (NICE, 2004). Nurses may also educate the individual about anorexia and provide more informal support and encouragement. In most patients with anorexia nervosa, an average weekly weight gain of 0.5 to 1kg in inpatients and 0.5kg in outpatients should be the aim of treatment. This usually requires about 3,500 to 7,000 extra calories a week (NICE, 2004).

Family therapy has been shown to be the treatment of choice for adolescents with anorexia nervosa (Carr, 2010). The 'Maudsley model' is the most researched form of family-based treatment (Dare and Eisler, 1997). Findings suggest a good outcome with significant rates of recovery (Eisler *et al.*, 2007; Lock and Le Grange, 2005; Eisler, 2011). Family therapy involves around 10 to 20 sessions over a 6- to 12-month period, where parents are taught to take control over their child's eating and weight. As the therapy continues the child's autonomy is linked explicitly to the resolution of the eating disorder.

Other psychological treatments for anorexia nervosa include individual therapies such as CBT which have been shown to be effective in improving outcomes and preventing relapse in weight-restored anorexia nervosa (Carter *et al.*, 2009). Also in a randomised trial of 33 patients with anorexia, Pike *et al.* (2003) found preliminary evidence that individual CBT was superior to nutritional counselling in preventing relapse following inpatient weight restoration.

Think about this

Can you identify what may have caused Lisa's eating behaviour? How would you try and confront this behaviour?

Treatment for bulimia nervosa

The National Institute for Health and Clinical Excellence (NICE, 2004) recommends CBT for the treatment of bulimia nervosa. CBT for bulimia nervosa is usually based on the cognitive model proposed by Fairburn *et al.* (1999), which comprises around 16 to 20 sessions over a period of four to five months (Wilson and Shafran, 2005). This is usually centred on three core areas which are required to deal with both the symptoms of bulimia and the dysfunctional cognitions that underlie these symptoms. These include: meal planning and stimulus control, cognitive reconstruction to address dysfunctional beliefs about shape and weight, and developing relapse prevention methods.

Another treatment for bulimia nervosa is through pharmacological methods. Although this is not the first line of treatment, there is some evidence to suggest that antidepressants, particularly SSRIs, contribute to the cessation of purging behaviours. However, there seem to be high drop-out rates due to side effects, as well as significant relapse rates of between 30 and 45 per cent between four and six months after stopping the treatment (Bennett, 2011).

8.10 Substance misuse

The criteria for harmful use (ICD-10) and substance misuse (DSM) are presented in Table 8.5. We should make it clear that 'substance' refers to alcohol, illicit drugs and volatile substances (e.g. glue). Similarly, the term 'misuse' must be emphasised. Many people use prescription medication but, for some, this may turn to misuse and result in significant consequences. For example, excessive paracetamol use can result in liver failure.

The World Health Organization (WHO, 2007) estimated the extent of worldwide psychoactive substance use to be 2 billion alcohol users, 1.3 billion smokers and 185 million drug users (of course the definition of 'illicit' drugs differs between cultures and countries). As can be noted the major substances used are alcohol and tobacco, with drug use (or substance use, more correctly) being a distant third.

Key message

Alcohol abuse is a significant health issue worldwide.

Table 8.5 ICD-10 (1992) and DSM-IV-TR criteria for harmful use and substance abuse

ICD-10 criteria for harmful use	DSM-IV-TR criteria for substance abuse
A pattern of psychoactive substance abuse that is causing damage to health, either physical or mental. The diagnosis requires that actual damage should have been caused to the mental or physical health of the user. Socially negative consequences, or the disapproval of others, are not in themselves evidence of harmful use.	A. A maladaptive pattern of substance use leading to clinically significant impairment or distress, as manifested by one (or more) of the following, occurring within a 12-month period: 1. Recurrent substance use resulting in a failure to fulfil major role obligations at work, school, or home (e.g. repeated absences or poor work performance related to substance use; substance-related absences, suspensions or expulsions from school; neglect of children or household) 2. Recurrent substance use in situations in which it is physically hazardous (e.g. driving an automobile or operating a machine when impaired by substance use) 3. Recurrent substance-related legal problems (e.g. arrests for substance-related disorderly conduct) 4. Continued substance use despite having persistent or recurrent social or interpersonal problems caused or exacerbated by the effects of the substance (e.g. arguments with spouse about consequences of intoxication, physical fights) B. The symptoms have never met the criteria for substance dependence for this class of substance.

In the UK, some 10 per cent of the population report having taken illegal drugs in the preceding year (British Crime Survey, 2009). People aged between 16 and 24 years are more likely than older people to have used drugs recently and more than a quarter (28 per cent) of all 16- to 24-year-olds had used at least one illicit drug in the year. The use of Class A drugs (the most severe) in the last year among 16- to 24-year-olds has remained stable since 1995 and stands at around 8 per cent. There may be serious consequences of substance misuse – death at the most extreme. The impact on health differs according to the drug being misused (see Table 8.6).

Key message

Substance misuse can result in significant health concerns.

Table 8.6 Illicit drug use and health consequences

Drug	Consequences
Heroin and morphine	Short-term effects include a surge of euphoria followed by alternately wakeful and drowsy states and cloudy mental functioning. Associated with fatal overdose and – particularly in users who inject the drug – infectious diseases such as HIV/AIDS and hepatitis.
Cocaine (including crack)	A powerfully addictive drug, cocaine usually makes the user feel euphoric and energetic. Common health effects include heart attacks, respiratory failure, strokes and seizures. Large amounts can cause bizarre and violent behaviour. In rare cases, sudden death can occur on the first use of cocaine or unexpectedly thereafter.
Club drugs (the most common club drugs include GHB, Rohypnol, ketamine, methamphetamine)	Chronic use of MDMA (3, 4-methylenedioxymethamphetamine) may lead to changes in brain function. GHB abuse can cause coma and seizures. High doses of ketamine can cause delirium, amnesia and other problems. Mixed with alcohol, Rohypnol can incapacitate users and cause amnesia.
Cannabis	Short-term effects include memory and learning problems, distorted perception, and difficulty thinking and solving problems.
LSD	Unpredictable psychological effects. With large enough doses, users experience delusions and visual hallucinations. Physical effects include increased body temperature, heart rate and blood pressure; sleeplessness; and loss of appetite.
Ecstasy	Short-term effects include feelings of mental stimulation, emotional warmth, enhanced sensory perception and increased physical energy. Adverse health effects can include nausea, chills, sweating, teeth clenching, muscle cramping and blurred vision.
PCP/Phencyclidine	Many PCP users are brought to emergency rooms because of overdose or because of the drug's unpleasant psychological effects. In a hospital or detention setting, people high on PCP often become violent or suicidal.
Alcohol	There are many consequences of excessive alcohol intake: CHD, stroke, diabetes, cancers, accidents, liver failure, psychiatric morbidity.

Why do people take illicit drugs?

Although there is no 'definitive list' of agreed risk factors supported by conclusive research evidence, there is general agreement that there is no single factor and that the origin of substance misuse is multi-factorial. Various psychosocial factors have been identified as significant correlates of substance use and these can vary across the lifespan (see Table 8.7). These factors range from the prenatal environment (including maternal behaviours) through to genetic factors and to wider social influences including school and socio-economic issues.

Key message

Psychosocial variables are risk variables for illicit drug use.

Table 8.7 Factors associated with illicit drug use (based on Fischer *et al.*, 2007)

Risk factor	Example
Personal factors	Gender
	Age
	Ethnicity
	Life events
	Self-esteem
	Hedonism
	Depression/anxiety
	Mental health factors
	Learning disabilities
	Genetic
Personal factors – behavioural or attitudinal	Early onset of substance use
	Other substance use
	Perceptions of substance use
Interpersonal relationships	Young parents
	Large families
	Parental divorce
	Low discipline
	Family cohesion
	Parental monitoring
	Family substance abuse/psychiatric conditions
	Peer behaviour and use
Structural-environmental and economic	Socio-economic
	Education, school performance and school management
	Drug availability

Think about this

Think about Jamie: what risk factors are present?

Treatment for substance misuse

At the outset, person-centred care is important: studies have shown that people given choices are more successful in treatment. Many of these treatments may be medical in nature, but there are a number of psychological approaches to assessing and preventing substance misuse and treating people with such problems.

In severe cases, detoxification and medically managed withdrawal will be required. Detoxification is the process by which the body clears itself of drugs and is often accompanied by significant and unpleasant side effects (some of which can be fatal). However, detoxification alone does not address the psychosocial problems associated with substance misuse and therefore does not produce long-lasting benefits.

Psychological approaches to substance misuse are many and varied but often have a cognitive-behavioural basis. A summary of the psychological interventions are presented in Table 8.8.

Table 8.8 A brief summary of the main psychological therapies used in treating substance misuse

Behavioural therapy (BT)

A structured therapy focusing on changing behaviour and the environmental factors that trigger maladaptive behaviour. Includes the following four approaches:

Cue exposure treatment (CET)

A structured treatment involving exposure to drug-related cues that have been associated with past drug use without consumption of the drug. This is intended to lead to a reduction (or habituation) of reactivity to drug cues and hence to a reduced likelihood of relapse.

Community reinforcement approach (CRA)

A behavioural approach that focuses on what the client finds rewarding in his/her social, occupational and recreational life. It aims to help him/her change their lifestyle and social environment to support long-term changes in behaviour whereby using substances is less rewarding than not using them.

Contingency management (CM)

Also known as voucher-based therapy, this aims to encourage adaptive behaviour by rewarding the client for attaining agreed goals (e.g. no use of illicit drugs as checked by urine screens) and not rewarding them when these goals are unmet (e.g. illicit drug use). Vouchers can usually be exchanged for consumer goods.

Cognitive therapy (CT)

A structured therapy using cognitive techniques (e.g. challenging a person's negative thoughts) and behavioural techniques (e.g. behavioural experiments; activity planning) to change maladaptive thoughts and beliefs.

(Continued)

Table 8.8 A brief summary of the main psychological therapies used in treating substance misuse (*Continued*)

Cognitive behavioural therapy (CBT)

A combination of both cognitive and behavioural therapies. Includes the following four approaches:

Relapse prevention (RP)

Uses several CBT strategies to enhance the client's self-control and prevent relapse. It highlights problems that the client may face and develops strategies he/she can use to deal with high-risk situations.

Motivational interviewing (MI)

A focused approach aiming to enhance motivation for changing substance use by exploring and resolving the individual's ambivalence about change.

Motivational enhancement therapy (MET)

A brief intervention based on MI which also incorporates a 'check-up' assessment and feedback.

Twelve-step approaches

Interventions used by self-help organisations like Alcoholics Anonymous. They are based on a philosophy that adopts an illness model and sees substance use as stemming from an innate vulnerability. An individual must acknowledge their addiction and the harm it has caused to themselves and others; they must also accept their lack of control over use and thus the only acceptable goal is abstinence.

Other approaches

The involvement of partners and family through marital and family therapy builds on the known social context of substance use. There are also various forms of counselling, group therapy and milieu therapy.

A number of cognitive-behavioural approaches have developed an evidence base for treating substance misuse and these include such interventions as those described in further detail below.

The National Institute for Health and Clinical Excellence (NICE) issued guidelines on psychosocial interventions for drug misuse in July 2007. It made recommendations for the use of psychosocial interventions in the treatment of people who misuse opioids, stimulants and cannabis in the healthcare and criminal justice systems. There were several key priorities for implementation:

✦ **Brief interventions:** Opportunistic brief interventions focused on motivation should be offered to people in limited contact with drug services (for example, those attending a needle and syringe exchange or primary care settings) if concerns about drug or alcohol misuse are identified by the service user or staff member.

✦ **Self-help:** Staff should routinely provide people who misuse drugs or alcohol with information about self-help groups. These groups should normally be based on 12-step principles.

✦ **Contingency management:** Drug services should introduce contingency management programmes. Contingency management is one form of behavioural therapy in which patients receive incentives for achieving specific behavioural goals. These approaches are based on operant conditioning whereby appropriate behaviour is rewarded with positive consequences and therefore more likely to be repeated. These forms of intervention have particularly strong and robust empirical support. For example, allowing a patient the privilege of taking home methadone doses, contingent on the patient providing drug-free urine specimens, is associated with significant reductions in illicit drug use (Stitzer *et al.*, 1992). Similarly, Budney, *et al.* (1998) demonstrated the efficacy of vouchers redeemable for goods and services, contingent on the patient providing cocaine-free urine specimens, in reducing targeted drug use and enhancing retention in treatment.

✦ **Contingency management to improve physical healthcare:** For people at risk of physical health problems (including transmittable diseases) resulting from their drug misuse, material incentives (for example, shopping vouchers of up to £10 in value) should be considered to encourage harm reduction.

Approaches to alcohol abuse follow the same pattern in severe cases. However, in addition, motivational interviewing approaches have strong empirical support for use in treating alcohol users and smokers, with several studies showing significant and durable effects (Dunn *et al.*, 2001; Burke *et al.*, 2003). Marijuana-dependent adults who received motivational interviewing had significant reductions in marijuana use, compared to a delayed treatment control group (Stephens *et al.*, 2000).

Quick check

List and explain the underlying reasons why people abuse substances. What can be done about these? Are some outside the scope of the healthcare professional?

8.11 The Mental Health Act

The Mental Health Act 1983, amended in 2007, is the law under which a person can be admitted, detained and treated in hospital against their wishes. It applies in England and Wales, although there are international versions available. You will hear people talking about sections of the Mental Health Act as well as people being sectioned. The sections refer to all the different parts within the Mental Health Act; these parts also include many subsections, which may become confusing. Being sectioned refers to when an individual has been admitted to hospital under force. You can be sectioned under a number of different parts of the Act for assessment or to receive treatment for a mental disorder. The term 'mental disorder' is very loosely defined under the Mental Health Act, as: 'any disorder or disability of mind'. This definition can encompass many different mental disordered conditions such as schizophrenia, anxiety disorders, depression, bipolar disorder, personality disorders, eating disorders, autistic-spectrum disorders, organic disorders such as dementia and mental disorders due to drugs. In the Act dependency on alcohol and drugs is not considered to be a mental disorder. As well as this, learning disabilities are only included in this definition when the behaviour is associated with abnormally aggressive or seriously irresponsible behaviour. The Mental Health Act also includes the rights of people while they are detained, how they can be discharged from hospital and what aftercare they can expect to receive.

Key message

The Mental Health Act (1983) was amended in 2007, and is the law under which a person can be admitted, detained and treated in hospital against their wishes.

Think about this

Why would the Mental Health Act be important in practice? Can you think about any times when this may have been used in your experience?

8.12 Conclusion

Mental health is an integral and essential component of health and encompasses a range of disorders, some of which are discussed in this chapter. Diagnosis of these is typically based on either the ICD or the DSM; however the DSM is a more widely consulted classification system for psychiatric disorders. A number of factors may contribute to the development of mental health disorders, including genetic and biological factors, socio-cultural and family factors and behavioural, cognitive and psychoanalytical factors. However, it is very likely that more than one of these is needed to explain the aetiology of a disorder, and some of these may be an effect of the disorder and not the cause, making it difficult and problematic to identify a specific cause to a disorder.

Research in Focus

Ledoux, T., Barnett, M.D., Garcini, L.M. and Baker, J. (2009) Predictors of recent mental health service use in a medical population: implications for integrated care. *Journal of Clinical Psychological Medical Settings* **16**, 304-310.

Background

Research suggests that medical patients under-utilise mental health services, even though it is estimated that 30-40 per cent of medical patients with a chronic illness experience psychological distress, typically in the form of anxiety or depression. The biopsychosocial model provides a useful framework for understanding patient factors that may predict mental health treatment rates among the medical population. This study aimed to test the ability of physical health, mental health, and psychosocial variables to predict mental health service use among medical patients. This was tested by three hypotheses. First, physical health variables including number of chronic medical conditions, bodily pain, physical functioning, and frequency of medical appointments would predict recent mental health service use among medical patients. Second, mental health variables including symptoms of anxiety and depression, and prior use of

→

mental health services would predict recent mental health service use among medical patients. And finally, psychosocial variables including referrals from a health service provider, and referrals from a non-professional (e.g. friends, family), attitudes toward mental health professionals, and perceived need for mental health services would predict recent mental health service use among medical patients.

Method

Participants: A convenient sample consisted of 240 medical patients who were recruited from general and speciality outpatient clinics. Participation required the individual be 18 years of age or older and be an outpatient in one of the clinics for which the researchers had permission to recruit participants. Participants' age ranged from 19 to 88, with a mean age of 53.

Measures: A *Demographic Questionnaire* was completed which included items about age, gender, income, education, ethnicity, and past medical history. *Prior help-seeking* was assessed which required participants to state any prior mental health treatment (i.e. psychotropic medication, individual psychotherapy, and/or group psychotherapy). *Recent mental health treatment* was assessed by participants' indication whether they had some form of mental health treatment (i.e. psychotropic medication, individual psychotherapy, or group psychotherapy) in the last 12 months. *Chronic medical illness* was determined by asking participants if they had or believed they had a chronic illness (e.g. cancer). *Referral for mental health treatment* was assessed by asking participants if they had been suggested by a GP or by a friend to receive treatment for an emotional or mental health problem. *Inventory of attitudes toward seeking mental health services* was also assessed by asking questions on attitudes towards mental healthcare. *Short Form-12* was used as a measure of physical and mental health and well-being. Finally, the *Hospital Anxiety and Depression Scale* was used to measure psychological distress, specifically anxiety and depression.

Results

43.3 per cent of the participants reported recently receiving mental health services in the form of psychotropic medication (75 per cent), psychotherapy (2 per cent), or a combination of these treatments (20.2 per cent). 16.3 per cent of participants reported having severe symptoms of depression, 23.8 per cent had moderate symptoms, and 59.6 per cent reported minimal symptoms of depression. Among patients with moderate to severe symptoms of anxiety or depression, approximately two-thirds (61.9 per cent) were receiving mental health treatment. Moreover, four variables (healthcare provider referral for mental health services, perceived need for mental health services, prior use of mental health services, and frequency of medical appointments) were significant unique predictors of recent mental health service use.

Implications

This study points out the importance of integrated healthcare that emphasises collaborative relationships between patients and medical and mental healthcare providers. Research needs to be completed to determine how best to identify those medical patients in need of mental health services in order to provide needed and more effective treatment.

8.13 Summary

- ✦ Mental health is an integral and essential component of health.

- ✦ People with mental health problems can experience problems in the way they think, feel or behave, which can affect their relationships, work and quality of life.

- ✦ There are two diagnostic classification systems used to diagnose mental illness: the DSM and the ICD. The DSM is more widely used.

- ✦ Schizophrenia is one of the most disabling mental health disorders.

- ✦ An alternative classification system identifies two clusters of symptoms: positive and negative.

- ✦ Schizophrenia can be caused by a combination of factors such as genetics, brain abnormalities, or psychosocial factors.

- ✦ Treatments for schizophrenia are largely medication-based. However, CBT and family therapies have also been shown to be effective.

- ✦ Anxiety disorders encompass specific phobias, social phobias, panic disorders, general anxiety disorder, obsessive compulsive disorder and post-traumatic stress disorder.

- ✦ Specific phobias can be explained by psychoanalytical, behavioural and evolutionary approaches and are usually treated using exposure therapy.

- ✦ The aetiology of social phobias can be explained by a genetic, developmental or cognitive perspective. Treatment mostly focuses on CBT in the form of social skills training and exposure therapy.

- ✦ Panic disorders can be explained as arising from biological, behavioural or cognitive models. CBT is widely used and is the most effective treatment.

- ✦ GAD appears to be associated with over-activation in part of the brain system as well as cognitive explanations. CBT which includes self-monitoring, relaxation, cognitive reconstruction and behavioural rehearsal is effective.

- ✦ OCD can be explained by a psychoanalytical approach; the most effective treatment is ERP.

- ✦ PTSD can be caused by experiencing a major traumatic event. PE and EMDR have shown to be effective in treating PTSD.

- ✦ Mood disorders are defined as significant disturbance in mood, and include major depression and bipolar disorder.

- ✦ Major depression is a condition where the individual experiences a significant degree of impairment. It can be explained by cognitive, behavioural and socio-cultural perspectives.

- ✦ Bipolar disorder is a condition where individuals fluctuate between periods of profound depression and manic behaviour. It can be explained by biological and psychoanalytical approaches.

- ✦ A personality disorder can be identified in three clusters: A – odd or eccentric; B – dramatic or emotional; C – fearful and anxious.

- ✦ Borderline personality disorder seems to be largely linked to experiences in childhood rejections and is difficult to treat.

+ Antisocial personality disorder seems to arise particularly from adverse social circumstances.

+ Anorexia nervosa is defined as the desire to achieve a body weight that is significantly below normal. Treatment is usually focused around family therapy and individual CT.

+ Bulimia nervosa is characterised by recurrent episodes of binge eating and compensatory behaviour.

+ The Mental Health Act is a law under which an individual can be admitted, detained and treated in hospital against their wishes.

Your end point

Answer the following questions which were asked at the beginning of this chapter to assess your knowledge and understanding of the psychology of mental health.

1. How many axes are present in DSM-IV-TR:

   (a) 1
   (b) 2
   (c) 3
   (d) 4
   (e) 5?

2. Which form of schizophrenia is characterised by 'delusions and hallucinations with themes of persecution and grandiosity':

   (a) paranoid
   (b) disorganised
   (c) catatonic
   (d) undifferentiated
   (e) residual?

3. Freud suggested what was a defence against the anxiety experienced by repressed id impulses, which results in displacement of the repressed feelings onto an object or situation:

   (a) major depression
   (b) phobia
   (c) personality disorder
   (d) bipolar disorders
   (e) schizophrenia?

4. What is the most common and effective treatment for OCD:

   (a) eye movement desensitisation
   (b) flooding
   (c) prolonged exposure
   (d) anti-depressants
   (e) exposure and response prevention?

→

5. The abuse of which substance causes the most health problems:
   (a) glue
   (b) cannabis
   (c) heroin
   (d) alcohol
   (e) Ecstasy?

Further reading

Bennett, P. (2011) *Abnormal and Clinical Psychology: An introductory textbook*. (3rd edn) New York: Open University Press.

Clarke, V. and Walsh, A. (2009) *Fundamentals of Mental Health Nursing*. New York: Oxford University Press.

Corrigan, P.W. (2007) How clinical diagnosis might exacerbate the stigma of mental illness. *Social Work* **52**(1), 31–39.

Davey, G. (2008) *Psychopathology, Research Assessment and Treatment in Clinical Psychology*. Chichester: BPS Blackwell.

Flanagan, E.H. and Blachfield, R.K. (2010) Increasing clinical utility by aligning the *DSM* and ICD with clinicians' conceptualizations. *Professional Psychology, Research and Practice*, **41**(6), 474–481.

Harvey, I. (2010) Implementation of the Mental Health Act 2007. *Nursing Standard* **24**, (51), 42–45.

Keyes, C.L., Dhingra, S.S. and Simoes, E.J. (2010) Change in level of positive mental health as a predictor of future risk of mental illness. *American Journal of Public Health* **100**(12), 2366–2371.

Nolen-Hoeksema, S. (2011) *Abnormal Psychology* (4th edn). New York: McGraw-Hill.

Shih, R.A., Belmonte, P.L. and Zandi, P.P. (2004) A review of the evidence from family, twin and adoption studies for a genetic contribution to adult psychiatric disorders. *International Review of Psychiatry* **16**(4), 260–283.

Smaldone, A. and Cullen-Drill, M. (2010) Mental health parity legislation: Understanding the pros and cons. *Journal of Psychosocial Nursing & Mental Health Services* **49**(9), 26–34.

Weblinks

www.mentalhealth.org.uk/
Mental Health Foundation. General information about mental health, specific problems, issues and treatment options.

http://www.mind.org.uk/
Mind. A leading mental health charity for England and Wales, which gives advice on how to promote and protect good mental health.

http://www.who.int/classifications/icd/en/
World Health Organization. Gives information and guidance on the use of the International Classification of Diseases (ICD).

http://www.dsm5.org/Pages/Default.aspx
American Psychiatric Association. Diagnosis and statistical manual, gives useful information about the future of psychiatric diagnosis in the DSM-5.

http://www.nice.org.uk/
National Institute for Health and Clinical Excellence. This website provides national guidance on promoting good health and preventing and treating ill health.

http://www.dh.gov.uk/
Department of Health. Information about public health, adult social care and the NHS.

Check point

Your starting point		Your end point	
Q1	B	Q1	D
Q2	E	Q2	A
Q3	D	Q3	B
Q4	D	Q4	E
Q5	E	Q5	D

Chapter 9

Developmental disorders: learning disability

Learning Outcomes

At the end of this chapter you will be able to:

✦ Understand and define both specific learning disabilities and pervasive learning disabilities

✦ Define and understand the causes of a specific learning disability: dyslexia

✦ Define and understand the causes and treatment of ADHD

✦ Define and understand the causes and treatment of autism

✦ Understand the importance of and have the knowledge to use appropriate communication with individuals with learning disabilities

✦ Have the knowledge to promote and facilitate the quality of life and emotional well-being of an individual with learning disabilities

✦ Understand psychological interventions to learning disabilities and their application.

Your starting point

Answer the following questions to assess your knowledge and understanding of learning disabilities.

1. What is the definition of learning disabilities according to the ICD?

   (a) A physical disability which renders an individual incapable of caring for themselves.
   (b) Lack of intelligence which is apparent from birth.
   (c) A condition of incomplete development of the mind.
   (d) Impairment of skills which are established through development.
   (e) Both (c) and (d).

2. How is dyslexia characterised?

   (a) A hyperactivity disorder where an individual is uncontrollable.
   (b) A disorder where one has no means of communication due to severe cognitive impairments.
   (c) A specific learning disability where the individual has specific deficits with particular skills.
   (d) A general learning disability where the individual has general deficits with intelligence.

3. How is autism characterised?

   (a) A specific learning disability where an individual has specific deficits with particular skills.
   (b) A pervasive learning disability where an individual has severe abnormalities.
   (c) A condition with communication, language and emotional disturbances.
   (d) A condition where the individual cannot concentrate on a specific task for long periods of time.
   (e) Both (b) and (c).

4. Which of the following can cause a barrier or difficulty to good communication:

   (a) cognitive impairments
   (b) speech disorders
   (c) social learning
   (d) undetected hearing loss
   (e) all of the above?

5. Which of the following statements are FALSE in relation to learning disabilities?

   (a) Individuals with learning disabilities do not have a quality of life.
   (b) Individuals with learning difficulties have experiences of quality of life.
   (c) We can measure the quality of life an individual experiences.
   (d) Quality of life is important for the well-being of an individual with learning disabilities.
   (e) Social support and inclusion are essential for quality of life.

Case Study

Judith has severe autistic spectrum learning disabilities which require a high degree of support. Judith is unable to communicate verbally and relies on other formats and processes of communication when trying to present her feelings or emotions. However, despite this, she finds it difficult to use non-verbal cues when communicating, making it very difficult for others to know when she may want something, or what that thing is.

Judith has been feeling very down lately and seems to be suffering with some form of depression. When her social worker, Kerry, goes to see her, she notices that Judith locks herself away in her room and doesn't even socialise with her family any more. Her family explain to Kerry that when she does come out of her room her behaviour becomes erratic and very challenging to deal with. Kerry is becoming increasingly worried about Judith's behaviour as it seems to be having a negative effect on her general mental health.

Kerry suggests some interventions and approaches that could be useful to help the family, and Judith herself to help understand her behaviour and how to change it to more appropriate and acceptable behaviour. The family decide to do this and after around a month Judith's behaviour is improving and she is beginning to spend more time out of the house, socialising with others and enjoying the time spent with her family.

9.1 Introduction

Within this chapter we will discuss the psychological theory behind developmental disabilities. First we will consider the disorders grouped under the broad category of learning difficulties and the problems associated with these. We will then move on to consider three specific conditions: **dyslexia, attention-deficit/hyperactivity disorder (ADHD)** and **autism**. Furthermore, we will examine the aetiology and treatment of these conditions. Once we have gained an understanding of these disorders we will proceed in considering how they may affect an individual in various ways. In particular, we will examine the effects in relation to communication, quality of life and emotional well-being. Finally, we will consider psychological ideas and approaches in developing interventions for learning difficulties and the effectiveness of these.

You are probably thinking, 'What has this got to do with me'? 'I'm not specialising in this area'. Well, the number of people in the UK who have a learning disability is estimated to be around 1,198,000, which is calculated as approximately 2 per cent of the general population (Gates, 2010). Furthermore, it is calculated that almost 298,000 children in England have a learning difficulty (Emerson *et al.*, 2010). Additionally, it is postulated that the number of children diagnosed with autism spectrum disorder and ADHD is continually increasing. For instance, the total number of individuals with profound and multiple learning disabilities increased by almost 120 per cent in the ten years between 1998 and 2008 (Glasper, 2011). Hence, it can be understood that there is an increasing need for learning disability nurses. However, the number of registered nurses who hold a qualification in learning disability nursing is significantly decreasing with approximately only 3 per cent (18,745) registered in the UK (Glasper, 2011). In addition to this, it is posited that the learning disability nurse workforce is significantly ageing. Because of this, the 2010 Nursing and Midwifery Council (NMC) standards for pre-registration training have made new curriculums adopt mandatory threads in relation to the sufficient care of people with learning disabilities throughout their courses (Glasper, 2011). All nurses will now be equipped with the skills and knowledge in order to provide care to patients with learning disabilities in line with the expectations of the NMC.

Key message

It is now essential for all nurses to have the skills and knowledge to provide excellent care to patients with learning disabilities.

Terminology

One thing that is worth mentioning is the terminology used in relation to learning disabilities. The term 'learning disability' is relatively new (Gates, 2007) and is often used within service provision and adopted by healthcare professionals (Pawlyn and Carnaby, 2009). However, another term used, specifically, within academic literature and posited to move into the professional area is 'intellectual disability'. This has been defined by the ICD-10 (WHO, 1996: 1) as: 'A condition of arrested or incomplete development of the mind, which is especially characterised by impairment of skills manifested during the developmental period, which contribute to the overall level of intelligence'.

These terms are generally adopted in describing a group of people who have significant delays in development which result in global difficulties in living and coping on a daily basis (Gates, 2007; Pawlyn and Carnaby, 2009). Therefore these terms will be used synonymously throughout this chapter.

9.2 Learning disabilities

The term learning disabilities is very broad and encompasses numerous conditions. These conditions are usually characterised by a significant impairment in an individual's intellectual functioning. IQ testing is one assessment adopted in helping to diagnose learning disabilities. The criteria an individual has to meet to be diagnosed as having a learning disability are as follows (Bennett, 2011):

✦ Its onset must be before the age of 18 years.

✦ There must not be any relation to the effects of trauma or other neurological illness,

✦ The individuals will need to score significantly below the population mean of an intelligence test (see Figure 9.1).

In addition, an individual must show evidence of an inability or failure to develop specific key skills essential for coping with the increasing demands of growing older (Bennett, 2011). However, the effectiveness of IQ testing has been criticised substantially regarding the

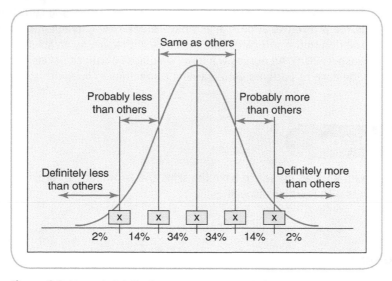

Figure 9.1 Normal distribution curve: IQ scores below the population mean

appropriateness of gaining accurate results (Barber, 2011). Thus, it has been argued that this form of measurement may not be the most efficient in determining whether, and to what extent, an individual may or may not have a learning disability.

However, the criteria used most extensively by healthcare professionals are those posited by the Department of Health (DoH, 2001a). It indicates that in order for an individual to be diagnosed with a learning disability the following have to be met:

✦ Reduced ability in understanding new and complex information,

✦ A reduced ability to develop or learn new skills,

✦ An inability to cope independently which was apparent in childhood and has had a significant effect on development.

Although this definition and criteria are the most widely accepted and used within healthcare, there are still issues that need to be considered when adopting these guidelines.

Key message

Defining learning disabilities involves the observation of reduced abilities in understanding new concepts, learning new skills and an inability to cope independently.

Quick check

What characteristics have to be apparent for a diagnosis of learning disability in an individual?

Table 9.1 Causes of learning disabilities

Causes of learning disability	Example
Genetic conditions	Down's syndrome, Fragile X syndrome
Infectious diseases	Rubella, parental syphilis, encephalitis
Environmental hazards	Lead paint and exhaust fumes in lead petrol
Antenatal events	Parental infection (including rubella), endocrine disorders such as hypothyroidism
Prenatal trauma	Asphyxia during birth

Aetiology

Research concerning the identification of the causes of learning disabilities has only accounted for approximately 25 per cent of cases – see Table 9.1.

Many researchers suggest that there is no biological cause to learning disabilities and that the environment is what predominantly influences their development. However, research concerning genetic causes (e.g. Filges *et al.*, 2011) has found that parents who may carry genes directly related to learning disabilities have a 50 per cent chance of passing it on to their children (Ghali and Josifova, 2009). Furthermore, substantial research illustrates how males tend to be more commonly affected by learning disabilities. This could be explained in relation to genetics due to the presence of genes which are involved in learning disabilities found in the X chromosome (Ghali and Josifova, 2009). However, it has been found that some of these disorders are predominantly apparent within females.

Tunnicliffe and Oliver (2011) conducted a literature review considering both biological and environmental theories in relation to individuals with learning disabilities. The authors indicate that these two theories remain quite distinct despite them being insufficient in explaining the challenging behaviours in genetic syndromes. Therefore, it was concluded that in order to gain a better insight into the underlying biological causes and the influential nature of environment, it is essential for us to adopt an integrated approach. Additionally, research concerning males who were diagnosed with learning disabilities discovered that they were most commonly from backgrounds which were economically deprived or adverse (Roeleveld *et al.*, 1997). Hence, it is essential to consider both biological and environmental influences on the development of learning disabilities.

Think about this

Thinking back to Judith, what causes could you attribute to her learning disabilities?

9.3 Dyslexia

Within this section we will discuss one form of **specific learning difficulties (SpLDs)**, namely dyslexia. Although we will be examining only dyslexia we need to acknowledge that there are many other conditions also referred to as SpDLs – see Table 9.2.

Table 9.2 Conditions associated to the term Specific Learning Difficulties

Specific Learning Difficulties	
	Dyslexia – reading, writing, automatic information processing
	Dyspraxia – motor skills
	Dyscalculia – mathematical skills
	Asperger's Syndrome – social skills
	Dysgraphia – handwriting skills
	Attention-deficit hyperactivity disorder – attention/inhibition
	Semantic pragmatic disorder - language

So, how are SpLDs any different to general learning disabilities? Well, there is an important distinction to be made between general learning disabilities and SpLDs. For instance, in the UK, learning disabilities are referred to as general difficulties in acquiring new knowledge and skills measured using an IQ test to determine cognitive ability and potential to learn. Conversely, an IQ assessment for individuals with specific learning disabilities will indicate a profile of ability where the individual may score high for many skills but poorly in others. These poor deficits are regarded as specific difficulties (Wood *et al.*, 2006). One example may be the inability to read and write efficiently, which could cause frustration for an individual.

Key message

Specific learning difficulties are defined as concerning specific difficulties rather than general cognitive ability.

Quick check

What are the differences between specific learning disabilities and general learning disabilities?

Dyslexia is a SpLD characterised as a persistent, chronic condition in which an individual's reading ability is significantly below that of the non-impaired individual (see Table 9.3 for characteristics related to dyslexia). There are a number of factors associated with dyslexia, including the inability to recognise rhymes and having difficulty naming familiar everyday objects in infancy (Araujo *et al.*, 2011; Bradley and Bryant, 1985; Wolf *et al.*, 1996). Recent research has indicated that risk factors include the slow progression through phonic phases (within school age children) (Snowling *et al.*, 2011) and even the season the infant was born in (Donfrancesco *et al.*, 2010). However, it has been indicated that there are strong genetic components underlying dyslexia, with the condition being highly heritable (Poelmans *et al.*,

Table 9.3 Characteristics found in individuals with dyslexia

Reading	Writing difficulties	Spelling	Memory	Oral and written word association
Slow reader	Freezing up when trying to write	Reverse letters in words	Poor short-term memory	Difficulty transferring talk into text.
Can't remember what you have just read	Forget sentences when trying to write them	Add or drop letters when writing	Difficulty in finding words from memory	When in higher education settings may have difficulty taking notes and listening simultaneously.
Reading out of sequence and omitting words	Miss errors when proofreading work	Inability to spell common words	Difficulty in learning sequences such as months of the year	Difficulty in comprehending words.
Mistaking words for others	When in school, teachers say your ideas are good but you have poor structure with work	Difficulty with sequence – letters and words often mixed up		Difficulty in recognising rhyme.
Skipping over words or lines – difficulty with tracking	Reduced ability in using cursive script			

2011) and it has now been argued that the main causes of dyslexia tend to be abnormalities within areas of the brain such as the temporo-parietal region (Shaywitz and Shaywitz, 2005).

We will now move on and look at theories of the aetiology of dyslexia with evidence related to genetic inheritance, cognitive impairments and brain abnormalities.

Genetic factors

It was reported as early as 1950 that a large majority of children with dyslexia also had another relative within their family with the disability (Davey, 2008). Studies have further illustrated the heritable component of dyslexia and suggest that the disability runs in almost all families pointing to a strong genetic relation (Miller, 2005). These findings have also been supported by research concerning twins which has illustrated that monozygotic (MZ) twins are significantly more likely to have dyslexia than dyzygotic (DZ) twins (Stevenson et al., 1987; Bishop, 2009). As well as this, many particular genes have been identified which are said to participate in brain development and can lead to the brain abnormalities associated with dyslexia (see Bates *et al.*, 2007; Elbert *et al.*, 2011; Scerri and Schult-Korne, 2010).

Cognitive factors and brain abnormalities

The **phonological theory** of dyslexia posits that reading disabilities evident in dyslexia are due to the individual's inability to differentiate differing elements of speech. Thus, the individual is unable to separate the spoken word in order to link the letters to its corresponding sound (Shaywitz, 2003; Shaywitz and Shaywitz, 2005). It has also been demonstrated that brain functioning may be attributed to difficulties in recognising sounds and linking them to letters. For instance, functional magnetic resonance imaging (fMRI) of children with dyslexia illustrates how they have less activation in a number of sites in their left hemisphere related to language when reading. Therefore it has been concluded that impaired functioning within the left hemisphere posterior brain systems causes the deficits associated with impaired reading (Galaburda, 1993; Shaywitz *et al.*, 2002).

Key message

There are many factors said to cause dyslexia. These include genetic, cognitive and brain structural abnormalities. Phonological theory suggests that the reading deficit associated with dyslexia is caused by difficulties in linking sounds of letters to written letters.

Quick check

What does the phonological theory suggest about dyslexia?

9.4 Attention-Deficit/Hyperactivity Disorder (ADHD)

Another learning disability we need to pay attention to is Attention-Deficit/Hyperactivity Disorder (ADHD). ADHD is mainly characterised as a persistent pattern of hyperactivity, impulsivity and inattention which is at a higher level than is appropriate for the level of development (Davey, 2008). The DSM-IV-TR has illustrated three categories in which this disorder falls: hyperactive-impulsive behaviour, poor attention and a combination of both of these, and further suggests that most children with ADHD will display both of these. In order for a child to be diagnosed with ADHD, they must have begun displaying problem behaviours before the age of seven within both school and home environments. They also have to have engaged, over the past six months, in at least six behaviours presented in Table 9.4.

Table 9.4 ADHD behaviours associated with diagnostic categories

Inattention	Hyperactivity/Impulsivity
Often fails to pay attention to detail resulting in careless errors in schoolwork, work or other activities.	Squirms in seat and often fidgets with their hands or feet.
Difficulty sustaining attention to tasks or play.	Inappropriately leaves their seat when in the classroom or other situation where remaining seated is essential.
Often appears as not listening when being told something.	Running and climbing excessively which is inappropriate within the situation. Adolescents and adults may be limited to excessive feelings of restlessness.
Often fails to complete tasks such as schoolwork, chores and duties in the workplace, and fails to follow through instructions given to them (not due to oppositional behaviour or failure to understand).	Has difficulty playing and engaging in leisure activities in a quiet manner.
Has difficulty organising tasks and activities.	Often appears driven and 'on the go'.
Avoids and is reluctant to participate in tasks which require sustained mental effort (e.g. schoolwork and homework).	Talks excessively.
Loses items and materials necessary for the completion of task or engagement in activities (e.g. toys, pencils, tools, school assignments).	Often answers questions which have been asked before they are completely asked.
Easily distracted by extraneous (irrelevant) stimuli.	Has great difficulty awaiting their turn.
Forgetful in their daily activities.	Interrupts or intrudes on others (e.g. interrupts in conversations which do not involve them).

Children with ADHD tend to have difficulty engaging with peers and developing friendships. This is often due to their inability to recognise that their behaviour is disruptive and a nuisance to others, resulting in them making social mistakes (Kofler *et al.*, 2011; Rich *et al.*, 2009). Infants with this disorder will exhibit fidgetiness and may engage in excessive activity such as running and climbing (Auerbach *et al.*, 2008; Ilott *et al.*, 2010). Conversely, they will display dislike for tasks which may be mentally demanding and find it extremely difficult to participate in calm, sedentary activities. ADHD is one of the most common disorders in the UK with approximately 25 per cent of children with ADHD suffering with some form of learning difficulty (Bennett, 2011). Consequently, due to their disruptive behaviour, these children have to attend special educational classes.

Key message

There are three categories of ADHD:

1. ADHD, predominantly inattentive type
2. ADHD, predominantly hyperactive-impulsive type
3. ADHD, combined type.

Aetiology of ADHD

There are two headings in which the causes of ADHD can be placed, namely biological and psychological. First we will discuss biological implications in ADHD as inherited factors, in particular, have been found to play a significant role in the prevalence of ADHD (Faraone and Khan, 2006).

Biological factors

First, we will discuss genetic factors which have been apparent throughout research concerning ADHD. For instance, a number of researchers have supported the supposition that there is an inherited susceptibility to ADHD. These include twin studies (see Waldman and Rhee, 2002), parent–infant studies (Quinn, 2009) and adoption studies which have found that children are more likely to present with ADHD if a birth parent has the condition than if their adopted parent has it (see Van den Oord *et al.*, 1994). However, research has met with great difficulty when trying to determine the genes that are inherited that underlie the disorder (Neale *et al.*, 2010). Nonetheless, there has been identification of particular genes related to abnormalities, in particular, the neurotransmitter systems such as dopamine have been found to be linked to ADHD (Sagvolden *et al.*, 2005). Although the genetic component has a significant stance regarding the aetiology of ADHD, it has been suggested that environmental factors may also be at play in converting a vulnerability to ADHD into the actual condition (Nikolas *et al.*, 2010).

Brain abnormalities are another area in biological factors worth mentioning. Magnetic resonance imaging (MRI) scans have revealed that children with ADHD tend to have slightly smaller brains than children without the condition (Castellanos, 2002; Durston *et al.*, 2004). It has been specified that the main areas of the brain affected include the frontal, parietal, temporal, occipital lobes, frontal cortex, basal ganglia and the cerebellum (Liston *et al.*, 2011). Furthermore, children with ADHD tend to show impairment in **executive functioning**, which is controlled by the frontal lobes (Trani *et al.*, 2011). Finally, it is further supported that abnormalities within the frontal lobes, caused by decreased volume, may be responsible for some of the symptoms of ADHD (Thorell, 2007).

Lastly, environmental toxins have previously been implicated in early accounts of ADHD. For instance, many believed that additives in children's food caused biochemical imbalances which resulted in the hyperactivity displayed in children with ADHD (see Feingold, 1979; Goyette *et al.*, 1977; Thompson *et al.*, 1989). It has also been suggested that the toxin lead is associated with the cause of ADHD (Biederman and Faraone, 2003; Waldman and Gizer, 2006; Yousef *et al.*, 2011).

> ## Key message
>
> There are many biological factors implicated in the cause of ADHD. These include genetic factors, which seems to hold most support, and abnormalities within the brain. Although environmental toxins have been said to cause biochemical imbalances, this assumption has very little empirical support.

Psychological factors

We now move on to psychological factors related to the cause of ADHD. Psychodynamic models have suggested that the parent and child interaction can play a large role in ADHD (Davey, 2008). For instance, it has been found that the parenting of children with ADHD tends to be ineffective and inconsistent. Bettelheim (1973) posited that when a predisposition is accompanied by an authoritarian parenting method, this resulted in the child displaying hyperactivity. Conversely, learning theorists have suggested that the disruptive behaviour exhibited by a child with ADHD requires attention from parents in order to control it (e.g. Healey et al., 2011). However, this attention results in reinforcement or rewarding such behaviours, increasing their occurrence (Gumpel, 2007). However, although this relationship between parent and child may exacerbate symptoms associated with ADHD, it cannot be said that it alone causes these behaviours (Johnston and Mash, 2001).

Another psychological explanation postulated is the **theory of mind** (TOM) deficits. Theory of mind is a person's ability to understand their own and others' mental states (Premack and Woodruff, 1978). A child with ADHD has great difficulty forming relationships with peers (as noted previously) and they often react in inappropriate ways due to this deficit. Although evidence has supported this theory and its relation to ADHD (Buitelaar et al., 1999), the research has not been consistent, often finding no impairment in children's TOM or any significant differences on TOM tasks (Geurts et al., 2010; Perner et al., 2002).

Treatment

How do we treat children and adults with ADHD? Approximately 90 per cent of children with ADHD are prescribed stimulant medication in order to control their behaviour (Denney, 2001). These stimulants include medications such as Adderall and Ratalin – Ratalin has been linked to side effects. When thinking of ADHD we think of hyperactivity and when thinking of stimulants, we think of hyperactivity. So, how can it be used to control the behaviour of an individual with ADHD? Well, although stimulants increase nervous system activity and behaviour in most people, when given to children with ADHD it only speeds up underactive areas which control attention, impulsivity and planning (Raphaelson, 2004). Hence, this increase in attention and focus results in an individual's hyperactivity and impulsivity naturally decreasing (Reeves and Schweitzer, 2004).

Although stimulant medication has been found to have significantly positive effects, particularly when used in conjunction with behaviour management (Chronis et al., 2004), it is not always successful in cases of ADHD. For example, children who are older, have high anxiety levels, or have less severe symptoms tend to have no effects on behaviour when prescribed medication (Gray and Kagan, 2000). In addition to this, the effects of stimulant medication have been found to increase the possibility of a cardiovascular event due to increased heart rate and blood pressure. Furthermore, it has been indicated that individuals with ADHD have a higher prevalence of cardiac pathology, which may be compounded when combined with multiple medication treatments (Elia and Vetter, 2010).

Recently, research has indicated the success of approaches which employ directed play and physical exercise in treating ADHD (Halperin and Healey, 2011). It is argued that widely used treatments such as medication and behaviour modification are, although success-ful, rarely maintained beyond the initial intervention (Halperin and Healey, 2011). However, these new approaches are successful and are potentially more enduring forms of treat-ment which promote positive brain growth in children. Furthermore, Azrin *et al.* (2006) discovered that the use of physical exercise as a reinforcer was highly effective in promot-ing attentiveness and calmness in children with ADHD. Subsequently, many mental health professionals are now recommending physical exercise several times a day for individuals with ADHD (Ratey, 2006).

Key message

Stimulant medication is the most widely used form of treatment for ADHD. However, research has indicated side effects – increased heart rate and higher blood pressure.

Exercise is a new alternative form of treatment for ADHD which is suggested to have more enduring, long-lasting effects.

9.5 Autism spectrum disorders

Finally, before moving on to communication, quality of life and emotional well-being, we will examine **autism spectrum disorders (ASD)**. These particular disabilities are characterised as pervasive developmental disorders (PDD) due to the serious abnormalities associated with them. Children with PDDs display a spectrum of impairments and delays within their devel-opment, including social and emotional disturbances, difficulty with regard to language and communication, intellectual disabilities and self-injurious behaviour patterns (Davey, 2008). The term ASD is a heading under which many disorders of differing severity and displaying autistic-style symptoms are clustered. See Table 9.5 for an example of some of the disorders associated with ASD. Within this section we will be examining one of these disorders in depth, namely **autistic disorder (AD).**

Think about this

Looking back to Judith and her behavioural characteristics, what type of autistic spectrum disorder would you diagnose her as?

Table 9.5 Autistic spectrum disorders

Disorder	Description	Estimated prevalence rate
Autistic Disorder	✦ Social interaction and communication are abnormally impaired. ✦ Activities and interests are restricted. ✦ Characterised by behaviour patterns in a significant number of cases and by intellectual disability in 70 per cent of cases.	Approximately 5 to 13 per 10,000 births
Rett's Disorder	✦ Multiple specific deficits become apparent at around 5 months of age. ✦ Previously learned hand skills are forgotten and head growth decelerates. ✦ Stereotypes: behaviour such as hand wringing and washing gestures develop at approximately 30 months. ✦ Expression is significantly impaired and apparent intellectual disability. ✦ It is a disorder which is apparent mostly in females.	
Childhood Disintegrative Disorder	✦ First two years – seemingly normal development – followed by regression in multiple areas of functioning. ✦ Regression in acquired language, social skills and adaptive behaviour. ✦ Majority of symptoms resemble symptoms of Autistic Disorder.	Approximately 0.2 per 10,000 births.
Asperger's Syndrome	✦ Social interaction is severely impaired. ✦ Develops restricted, repetitive patterns of behaviour, interests and activities. ✦ There are no apparent delays in language and communication or early cognitive development.	Approximately 3 per 10,000 births.

Autistic Disorder

Autism is a disorder with profound disruptions in an infant's development which can become apparent before the age of one. The infant will show signs of withdrawal, lack of communication and skills, and will often be unaware of or uninterested in their surrounding environment. Approximately 50 per cent of infants with autism cannot speak and never learn to but those who do have severe abnormalities. For instance, one characteristic of the speech of an autistic child is called **echolalia**. This is a form of communication in which the child rapidly repeats words or phases which have been spoken to the child in the past (Bennett, 2011). Other characteristics evident in autistic children are obsessive-compulsive and ritualistic acts. This is characterised by the child engaging in repetitive, seemingly meaningless behaviour which, if prevented, will result in displays of extreme distress (Bennett, 2011). Two significant features of this disorder are the severe impairment of an infant's social skills and their communication skills, in which the severity of impairment is dependent on the development level of the child (Davey, 2008). However, according to the DSM, in order to make a diagnosis of autism it is essential for a total of six symptoms (see Table 9.6) to be present before the age of three. Furthermore, there have to be at least two symptoms from the first section, and at least one from section two and three.

Aetiology of autism

Biological factors

Research consistently suggests that the social and language deficits, and the psychological problems associated with autism are ongoing throughout family history (Piven and Palmer, 1999; Atladóttir *et al.*, 2009). There is significant evidence to support the findings for a strong familial aggregation of symptoms related to autistic disorders. For instance, Bailey *et al.* (1996)

Table 9.6 DSM diagnosis criteria

Sections	Behaviours/symptoms
Impairment in social interaction	✦ Non-verbal communication is significantly impaired, resulting in an inability to regulate social interaction. ✦ Inability to develop peer relationships. ✦ Lacks seeking behaviour for enjoyment, interests or achievements with other people. ✦ Lack of social and/or emotional reciprocity.
Abnormalities in communication	✦ Inability or delay in acquisition of language. ✦ Individuals who are able to speak cannot initiate or sustain a conversation adequately. ✦ Repetitive use of language or idiosyncratic language. ✦ Lacks the ability to participate in make-believe play or social imitative play.
Restricted, repetitive and stereotyped patterns of behaviour, interests and activities	✦ Inflexible adherence to specific, non-functional routines or rituals. ✦ Stereotypes and repetitive motor mannerisms. ✦ Persistent preoccupation with parts of objects.

demonstrated how siblings of a child with autism have approximately a 2–14 per cent chance of also having the disorder. Twin literature has provided further support for the genetic component as concordance rates for monozygotic (MZ) twins are reported from approximately 60 per cent and sometimes as high as 90 per cent, whereas dizygotic (DZ) twins seem to be at a significantly lower rate of 5–20 per cent (see Bohm and Stewart (2009) for a review).

Autism has also been found to co-occur with other disorders which have been proposed to be genetically related. This is also supportive of an underlying genetic component (Reiss and Freund, 1990). However, despite these findings supporting the genetic predisposition, there is very limited research demonstrating which gene is responsible for the disorder. Therefore, some researchers, such as Santangelo and Tsatsanis (2005), believe that multiple genes must be accountable for the disorder – as many as 15 differing genes. It is evident that this particular disorder is highly complex and involves many differing genes which, consequently, differ in their effects on the expression and severity of the disorder.

Chromosomal disorders such as Fragile X syndrome and tuberous sclerosis have been found to have a link with autistic disorders. Thus, it is suggested that ASD can be linked to chromosomal problems, such as chromosomal duplications and inversions found within each of these disorders (Piton *et al.*, 2011; Hogart *et al.*, 2010). However, this link seems to account for less than 10 per cent of ASD cases (Folstein and Rosen-Sheidley, 2001; Reddy, 2005).

It has also been illustrated how the neurotransmitters which regulate and facilitate normal adaptive brain functioning can be linked to ASD. For instance, early research concerning children with ASD discovered that they exhibited very low levels of the neurotransmitters serotonin and dopamine, which are both associated with the efficient development of cognitive, behavioural and motor functioning (Chungani *et al.*, 1999). Nonetheless, studies within this area seem to provide inconsistent results and are plagued by methodological difficulties, making it extremely hard to obtain valid and reliable results (Lam *et al.*, 2006).

It has also been established that ASD can occur due to aberrant brain development, with autopsy studies revealing that the brains of individuals with ASD have significant abnormalities evident in numerous areas of their brain, including (Davey, 2008):

✦ **Limbic system** – neurons within this area are smaller and denser. Dendrites are shorter and underdeveloped.

✦ **Cerebellum** – abnormalities within this area correspond to difficulties in motor skills evident within individuals with ASD.

✦ **Overly large brain** – individuals with ASD tend to have larger than usual brains and enlarged ventricles.

✦ **Abnormal pattern in frontal and temporal lobes** – usually individuals have displayed clinical seizures.

These abnormalities tend to be both anatomical and functional and seem to appear within the first two years of life, where there is evidence of abnormal overgrowth (Davey, 2008).

Key message

Many factors can be attributed to the cause of ASD. Brain abnormalities such as an overly large brain, and abnormalities within the limbic system and cerebellum are becoming increasingly supported within the literature.

Psychodynamic explanations

Historically, psychological theories in relation to autism tended to focus on processes of a psychodynamic nature. For instance, it was argued that individuals adopted autism as a form of escape from hostile or uncaring settings. One of these theorists was Bettelheim (1967). The author argued that children developed autism in reaction to rejecting and unloving parents when the child could perceive their parents' negative feelings. Due to this, the child accepts that their behaviour and actions seem to have no effect on the reactions they receive from their parents. Thus, they isolate themselves believing that they have no power or influence in their world in order to protect themselves from any pain or disappointment they may incur.

As you have probably noticed, this perspective is highly irregular and insensitive to the parents of autistic children. It is also unsupported by the literature. For example, Cox *et al.* (1975) conducted a study with the parents of children who had autism and children who only had problems in understanding speech. The authors discovered that they did not differ at all in their emotional demonstrativeness, responsiveness to their children and their sociability towards their children. However, evidence has been presented which suggests that treatments of autism grounded in a psychodynamic approach can have a positive impact (Sherkow, 2011).

Key message

Early psychodynamic theories of autism believed that it was caused by the child's reaction to parents who were unresponsive and uncaring.

The biopsychosocial model of autism

Another theory postulated in explanation of autism is the psychobiological theory. Koegel *et al.* (2001) suggested that children with autism tend to withdraw from society due to their inability and lack of motivation to engage with their peers and others around them. It is suggested that this withdrawal begins early in a child's life as a result of some form of neurological dysfunction but can be intensified by parents when trying to 'help'; as whatever the child does, however they behave, they are responded to in the same way. This, and their inability to communicate socially, leads to the child using immature forms of communication, including crying for attention and pulling tantrums.

Treatment of autism

So how do we treat autism? There are many psychoactive drugs and dietary aspects that can be implemented in order to treat autism. These all cluster around a pharmacological approach to treatment. Another approach to treatment includes behavioural approaches (these will be discussed later in the section) which tend to adopt reinforcement strategies in order to establish behaviour change.

Pharmacological approaches

So what psychoactive drugs are used when treating symptoms of autism? Neuroleptics, which block the effects of dopamine, tend to be the drug most commonly used for treatment. For example, an early study which used neuroleptics, in particular haloperifol, demonstrated its effectiveness in decreasing levels of stereotypical behaviour and withdrawal in autistic children when compared with a condition group prescribed a placebo (Campbell *et al.*, 1988). In addition to this, recent research has demonstrated the positive effects of aripiprazole in improving irritable behaviour, including aggression, self-injury, and severe tantrums (Erickson *et al.*, 2011). However, there are some side effects associated with these drugs – akathisia, drooling, tiredness and so on – therefore, they need to be used in relatively low dosages and episodes (Erickson *et al.*, 2011).

Alternatively, another biological approach adopted as treatment is that of dietary control, in which the levels of casein and gluten are reduced resulting in a reduction in the amount of opiates absorbed by the gut (Bennett, 2011). For example, Harrison *et al.* (2006) conducted a study to test the efficacy of a gluten- and casein-free diet with 15 autistic children aged 2 to 16. The authors reported that parents of the children found an improvement in their children's behaviour. Furthermore, Knivsberg *et al.* (1998) studied 20 children who were split into diet and non-diet conditions and reported significant improvement in the treatment group in relation to behaviour and communication. However, both of the above studies are relatively small and preliminary (Millward *et al.*, 2004). Hence, the reliability and effectiveness of this approach is not yet convincing.

Behavioural approaches to treatment

An alternative approach to treatment is that grounded in behaviourism, in particular the concepts of classical and operant conditioning. Behavioural approaches assume reinforcement strategies in order to implement a change in behaviour. These may include behaviours such as speech or pro-social behaviours. A therapist may provide a **cue** in which they ask a question or a command of the autistic child and if the desired behaviour is displayed, will reward the child with, for example, a sweet. Alternatively, undesirable behaviours such as self-harming behaviour can be followed by aversive responses in the hope that the behaviour will decrease (Koegel *et al.*, 2001). For instance, Reichle *et al.* (2010) evaluated the effectiveness of reinforcement on increasing task engagement and decreasing challenging behaviours exhibited by autistic children. It was discovered that participants increasingly demonstrated engagement with concurrent decreases in challenging behaviour, supporting the use of reinforcement strategies.

Ivar Lovaas was a key researcher within this area and developed an intensive operant programme for children over a period of two years (Lovaas, 1987). The programme was implemented during much of the child's waking hours in which the child was continually rewarded for social behaviour and showing less aggression and punished for undesirable behaviour. When compared with another 10-hour-a-week intervention it was discovered that the IQ of the children within the two-year programme was significantly higher than those from the 10-hour treatment. In addition to this, when the children from the intensive programme were followed up four years later, the advances they had made were still evident.

Due to the considerable criticisms targeted at the study, Koegel *et al.* (2001) refined the operant condition in order to target primary factors associated with ASD. For example, the authors suggested that it was essential to target these primary factors in order to avoid the development of secondary factors (i.e. lack of communication skills may lead to severe behavioural problems). In order to do this, it was argued that reinforcement should be targeted at numerous pro-social behaviours in order to facilitate the development of communication skills. This was later adapted to allow the child to have some form of control over the reward they would receive as reinforcement (Bennett, 2011).

Key message

Autistic disorders are generally treated using psychoactive drugs. However, these can have undesirable side effects. Alternatively, behavioural approaches have been found to be effective and have no known side effects.

9.6 Communication

During Chapter 5 we discussed the importance of communication when working with our patients. We also considered the importance of understanding non-verbal communication in relation to both our own and our patients' signals. Within this section we will explore the nature of communication with patients who have learning disabilities and the barriers which we, as healthcare professionals, may encounter.

Many individuals who have learning disabilities can have difficulties with communication (Feiler and Watson, 2010; Tait and Genders, 2002). This can range from relatively minor difficulties to severe problems. For example, think back to dyslexia – one area individuals with dyslexia sometimes find difficult is in comprehending a message which has been communicated to them. Hence, we have to present the information in a manner which is more appropriate for them, be it chunking information (see Chapter 4) or providing written information. However, we know that some individuals with autism have no spoken language ability. When dealing with an individual in this situation it can be extremely difficult to grasp how that person is feeling and whether they understand the information you have provided. Therefore, it is imperative for a nurse to have an understanding of their patients' non-verbal cues. In order to build good relationships with our patients we need to have good communication skills; however, we also have to be aware of the barrier which we can encounter. Table 9.7 presents some of the difficulties and barriers which may prevent good communication.

Maximising our communication

Communication is very important in the progression to a fulfilling life – which, in turn will affect an individual's emotional well-being. Hence, it is important for you, as a nurse, to maximise your communication in relation to yourself and in looking for appropriate and comfortable ways for your patient to communicate. First, due to the complex nature of communication difficulties apparent in differing disabilities (i.e. some may have excellent verbal skills but have severe deficits in understanding and cognition and some may have difficulties with abstract concepts) it is essential that you are fully aware of your patient's communication abilities. This will enable you to begin to meet their needs in an appropriate manner and in relation to their communication. In order to fully understand your patient's communication ability you may want to have a full assessment carried out by a professional speech and language therapist (Tait and Genders, 2002). Furthermore, there are various techniques you may wish to adopt. For instance:

✦ **Sign shapes** – the use of hand shapes such as the British Sign Language or 'Makaton' Sign Language.

✦ **Symbol systems** – using symbols and pictures to represent feelings and objects.

Table 9.7 Communication difficulties and barriers

Cognitive impairment	✦ Thought processes are impaired, resulting in difficulties with understanding and perception. ✦ A large majority of individuals with a learning disability have some degree of cognitive impairment – the degree to which they have this may affect their ability to communicate effectively.
Undetected hearing loss	✦ Approximately 40 per cent of individuals with a learning disability are affected, unknowingly, with hearing loss. ✦ When this hearing loss is apparent in children, there is a significant chance that their speech will also be affected.
Speech disorders	✦ Speech disorders can vary from mild to severe disorders – often affecting individuals with profound and complex disabilities. ✦ These speech disorders can sometimes be caused by physical problems, such as a cleft lip. ✦ Speech disorders can also be due to motor disorders – affecting the nerve supply and/or muscles needed for speech production.
Social learning	✦ Individuals who have not had the opportunity to learn about communicating with others through family, friends, play and talk may behave inappropriately within a new situation. ✦ Individuals who have learning disabilities may not have been exposed to the same social learning as others, or they may not have the ability to transfer what they have learnt to different situations. ✦ Social learning is key to non-verbal communication – we learn body posture, social distance and so on. An individual who has not learned these may have significant effects on their ability to communicate.

✦ **Objects of reference** – using everyday objects to represent some other activity.

✦ **Multi-system** - mixing different techniques and systems in order to meet the needs of your patient in differing settings.

Table 9.8 presents some tips from Gates (2007) to ensure successful communication.

Think about this

Thinking about Judith and her difficulties with communication . . . knowing what you now know from reading the last section, what techniques would you adopt in order to communicate effectively with Judith?

Table 9.8 General principles for good communication practice

Principle	Action/example
Learn to step back	Allow the individual to take the lead. This includes the ability to notice small signals which your patient may make and acting upon them, or perceiving what it is that your patient wants to talk about.
Monitor	It is important that you monitor your speech in relation to the speech of your patient. Make sure you avoid dominating the conversation or talking over your patient.
Consideration	Make sure you consider the type of speech you adopt. Aim for conversational rather than controlling speech.
Adapt	Make sure you adapt the pace of your communication in a way that is suitable and comfortable for your patient. Allow plenty of time for your patient's responses.
Create opportunities	Try to provide situations where your patient may have contact with positive role models or other individuals with communication problems.
Inclusion	Try to ensure that your patient is included within a conversation – do not ignore their presence or talk for them because you think it would be easier. Inform others of how your patient communicates.
Be a role model	The way you communicate with your patient will provide others within the general public, and even within the healthcare environment, with a role model from which they can take their lead.

9.7 Quality of life

Within this section we will discuss the importance of promoting the quality of life (QOL) of individuals with learning disabilities. How can we, as nurses, support our patients in improving their QOL? Do we need to measure their QOL in order to explore ways in which it can be improved?

Quality of life (QOL)

Historically, the idea that individuals with learning disabilities had a QOL was considered scientifically suspect (Pawlyn and Carnaby, 2009). However, today, the main priority is not to determine whether individuals with learning disabilities actually have experiences of QOL but how we can learn and measure these experiences. This measurement of QOL continues to be one of the most difficult and challenging areas faced by healthcare professionals (Lyons, 2005). It is a subjective form of measurement which cannot be verified by another person alone (Colver, 2006). Nonetheless, it is an area that is significant within this field and it has been argued that it is essential for nurses to have a role in improving and promoting their patients' QOL especially in relation to promoting social skill development and social inclusion (Madden and Parkes, 2010). Quality of life has been defined as (WHO, 1997):

'an individual's perception of their position in life in the context of the culture and value systems in which they live, and in relation to their goals, expectations, standards and concerns'

QOL has been found to be a useful application within numerous areas of people with learning disabilities lives. This includes:

✦ mental health and health in general (Prasher and Janicki, 2002; Davidson *et al.*, 2003)

✦ education (Brown and Shearer, 2004)

✦ social service programmes – in particular with ageing (Bigby, 2003)

✦ accommodation (McVilly, 1995).

The ecological model and the social model both increasingly form the concept of QOL (Brown *et al.*, 2009). These models view disability as the expression of limitations one may have within a particular social context and as a core aspect which should be fully accommodated within society, retrospectively (Brown *et al.*, 2009). Thus, it is suggested that all individuals, including those with learning disabilities, have the right to live a life of quality and in order to achieve this, it is essential that the main goal is to enhance both the QOL of individuals with learning disabilities and their families (Brown *et al.*, 2009).

So how do we achieve this in our day-to-day practice? Although it is continually agreed that the measurement of QOL is a highly complex and challenging procedure, when promoting QOL it is necessary to first measure one's own QOL (Pawlyn and Carnaby, 2009). We can do this by using one of the scales, questionnaire or interview methods which have been developed. Historically, there are six approaches which have been developed within this area. These are presented in Table 9.9.

Key message

Measuring the quality of life of your patient is a very complex and challenging phenomenon.

We know about the measurements of QOL, but what about promoting QOL in individuals who have learning disabilities? First, research concerning QOL in individuals with learning disabilities consistently supports the positive effects of choice (Verdugo and Schalock, 2009). For instance, QOL is significantly improved if opportunities, decision-making and choice are made available both for patients with learning disabilities and for their families (Verdugo and Schalock, 2009). Second, it is also important to strengthen the proactive role taken by family members which will strengthen the support you give and the support network in general (Verdugo and Schalock, 2009). In addition to this, Brown *et al.* (2009) posited six principles which we should follow in applying QOL:

✦ We need to use QOL as a sensitising concept.

✦ We need to consider lifespan when applying QOL as what is done at one period of an individual's life can influence subsequent periods.

Table 9.9 Approaches to QOL measurement

Approach	Description
Multidimensional scaling approaches	These approaches measure the individual's reactions to their life experiences using psychological well-being, happiness and personal satisfaction.
Ethnographic approaches	This particular approach departs from the idea that the best way to assess one's QOL is through longitudinal research that uses naturalistic, unobtrusive observation in order to view a person's life within their natural context.
Discrepancy analysis	This approach determines the goodness of fit between one's needs and personal satisfaction of those needs. It also examines the nature of fit between a person and their environment.
Behavioural measures	This is a direct approach in which behaviours are measured in relation to changing challenging behaviour, engagement in activity, social interaction and personal freedom and autonomy.
Social indicators	This approach focuses on applying social indicators within QOL measurement. These may include indicators such as health, social welfare and standard of living.
Self-assessment	This approach allows the individual with learning disabilities to assess their own QOL. The most commonly used by QOL researchers is Participatory Action Research.

✦ Examine the perception of the people who are involved (i.e. family members) but make sure you focus on the individual's own perception in order to drive their behaviour.

✦ Determine, using observation and measurement, the choices and decisions which are important to your patient.

✦ Make sure that you take into consideration all the small aspects and recognise that these can be critical for the individual.

✦ Adopt holistic approaches which enhance the patient's (and their family's) well-being.

It is also important for you to take into account the possible need for the individual's self-image to be enhanced. For example, create opportunities for personal empowerment.

Key message

It is essential to allow your patients to take control of their choice and decisions; create opportunities for them to gain personal empowerment.

Think about this

?

After reading this section, how would you explain Judith's behaviour and depression? What could be done to avoid this in the future?

9.8 Emotional well-being

We now know about the importance of quality of life in an individual with learning disabilities, and we should have an understanding of how we can measure and promote this within our practice. Now we need to consider a factor very closely linked to QOL: emotional well-being.

Emotional well-being has been defined as:

A holistic, subjective state which is present when a range of feelings, among them energy, confidence, openness, enjoyment, happiness, calm, and caring are combined and balanced **(Pawlyn and Carnaby, 2009).**

Emotional well-being is bound up closely with issues surrounding quality of life (as noted above) (Moss *et al.*, 2000). There are many strong overlaps in concepts and defining aspects apparent within the two with emotional well-being being closely associated with one's ability to establish meaningful relationships and self-control. Thus, it is a very important aspect in relation to one's health and mental health. We need to note that this aspect is of high importance in relation to individuals with learning disabilities as it has been demonstrated that these people are at more risk of experiencing mental health difficulties than the general population (Hunt and Tarleton-Lord, 1998).

Key message

🔑

Emotional well-being is very important in people with learning disabilities due to their susceptibility towards mental health difficulties.

9.9 Psychological approaches

In Chapter 2 we discussed, in detail, the main psychological theories developed in order to explain human thought and behaviour. We will now move on and examine how psychological approaches can be applied within the area of learning disability nursing. We will consider how these theories can be applied both to our patients and to ourselves, as healthcare professionals, in order to improve individuals' health and healthcare in general.

Promoting health and healthy lifestyle choices

Psychological knowledge and understanding can have a huge influence in helping people to adopt healthier choices in relation to the identification of key areas critical for promoting behaviour change. Berry (2004) identified five models of health belief through her exploration of cognitive factors such as knowledge and beliefs in decision-making about health. She names three of these as expectancy models, which assumes that an individual does not choose a particular course of action on their knowledge alone, but also considers actions needed to achieve the outcome and estimating how important the outcome would be. Let us look at an example of a gentleman who smokes:

✦ **Knowledge** – He may know that smoking will result in serious diseases. However, this alone will not be enough to make him quit smoking.

✦ **Action** – He may not believe that he has the willpower to quit smoking. However, if he does believe that he can persist with quitting he will go on to the next step.

✦ **Outcome** – He may or may not believe that the outcome is worthwhile. For instance, he may believe that the money that could be saved will only be spent on other unnecessary products.

This model has produced much support for its explanations of how an individual will make a choice. However, when applied within health promotion activity it does not seem to yield consistent results (Rutter and Quine, 2002). Nonetheless, Berry (2004) has indicated that this may be due to the model only considering behaviour in relation to health while completely ignoring other influencing factors, such as wanting to look good and avoid putting on weight. Hence, in order for the application of this model to prove fruitful it is essential that we modify incentives appropriately for an individual.

So, how can we apply these general models to our healthcare with individuals with learning disabilities? As far as the literature is concerned, there is a large and growing amount of information which supports the idea that it can work. However, there are some additional points that have been suggested in order to gain successful results. First, we must assume that individuals with learning disabilities have the same interest in their health as the rest of the population (Gates, 2007). It is also essential that, as do the general population, we do not ignore that individuals with learning disabilities also have other persuasive factors influencing their behaviour. Second, we need to be aware that we may need to take additional steps to ensure that the needs of our patients with learning disabilities are met. This includes us having the understanding to take into account our patients' experiences when considering the role of self-efficacy in influencing behaviour change (Gates, 2007). Thus, it may be appropriate for you, as a healthcare professional, to enquire into your patient's decision-making experiences – as many individuals with learning disabilities have not had the opportunity to make decisions about their health (Shaughnessy and Cruse, 2001; Alaszewski et al., 1999; Feiler and Watson, 2011). Finally, we need to take into consideration the communication skills of our patient in order to adapt the way we communicate any information, while making it relevant to the patient's life (Turnbull et al., 2005). Once considered, these factors should all contribute to the successful application of health promotion to individuals with learning disabilities.

Behavioural theory – promoting behavioural change

Psychological knowledge is most often used to implement behaviour change with a patient with regard to health promotion. Behavioural approaches are by far the most widely used approach when targeting challenging behaviours and improving self-esteem within patients with learning disabilities. Challenging behaviours displayed by patients with learning disabilities are characterised by numerous behaviours which may put people's safety at risk, resulting in mainstream services being denied (Emerson *et al.*, 1998). Behavioural approaches assume that the challenging behaviour that one might display has a function or a purpose for that person – becoming loud by shouting and screaming may gain attention for that individual. In addition, behaviourists emphasise the importance of an individual's environment in establishing or provoking challenging behaviour (Gates, 2007). This assumption has been supported by findings which demonstrated that approximately 90 per cent of challenging behaviour was explained by the environment (Iwata *et al.*, 1994).

So how do behavioural approaches translate into interventions? It is essential to start with a process of assessment in which we determine what the function of a particular behaviour is to that individual. It is important to focus on what is influencing and maintaining that particular behaviour at a particular time; this is due to the finding that one particular behaviour may have a different function at various times (Kiernan *et al.*, 1997). In order to do this, behaviourists may observe the behaviour directly as it happens, and conduct interviews with parents or care staff (Gates, 2007). This entails the completion of a simple form called the ABC chart (see Figure 9.2) – Antecedent, Behaviour and Consequence.

Second, an explanation for the behaviour will be determined, which will vary dependent on the individual. Table 9.10 displays the four main categories which have been developed to explain the function of behaviour (O'Neill *et al.*, 1990).

Finally, after taking these factors and the environment into consideration, we are able to develop a functional hypothesis from which an intervention plan can be constructed. These interventions must be constructive in nature, aiming to replace challenging behaviour with subsequent functional behaviour (Goldimond, 1974). This approach is arguably the most ethical and empirically founded approach (Gates, 2007). In addition, self-management approaches have now become more common in relation to individuals with learning disabilities. Here, an individual is taught how to develop alternative antecedents and consequences for a particular challenging behaviour (see Turnbull, 1994). This particular approach has been found to produce long-lasting changes in which the individual is involved with both their targets and reinforcement (Korinek, 1991).

Cognitive-behavioural theory

We have examined how behavioural approaches are used in order to change the way individuals act. But what about their thought processes and the way they think about that

Antecedent	Behaviour	Consequence
The teacher places James' work folder on his desk in front of him.	James sweeps his folder and pencil onto the floor.	The classroom aide puts James in the time out corner. He escapes doing his work.
At lunch, James sees that Martin has yogurt.	James bangs himself on the head with his fist at the lunch table.	Martin gives James his yogurt. He acquires the desired object.

Figure 9.2 ABC (Antecedent-Behaviour-Consequence) chart

Table 9.10 O'Neill *et al.* categories for functions of behaviour

Category	Description
Escape or avoidance of aversive situations	They adopt a particular behaviour as it may help them to escape the demands to take part in an activity or avoid being asked to do them altogether.
Increased social contact	They adopt a particular behaviour as it results in greater social contact.
Adjustments of levels of sensory stimulation	Adoption of a particular behaviour will result in either the increase or decrease of the level of stimulation (decreasing the level overlaps with the category of escape from demand situations).
Increased access to preferred objects or activities	They adopt a particular behaviour as it results in access to a preferred activity.

Source: based on O'Neill *et al.*, 1990

behaviour? Cognitive-behavioural approaches are combined in order to produce a therapeutic technique which targets the way individuals act as well as how they think. These particular approaches assume that cognitive events (such as thoughts and expectations) underlie all human behaviour. Because of this, cognitions are the main target of intervention.

Cognitive behaviourists posit that a large majority of people tend to display problematic thoughts and assumptions; however these only become a problem in relation to their behaviour when the individual reacts in an extreme manner (Gates, 2007). For instance, an individual may lose their job and feel sadness for a few days. However, if these feelings intensify and are prolonged over weeks or even months, then therapeutic help may be advantageous to that individual.

This particular approach is characterised by a collaborative relationship in which the therapist and their patient share information and discuss any options available to them. Initially, the therapist may use a range of paper-based and conversation-based assessments; this enables the therapist to gain an insight into how the individual might perceive their world. The sessions then create opportunities where the individual and the therapist may identify and challenge their patterns of behaviour. This involves role-playing and homework tasks which will eventually lead to the individual being able to become their own therapist (see Turnbull *et al.* (2001) for an example).

Think about this

Think about each of these approaches and how they could be adapted to Judith's situation. Are there any barriers that you can think of? How do you think these could be overcome?

So what difficulties are associated with this approach? How can it be applied to individuals with learning disabilities? Obviously, due to the difficulties some people with learning disabilities may have with communication, it has been argued that these talking therapies may not produce the most effective results. However, Hurley *et al.* (1998) adopted an adapted version of this approach suitable for individuals with learning disabilities where ideas and language were simplified to an appropriate level. Thus, the effectiveness of these approaches has now been supported empirically (e.g. Taylor *et al.*, 2002; Sturmey, 2006).

Key message

The ability of individuals to have access to a greater range of therapeutic approaches is a significant positive development.

Research in Focus

Marshall, D., McConkey, R. and Moore, G. (2003) Obesity in people with intellectual disabilities: The impact of nurse-led health screenings and health promotion activities. *Journal of Advanced Nursing* **41**(2), 147-153.

Background

Although obesity tends to be more apparent among individuals with learning disabilities, few studies have aimed to achieve weight reduction. Therefore, this research aimed to: first, follow up on individuals who had previously been identified as overweight at a special health screening clinic and identify the actions which were taken. Second, to provide an evaluation of any impact of health promotion classes on the individuals.

Methods

Four hundred and sixty-four participants aged 10 years and above were recruited to a clinic held by two learning disability nurses in accordance with one Health and Social Services Trust in Northern Ireland. A second study recruited 20 participants to take part in health promotion classes.

Findings

Following the health screening 64 per cent of adults and 26 per cent of 10- to 19-year-olds were identified as being overweight. However, a follow-up questionnaire revealed that only 34 per cent of participants reported having lost weight after being identified for weight reduction action. Alternatively, the health promotion classes led to significant reduction in weight and body mass index scores.

Conclusions

Due to the limited impact of health screening on reducing obesity levels, health personnel need to work in conjunction with other service staff and the individuals with learning disabilities to promote active lifestyles.

9.10 Conclusion

It has now become essential for all nurses, regardless of their speciality, to learn and have an understanding of how to care for an individual with learning disabilities. This has led to the integration of mandatory modules regarding patients with learning disabilities into all nursing courses. Due to the communication difficulties associated with patients with learning disabilities, it is essential for nurses to have the ability to adjust information within an appropriate format. Although it was previously suggested that individuals with learning disabilities did not experience QOL, the importance of promoting QOL for all patients is now highly regarded within professional practice.

9.11 Summary

✦ The number of people in the UK who have a learning disability is currently approximately 1,198,000 – around 2 per cent of the general population.

✦ The number of children diagnosed with autism spectrum disorder and ADHD is continually increasing; the total number of individuals with profound and multiple learning disabilities increased almost 120 per cent from 1998 to 2008.

✦ The 2010 NMC standards for pre-registration nursing training have created the need for new curriculums to adopt mandatory threads in relation to the sufficient care of people with learning disabilities evident.

✦ The terms 'learning disability' and 'intellectual disability' are used synonymously.

✦ These terms are generally adopted in describing a group of people who have significant delays in development which result in a whole range of difficulties in living and coping on a daily basis.

✦ IQ testing is one assessment for diagnosing learning disabilities.

✦ The Department of Health indicates that for an individual to be diagnosed with a learning disability they have to have: reduced ability in understanding new and complex information; a reduced ability to develop or learn new skills; an inability to cope independently which has a significant effect on development.

✦ Defining learning disabilities involves the acknowledgement of reduced abilities in understanding new concepts, learning new skills and an inability to cope independently.

✦ Specific learning difficulties are defined as concerning specific difficulties rather than general cognitive ability.

✦ Dyslexia is a SpLD characterised as a persistent, chronic condition in which an individual's reading ability is significantly below that of the non-impaired individual.

✦ ADHD is mainly characterised as a persistent pattern of hyperactivity, impulsivity and inattention which is at a higher level appropriate for the level of development.

✦ Autism spectrum disorders are characterised as pervasive developmental disorders due to the serious abnormalities associated with them.

✦ Many factors can be attributed to the cause of ASD. Brain abnormalities such as an overly large brain, and abnormalities within the limbic system and cerebellum are becoming increasingly supported within the literature.

✦ Many individuals who have learning disabilities can have difficulties with communication.

✦ In order to build good relationships with our patients we need to have good communication skills; however, we also have to be aware of the barriers we can encounter.

✦ Measuring the Quality of Life of your patient is a very complex and challenging phenomenon.

✦ It is essential to allow your patients to take control of their choice and decisions; create opportunities for them to gain personal empowerment.

✦ Emotional well-being is very important in people with learning disabilities due to their susceptibility towards mental health difficulties.

✦ Behavioural approaches and cognitive-behavioural approaches are both psychological approaches which are used in order to treat learning disabilities.

Your end point

Answer the following questions to assess your knowledge and understanding of learning disabilities.

1. According to the Department of Health, in order to be diagnosed with a learning disability which of the following have to be met?

   (a) Reduced ability in understanding new and complex information.
   (b) A reduced ability to develop or learn new skills.
   (c) An inability to cope independently which was apparent within childhood and has had a significant effect of development.
   (d) All of the above.
   (e) None of the above.

2. Somebody with Asperger's Syndrome has difficulty with:

   (a) motor skills
   (b) social skills
   (c) mathematical skills
   (d) handwriting skills
   (e) reading skills?

3. A child with ADHD will:

   (a) develop friendships with peers
   (b) develop friendships with adults only
   (c) have difficulty developing friendships
   (d) be sullen and uncommunicative
   (e) sit quietly and read?

→

4. Which is an approach to measuring QoL:

    (a) multi-dimensional scaling approaches
    (b) ethnographic approaches
    (c) discrepancy analysis
    (d) behavioural measures
    (e) all of the above?

5. What is the major determinant of challenging behaviour:

    (a) the environment
    (b) the food people eat
    (c) inappropriate communication
    (d) all of the above
    (e) none of the above?

Further reading

Barber, C. (2011) Understanding learning disabilities: An introduction. *British Journal of Healthcare Assistance* **5**(4), 168–169.

Bettelheim, B. (1967) *The Empty Fortress*. New York: Free Press.

Biederman, J. and Faraone, S.V. (2003) Current concepts on the neurobiology of attention-deficit/hyperactivity disorder. *Journal of Attention Disorder* **6**(1), 7–18.

Buitelaar, A.J., van der Wees, M., Swaab-Barneveld, H. and van der Gaag, R. (1999) Theory of mind and emotion-recognition functioning in autistic spectrum disorders in psychiatric control and normal children. *Development and Psychopathology* **11**, 39–58.

Curtis, K., Tzarnes, A. and Rudge, T. (2011) How to talk to doctors: A guide for effective communication. *Nursing Standard* **58**(1), 13–20.

Department of Health (2001) *Valuing people: A new strategy for learning disabilities for the 21st century*. London: The Stationery Office.

Gates, B. (2007) *Learning Diabilities: Toward Inclusion*. (5th edn.) Elsevier: Churchill Livingstone.

Jillian, P. and Carnaby, S. (eds) (2009) *Profound Intellectual and Multiple Disabilities*. Oxford: Wiley-Blackwell.

Miller, G. (2005) Genes that guide brain development linked to dyslexia. *Science* **310**(5749), 759.

Weblinks

http://tinyurl.com/learndis-england-2010
People with learning disabilities in England. A useful website giving a general discussion of learning disabilities within England and their prevalence.

http://www.mencap.org.uk/all-about-learning-disability/about-learning-disability
Mencap – Useful site with loads of information regarding many areas of learning disabilities, including information for parents, carers and family.

http://www.rcpsych.ac.uk/mentalhealthinfoforall/problems/learningdisabilities.aspx
Psychological website – discusses learning disabilities and the psychological assumptions behind them.

http://www.learningdisabilities.org.uk/
Informative website with publications and updated news regarding their work around learning disabilities.

Check point

Your starting point		Your end point	
Q1	C	Q1	D
Q2	C	Q2	B
Q3	C	Q3	C
Q4	E	Q4	E
Q5	C	Q5	A

Glossary

ABC model Model developed by Albert Ellis, characterised by a link between how an event is perceived and the behavioural and emotional consequences of that event.

Acupuncture The technique of using fine needles, positioned in specific areas of the body, as a means of stimulating the body's natural healing response in order to restore balance.

Acute pain A short-term pain arising from physical injury.

A-delta fibres Types of sensory fibres that relay pain information very quickly.

Alogia Literally wordless, but usually taken to mean impoverishment of thought inferred from poverty of speech or poverty of content.

Anal stage Second stage of psychosexual development in which the ego is developed.

Antigens Proteins on the surface of cells that identify them as native or foreign.

Anxiety A state of uneasiness, accompanied by dysphoria and somatic signs and symptoms of tension, focused on apprehension of possible failure, misfortune or danger.

Anxiety disorders An excessive or aroused state characterised by feelings of apprehension, uncertainty and fear.

Appraisal Thought processes used to evaluate potential stressors.

Asperger's Disorder A pervasive developmental disorder characterised by severe and sustained impairment in social interaction together with restricted, repetitive, or stereotypical patterns of behaviour, interests or activities, causing clinically significant impairment in everyday living, without the language and cognitive deficits characteristic of autistic disorder but in other ways similar to it, usually found in males.

Attention-Deficit/Hyperactivity Disorder (ADHD) A mental disorder of childhood affecting between 2 and 10 per cent of school-age children worldwide, at least three times as common in boys as in girls, characterised by persistent inattention, hyperactivity or impulsivity, with some of these signs and symptoms appearing before the age of seven, causing problems at school or work and in the home, and interfering significantly with social, academic or occupational functioning.

Attitude An enduring pattern of evaluative responses towards a person, object or issue.

Autism Spectrum Disorder (ASD) An umbrella term for a group of mental disorders ranging from Asperger's Disorder at the mild end to Autistic Disorder at the severe end.

Autism An alternative name for Autistic Disorder.

Autistic Disorder A pervasive developmental disorder characterised by gross and sustained impairment of social interaction and communication; restricted and stereotypical patterns of behaviour, interests and activities; and abnormalities manifested before age three in social development, language acquisition or play.

Autonomic nervous system (ANS) Part of the peripheral nervous system that participates in the regulation of the body's internal environment.

Avolition An inability to initiate or sustain purposeful activities.

Behaviourism Movement in psychology, also known as the learning perspective: everything we do is the result of learning. A perspective aimed at transforming psychology into an objective science through the omission of subject matter that is not observable.

Biofeedback The technique of using feedback on activities within the body as a means of training individuals to control these activities.

Biopsychosocial model A general model or approach that posits that biological, psychological and social factors all play a significant role in human functioning in the context of disease or illness.

Bipolar disorder (BD) A condition in which individuals fluctuate between periods of profound depression and manic behaviour.

Bottom-up processing Stimulus driven – directly affected by the stimulus you put in.

C fibres Slower sensory fibres.

Cartesian dualism Refers to Descartes' theory of duality of mind and body, or that the mind and soul are separate from the body but they work in harmony.

Castration anxiety Phenomenon referred to in Freud's theory of psychosexual development, in which the son fears castration by his father as a result of his feelings towards his mother being uncovered.

Catastrophising Refers to the beliefs that things are awful and can only get worse.

Catatonic behaviour Refers to behaviour characterised by a significant decrease in reactivity to the environment, maintaining rigid, immobile postures, resisting attempts to be moved, or purposeless and excessive motor activity that often consists of simple, stereotyped movements.

Catharsis The release of emotional tension.

Central nervous system (CNS) A division of the nervous system made up of the brain and spinal cord.

Cerebral artery Arteries supply blood to the cerebral cortex.

Childhood Disintegrative Disorder A pervasive developmental disorder characterised by at least two years of apparently normal development followed by significant loss of language abilities, social skills, bowel or bladder control, motor skills, or play, together with impairment in social interaction and communication, or restricted, repetitive or stereotypical mannerisms, interests or activities.

Chronic disorder A disorder such as back pain or arthritis that is persistent and long-lasting in nature.

Chronic pain A long-term pain, outliving any original tissue damage.

Chunking Combining smaller pieces of information into larger chunks of information.

Classical conditioning etc. Associative learning in which a behaviour is learnt through its pairing with an unconditioned stimulus, eventually resulting in the learnt stimulus evoking a conditioned response in the absence of the unconditioned stimulus.

Cognitions Thought processes in which information is perceived, acknowledged and/or processed.

Cognitive appraisal The personal interpretation of a situation.

Cognitive behavioural therapy (CBT) Form of therapy that emphasises the role of thought in changing our behaviour and emotional responses.

Cognitive dissonance Conflict or anxiety arising from the existence of two contradictory feelings, beliefs or actions.

Cognitive hypothesis model of compliance Was developed by Phillip Lay and explains that patient compliance can be predicted by patient satisfaction and understanding of a consultation and the ability to retain and recall this information.

Cognitive impairment A slight impairment in cognitive function with otherwise normal function in the performance of activities of daily living.

Cognitive psychology Division of psychology focused on internal mental processing.

Cognitive revolution Stage in the history of psychology in which behaviourism (focused on objective observable phenomena) was replaced with an acceptance of the role of internal processes.

Cognitive therapy (CT) A form of psychotherapy based on the belief that psychological problems are the products of faulty ways of thinking about the world.

Comorbidity Refers to the co-occurrence of two or more distinct disorders.

Compliance A form of social influence in which a person yields to explicit requests from another person or other people. Also called social compliance.

Conditioned response A learnt response.

Conditioned stimulus A previously neutral stimulus which through associations with an unconditioned stimulus has become a trigger for a conditioned response.

Conformity A form of social influence in which a person yields to group pressure in the absence of any explicit order or request from another person to comply.

Conscious A mental state in which events and thoughts are perceived.

Context-dependent learning Learning, the recall of which is dependent on the reproduction of certain aspects present in the context in which it was learnt.

Control The extent to which a person feels they are able to change their own circumstances.

Control methods A group that does not receive treatment in an experiment is known as the control group. This group receives a control method, a method similar to that of the treatment group but lacking the key component (e.g. a control method in an experiment looking at a new type of drug would be the distribution of a placebo to the control group).

Cortex The outer layer of the brain.

Cue A stimulus that provides information about what to do.

Defence mechanisms From Freudian theory, mental strategies for reducing the emotional distress experienced by the awareness of an unacceptable or traumatic thought or memory.

Demand characteristics Refers to the event in which a participant involved in experimental research interprets the purpose of the research and adjusts their response to the situation according to this interpretation.

Denial Rejection of information presented.

Deterministic Philosophical view that every event is caused by a preceding chain of events.

Dialectical behaviour therapy (DBT) A form of cognitive behavioural therapy specially designed for the treatment of bipolar disorder and sometimes to treat other personality disorders.

Displacement Emotions which cannot be directed at the person from whom they stem are directed towards a substitute target.

Distraction Diversion of attention away from a given stimulus.

Dorsal horns One of the two roots of a spinal nerve that passes dorsally to the spinal cord and that consists of sensory fibres.

Dysfunctional schemas In personality disorders, these refer to a set of dysfunctional beliefs that are hypothesised to maintain problematic behaviour characteristic of a number of personality disorders.

Dyslexia Impairment in ability to read, not resulting from low intelligence. It was first described in 1877 by the German physician Adolf Kussmaul who coined the term word blindness to refer to it.

Eating disorders Refer to disturbances or problems associated with eating.

Echoic stores (auditory store) Store for auditory information.

Echolalia A pathological, parrot-like repetition of overheard words or speech fragments, often with a mocking intonation, symptomatic of some mental disorders, including: catatonic schizophrenia, latah, pibloktoq and some tic disorders.

Ecological validity Reflects real-life situations and circumstances.

Egocentric/Egocentrism Self-centredness, a term given a technical meaning in 1926 by Jean Piaget to denote a cognitive state in which a child in the pre-operational stage of development comprehends the world only from its own point of view and is unaware that other people's points of view differ from its own. It implies a failure to differentiate subjective from objective aspects of experience, and it therefore imposes the unconscious personal bias on cognition.

Ego One part of the personality as divided by Freud. Based on the reality principle, this component works to achieve the aims of the id in the long term, identifying and overcoming likely obstacles to this goal.

Electra complex Female equivalent of the Oedipus complex.

Electroconvulsive therapy (ECT) A treatment for some depressions and other mental disorders by administering anaesthetic and a muscle relaxant drug and then passing an electric current through the brain to induce either convulsion or coma.

Electromyography (EMG) Measurement tool for assessing and recording activity levels in the muscles.

Emotion-focused coping Dealing with a problem by focusing on your emotional response to it.

Encoding The organisation of information into a form that can be retrieved and stored.

Executive functioning A part of the working memory containing both a short-term memory store and an executive processor that operates on and briefly stores information and plays an important part in language comprehension.

Existentialism A philosophy that emphasises the uniqueness and isolation of the individual experience in a hostile or indifferent universe, regards human existence as unexplainable, and stresses freedom of choice and responsibility for the consequences of one's acts.

Exposure and response prevention A treatment for obsessive compulsive disorder which involves graded exposure to the thoughts that trigger distress, followed by the development of behaviours designed to prevent the individual's compulsive rituals.

Exposure therapy Treatment where sufferers are helped by the therapist to confront and experience events and stimuli relevant to their trauma and their symptoms.

External LoC View that all actions are controlled by a force external to the individual such as luck.

Extinction Removal of a learnt response through a lack of reinforcement to the point that the association no longer exists.

Eye movement desensitisation and reprocessing (EMDR) A treatment for post-traumatic stress disorder where individuals are required to focus their attention on the traumatic memory while simultaneously visually following the therapist's finger moving backwards and forwards.

Family therapy A form of psychotherapy based on the assumption that psychological problems are often rooted in and sustained by family relationships, in which two or more members of a family participate simultaneously with the aim of improving communication and modes of interaction between them.

Feminine Oedipus attitude Renamed as the Electra complex by Jung, this refers to the young girl's fixation on her father as a love interest.

Fixation Event in which the ego's energy is tied up with a conflict at a particular stage in psychosexual development resulting in the presentation of behaviours typical of this stage.

Gate control theory Theory of pain in which pain is the result of pain messages negotiated by a gate, which in turn is opened or closed by various biological, psychological and social factors.

Genital phase The final stage of psychosexual development as outlined by Freud.

Grey matter Mass of neuronal cell bodies.

Health belief model (HBM) A psychological model attempting to explain health behaviour through a consideration of perceived susceptibility, severity, benefits, barriers, cues and self-efficacy.

Health LoC The location in which control for health is placed, e.g. externally or internally.

Health value The value people attach to their health and how it compares to other considerations in their life.

Hypnosis The act of producing a suggested state similar to that of sleep.

Iconic store (visual store) Store for visual information.

Id The earliest component of personality, as identified in Freudian theory. Working on the pleasure principle, the id is responsible for attempting to fulfil instincts or natural drives through any means.

Idiographic approach Focuses on people as individuals with the view that no two people are alike.

Imagery The formation of mental images.

Information processing approach An approach within cognitive psychology which views the brain's function as that of a computer in order to understand human thinking.

Internal LoC View that all actions are controlled by the individual.

Introspective approach The study of human consciousness which involves research participants reporting on their own internal thought processes.

Latency period Fourth stage of psychosexual development, a rest period for the libido.

Law of effect View that responses which elicit a positive outcome will increase in frequency as a result of that positive outcome.

Learned helplessness Situation in which individuals or animals have learnt to act helpless in response to a given stimulus.

Linear-biomedical model One line or pathway which is biological in nature.

Locus of control (LoC) The location in which control for something is placed (e.g. externally or internally).

Major depression A condition where the individual experiences a significant degree of impairment as a result of depression.

McGill pain questionnaire Multi-modal self-report pain survey.

Medical intervention Refers to medical procedures or applications that are intended to relieve illness or injury.

Medical literacy An individual's ability to read, understand and use healthcare information to make decisions and follow instructions for treatment.

Medical model Approach to an issue taken by Western medicine.

Memory The retention of and ability to recall information.

Mindfulness Refers to being completely in touch with and aware of the present moment, as well as taking a non-evaluative and non-judgemental approach to your inner experience.

Mindfulness-based cognitive therapies (MBCT) A form of treatment which has been developed to prevent relapse in recovered depressed individuals by making them aware of negative thinking patterns that may trigger subsequent bouts of depression.

Mindfulness meditation training (MMT) Teaches patients to increase awareness of their immediate experiences through intensive meditative practice.

Modelling Responding to a given stimulus based on behaviours observed by another, also known as observational learning.

Mood disorders A significant disturbance in mood.

Multi-modal methods Use of a combination of more than one approach or model.

Negative reinforcement The absence or avoidance of a negative outcome or activity.

Negative symptoms Symptoms of affect flattening, alogia and avoliation in schizophrenia.

Nervous system Network of nerves.

Neurons Cells in the nervous system which relay information.

Neuropathic pain Pain occurring from within the nervous system itself which may originate from the peripheral nervous system or from the central nervous system.

Neuroses Used to refer broadly to psychological disorders, such as anxiety, depression and irrational fears, but without psychotic symptoms such as delusions or hallucinations.

Nociceptive pain Pain resulting from the stimulation of specific pain receptors.

Nominal fallacy When you apply a label or name to something as explanation.

Non-nociceptive pain Pain arising from within the peripheral and central nervous system.

Non-verbal communication Any form of communication apart from language including paralanguage, facial expressions, communicative gaze and eye contact, kinesics and proxemics.

Obedience A form of social influence in which a person yields to explicit instructions or orders from an authority figure.

Object permanence The awareness that an object continues to exist even when it is not in view.

Observational learning Learning through observing someone.

Oedipus complex Conflict within the phallic stage of psychosexual development in which the young boy fixates on his mother as a love interest.

Operants An influence, having an effect on something.

Oral stage First stage of psychosexual development, the outcome of which is predicted to influence trust factors in adult personality.

Paradigm A set of beliefs that are taken as fact, the generally accepted perspective in a discipline.

Pattern theory Developed by Glodschneider and suggests that the pattern of nerve impulses determined the degree of pain and that messages from the damaged area were sent to the brain via these impulses.

Penis envy Reaction by young girls to their realisation that they do not have a penis.

Personal agency The humanistic term for exercising free will.

Personality disorders (PD) Categorised by pervasive, inflexible and enduring patterns of cognition, affect, interpersonal behaviour or impulse control that deviate markedly from culturally shared expectations and lead to significant distress or impairment in social, occupational, or other important areas of functioning.

Person-focused approach A non-directive approach to being with another, which believes in the other's potential and ability to make the right choices, regardless of the therapist's own values, beliefs and ideas.

Persuasion The process by which an attitude change is brought about. Usually persuasion takes the form of a message that contains arguments for and against a particular attitude and is targeted towards a particular audience.

Persuasive communication A process by which attitude change is brought about by a message intended to change an attitude and related behaviours of an audience.

Phallic stage Third stage of psychosexual development in which the Oedipus and Electra complexes supposedly occur.

Phantom limb pain Sensation emanating from an absent or removed limb suggesting the limb is still present.

Phonological theory Posits that the reason that reading disabilities are evident in dyslexia is the individual's inability to differentiate differing elements of speech.

Placebos An assumedly inactive substance or dummy treatment administered to a control group to serve as a baseline for comparison of the effects of an active drug or treatment.

Positive reinforcement Providing praise or reward for an action.

Positive symptoms The symptoms of delusions, hallucinations and disorganised speech in schizophrenia.

Power The capacity of one person to influence another individual to do what they would like whilst resisting the attempts of another to influence them; influence is power in action.

Powerful others An individual may regard their health as under the control of powerful others, for example 'I can only do what my doctor tells me to do'.

Pre-conscious thoughts Thoughts that are unconscious at a particular moment in time.

Pre-therapy The theory and practice of psychological contact practised with low-functioning persons; it is defined in terms of the therapist's work, the client's internal process, and behaviours for measurement.

Primacy effect A tendency for the items near the beginning of the series to be better recalled than those near the middle.

Problem-focused approach Coping style which focuses on methods of solving the problem.

Progressive muscle relaxation training (PMRT) A technique for reducing anxiety by alternately tensing and relaxing the muscles.

Projection A defence mechanism in which one's own feelings and unwanted thoughts are projected onto someone else.

Prolonged exposure (PE) Characterised by re-experiencing the traumatic event through remembering it and engaging with, rather than avoiding, reminders of the trauma.

Protection motivation theory Proposes that health behaviours can be predicted on the basis of severity, susceptibility, response effectiveness and self-efficacy.

Psychic determinism A philosophical doctrine stating that all psychological and behavioural phenomena, such as human cognition, behaviour, decision and action, are determined by the inevitable consequences of previous occurrences.

Psychoanalysis A system of ideas developed by Sigmund Freud, focusing on the development of abnormal personalities and developed through his work as a therapist.

Psychoanalytic theory Term referring to approaches to psychoanalysis based on empirical research.

Psychodynamic approach The theories and works of both Freud and his followers, all of whom view personality in relation to drives and instincts.

Psychoneuroimmunology The study of the interaction among psychological factors, the nervous system, and the immune system.

Psychopathology The study of mental illness or distress.

Randomised control trial (RCT) A research design used for testing the effectiveness of a drug, or any type of treatment, in which research participants are assigned randomly to treatment and control or placebo groups and the differences in outcomes are compared.

Rational emotive (therapy) Framework founded by Ellis and applying the ABC model of thoughts and behaviours to therapy.

Reaction formation Defence mechanism in which unwanted thoughts or feelings are masked by extreme expressions of the opposite view.

Recency effect A tendency for the items near the end of the series to be better recalled than those near the start.

Reconceptualisation The act or process of developing a new concept for something (e.g. viewing the same experience in a more positive light to elicit different beliefs about the event).

Reductionist The simplification of complex systems into interactions between smaller parts.

Reflexive response An instantaneous response sidetracking deep thought processes relating to how to respond.

Regression Refers to the movement backwards through the stages of psychosexual development.

Reinforcement An increase in the strength of a response as a result of the impact it has on the environment.

Reinforcement schedule When and how often a behaviour is reinforced. It can have a dramatic impact on the strength and rate of the response.

Reinforcement value The extent to which we prefer one reinforcer over another when the probability of obtaining each reinforcer is equal.

Reinforcer A stimulus that strengthens or weakens the behaviour that produced it.

Repression A form of defence mechanism in which unwanted or harmful information is removed from the conscious into the unconscious.

Retrieval The gathering of information.

Rett's Disorder A pervasive developmental disorder found only in girls, characterised by the appearance, between five months and four years of age, of accelerated head growth and psychomotor retardation, replacement of purposeful hand movements with stereotyped gestures.

Role schemas A collection of information relating to one's role within a given situation.

Scaffolding Adjusting the quality of support during a teaching session to fit the child's current level of performance. Direct instruction is offered when a task is new; less help is provided as competence increases.

Schema A collection of information relating to a particular group of topics, an organisational structure for cognitions.

Schizophrenia A major psychiatric disorder, or cluster of disorders, characterised by psychotic symptoms that alter a person's perception, thoughts, affect, and behaviour.

Script Information on the process of an action.

Self-actualisation A term to denote the motive to realise one's latent potential, understand oneself and establish oneself as a whole person.

Self-efficacy The belief that one is capable of performing in a certain manner to attain certain goals.

Self-fulfilling prophecy A prediction that becomes true as a consequence of having been made. For example, if the president of a large company predicts a fall in the company's share price, then the prediction is likely to bring about a fall in the share price irrespective of any other factors, because investors will be more inclined to sell their shares.

Self-schemas Organisation of information relating to the self.

Separation anxiety The normal fear of apprehension of infants when separated from their mothers or other major attachment figures, or when approached by strangers, usually most clearly evident between six and ten months of age or, in later life, similar apprehension about separation from familiar physical or social environments.

Serial processing Information units processed one after the other.

Social learning theory Theory focusing on the learning produced within a social context, seeing learning occurring through interactions and observations of others.

Somatic pain Detected with somatic nociceptors and present in ligaments.

Specific learning difficulties A learning disability in a circumscribed area of functioning such as specific learning developmental disorder of language, specific disorder of arithmetic skills, or a specific language disability, not caused by any general deficit.

Specificity theory Developed by Von Frey in 1894, assumes there are specific sensory receptors responsible for the transmission of sensation, warmth and pain.

Status The position of an individual in relation to another or others, especially in regard to social or professional standing.

Stereotyping Oversimplified descriptions of group members.

Stigma A mark of disgrace associated with a person, a personal quality, or a personal circumstance.

Stimulus generalisation The generalisation of a response to one stimulus to all stimuli that are similar to this conditioned stimulus.

Storage The holding of information.

Stranger Anxiety A form of anxiety occurring in response to the appearance of an unfamiliar person, normally developing in infants between six and eight months of age, manifested by avoidance of eye contact, hiding or crying. (Can sometimes be referred to as eight-month anxiety.)

Stress inoculation training A cognitive behavioural treatment with the basic goal to help a person gain confidence in their ability to cope with anxiety and fear stemming from reminders of their trauma.

Stress management techniques Techniques that are devised to try to reduce stress or at least teach people how best to cope with it.

Sublimation A defence in which unacceptable impulses are channelled through more acceptable behaviours.

Substantia gelatinosa Part of the posterior horn of the grey matter of the spinal cord.

Superego Final part of the personality to develop in Freud's personality theory. The superego refers to the conscience or inner parent that applies values and morality to the way in which we choose to act.

Sympathetic pain Pain that occurs due to possible over-activity of the sympathetic nervous system, and central/peripheral nervous system mechanisms.

Syndrome Refers to a pattern of signs and symptoms that tend to co-occur and may indicate a common origin, course, familiar pattern or indicated treatment of a particular disorder.

Systematic desensitisation Type of behavioural therapy in which individuals are gradually presented with stimuli that more and more closely resemble their fear, in an attempt to reduce the anxiety provoked by this stimulus.

Tabula rasa view of mind View that the mind is a blank slate on which the experiences of life are written.

Talking cure Developed from treatment first piloted by Dr Breuer, refers to the process of talking that eventually reduced his patients' hysteria.

Theory of infantile sexuality A Freudian theory, explaining the erotic life of infants and children, encompassing the oral, anal and phallic stages of psychosexual development.

Theory of mind The ability of one person to understand their own and others' mental states.

Top-down processing Concept driven and affected by what the individual contributes – information stored in the memory is used to interpret what is in front of you.

Transcranial doppler A test that measures the velocity of blood flow through the brain's blood vessels.

Transcutaneous electrical nerve stimulation (TENS) Application of electrical current through the skin for pain control.

Unconditioned response Innate response to a stimulus, such as fear or hunger.

Unconditioned stimulus Stimulus which naturally elicits a response such as food or a loud noise.

Unconscious Information to which we show no awareness.

Unstructured interview Interview with an individual, conducted without a requirement to stick to a plan of how content will be covered.

Validation theory The process of communicating with a disorientated older person.

Verbal rating scale (VRS) A categorical assessment that involves patients rating their pain on a scale.

Vicarious reinforcement Reinforcement observed in another which will influence the observer's probability of completing the same reaction.

Visceral pain Pain occurring from stimulation of receptors within internal organs of the main body cavities. This pain originates from ongoing injury to the internal organs or the tissues that support them.

Visual analogue scale (VAS) A numerical assessment, involving patients rating their pain on a scale.

Zone of proximal development Refers to a range of tasks that a child cannot yet handle alone but can do with the help of more skilled partners.

References

Abramowitz, C.S., Kosson, D.S. and Seidenberg, M. (2004) The relationship between childhood attention deficit hyperactivity disorder and conduct problems and adult psychopathy in male inmates. *Personality and Individual Differences* **36**, 1031–1047.

Action on Elder Abuse (2004) *Hidden Voices*. London: Age Concern.

Adams, J. and Neville, S. (2011) Resisting the 'condom everytime for anal sex' health education message. *Health Education Journal*, **70**(2), 1–9.

Adler, N. (2000) An international perspective on the barriers to the advancement of women managers. *Applied Psychology: An International Review* **42**, 289–300.

Adler, R. (1981) *Psychoneuroimmunology*. New York: Academic Press.

Adler, R., Felten, D.L. and Cohen, N. (eds) (2001) *Psychoneuroimmunology*, Vol. 2. San Diego, CA: Academic Press.

Agallia, I., Kirsh, V., Kreiger, N., Soskoline, C. and Rohan, T. (2011) Oxidative balance score and risk of prostate cancer: Results from a case-cohort study. *Cancer Epidemology* **35**(4), 353–361.

Age Concern (2006) How ageist is Britain? www.ageconcern.org.uk

Ainsworth, M.D.S. (1985) Patterns of infant-mother attachments: Antecedents and effects on development. *Bulletin of the New York Academy of Medicine* **61**(9), 771–791.

Ainsworth, M.D.S., Blehar, M.C., Waters, E. and Wall, S. (1978) *Patterns of Attachment*. Hillsdale, NJ: Lawrence Erlbaum.

Ajzen, I. (1985) From intentions to actions: A theory of planned behavior. In J. Kuhl and J. Beckmann (eds) *Action Control: From Cognition to Behavior*. Berlin, Heidelberg, New York: Springer Verlag.

Ajzen, I. (1988) *Attitudes. Personality, and Behaviour*. Milton-Keynes, England: Open University Press.

Ajzen, I. and Fishbein, M. (1970) The prediction of behavior from attitudinal and normative variables. *Journal of Experimental Social Psychology* **6**, 466–487.

Al-Shaer, D., Hill, P. and Anderson, M. (2011) Nurses' knowledge and attitudes regarding pain assessment and intervention. *MEDSURE Nursing* **20**(1), 7–11.

Alaszewski, H., Parker, A. and Alaszewski, A. (1999) *Empowerment and Protection*. London: Mental Health Foundation.

Albers-Heitner, C.P., Largro-Janssen, A.L.M., Venema, P.L., Berghmans, L.C.M., Winkers, R.A.G., De Jonge, A. and Joore, M.A. (2011) Experiences and attitudes in primary care regarding their role in care for patients with urinary incontinence. *Scandinavian Journal of Caring Science* **25**(2), 303–310.

Alden, L.E., Mellings, T.M. and Laposa, J.M. (2004) Framing social information and negative predictions in social phobia. *Behaviour Research and Therapy* **42**, 585–600.

Aldwin, C.M. and Park, C.L. (2004) Coping and physical health outcomes: An overview. *Psychology and Health* **19**(3), 277–281.

Alford, P., Kirk, M., Llewellyn, I., Lowe, K., McDermott, G., Meakins, B., Davies, N., Kilbane, G., Keel, N., and Fo, E. (1995) Should nurses wear uniforms? *Nursing Standard* **9**, 52–53.

Ali, U. and Hanson, S. (2010) The effectiveness of relaxation therapy in the reduction of anxiety related symptoms (a case study). *International Journal of Psychological Studies* **2**(2), 202–208.

Altman, C., Sommer, J. and McGoey, K. (2009) Anxiety in early childhood: What do we know? *Journal of Early Childhood and Infant Psychology* **5**, 157–175.

Alzheimers Society (2011) What is dementia? http://www.alzheimers.org.uk/site/scripts/documents_info.php?documentID=106 (accessed on 24/05/2011)

American Psychiatric Association (1994) *Diagnostic and Statistical Manual of Mental Disorders* (4th edn, Text revision) Washington, DC: American Psychiatric Association.

American Psychiatric Association (2000) *Diagnostic and Statistical Manual of Mental Disorders* (4th edn, Text revision, DSM-IV-TR). Washington, DC: American Psychiatric Association.

Anatchkova, M., Velicer, W. and Prochaska, J. (2005) Replication of subtypes for smoking cessation within the contemplation stage of change. *Addictive Behaviours* **30**(5), 915–927.

Anderson, T., Watson, M. and Davidson, R. (2008) The use of cognitive behavioural therapy techniques for anxiety and depression in hospice patients: A feasibility study. *Palliative Medicine* **22**(7), 814–821.

Andersen, S. and Teicher, M. (2009) Desperately driven and no brakes: Developmental stress exposure and subsequent risk for substance abuse. *Neuroscience and Biobehavioural Reviews* **33**(4), 516–524.

Anderson, W.G., Chase, R., Pantilat, S.Z., Tulsky, J.A. and Auerbach, A.D. (2011) Code status discussions between hospital physicians and medical patients at hospital admission. *Journal of General Internal Medicine* **26**(4), 359–366.

Andrasik, F. (2007) Efficacy of behavioural treatments for recurrent headaches. *Neurological Science* **28**, S70–S77.

Andre, E., Bevacqua, E., Heylen, D., Niewiadomski, R., Pelachaud, C., Peters, C., Poggi, I. and Rehm, M. (2011) Non-verbal persuasion and communication in an affective agent. In P. Petta, C. Pelachaud and R. Cowie (eds) *Emotion-Oriented Systems: The Humaine Handbook*. Springer/Berlin: Heidelberg, pp. 585–608.

Andreasson, S., Allebeck, P. and Engstrom, A. (1987) Cannabis and schizophrenia: A longitudinal study of Swedish conscripts. *Lancet* **2**, 1483–1486.

Andrews, G., Henderson, S. and Hall, W. (2001) Prevalence, comorbidity, disability and service utilization: Overview of the Australian National Mental Health Survey. *British Journal of Psychiatry* **178**, 145–153.

Ansari, F., Molavi, H. and Neshatdoost, H.T. (2010) Effect of stress inoculation training on general health of hypertensive patients. *Psychological Research* **12**(3-4), 81–96.

Araujo, S., Faisca, L., Bramao, I., Inacio, F., Petersson, K.M. and Reis, A. (2011) Object naming in dyslexic children: More than a phonological deficit. *The Journal of General Psychology* **138**(3), 215–228.

Archer, J. (1999) *The Nature of Grief: The Evolution and Psychology of Reaction to Loss*. London: Routledge.

Aretouli, E. and Brandt, J. (2010) Everyday functioning in mild cognitive impairment and its relationship with executive cognition. *International Journal of Geriatric Psychiatry* **25**, 224-233.

Argyle, M. (1988) *Bodily Communication*. London: Routledge.

Arkes, J.R., Boehm, L.E. and Xu, G. (1991) Determinants of judged validity. *Journal of Experimental Social Psychology* **27**, 576-605.

Arkon, B., Kerime, D. and Zekiye, C. (2011) Attitudes of health professionals towards mental disorders: Studies in Turkey during the last decade. *Current Approaches in Psychiatry* **3**(2), 214-231.

Arnett, J.J. (1999) Optimistic bias in adolescent and adult smokers and non smokers. *Addictive Behaviours* **25**(4), 625-632.

Aromaa, E., Tolvanen, A., Tuulari, J. and Wahlbeck, K. (2011) Personal stigma and use of mental health services among people with depression in a general population in Finland. *BMC Psychiatry* **11**(1), 52-57.

Asch, S.E. (1952) *Social Psychology*. Englewood Cliffs, NJ: Prentice Hall.

Ashmore, R. (2010) Section 5(4)(The nurse's holding power): Patterns of use in one mental health trust (1983-2006). *Journal of Psychiatric and Mental Health Nursing* **17**(3), 202-209.

Atkinson, R.C. and Shiffrin, R.M. (1968) Human memory: A proposed system and its control processes. In K.W. Spence and J.T. Spence (eds) *The Psychology of Learning and Motivation*, vol. 8. London: Academic Press.

Atladóttir, H., Pedersen, M., Scient, C., Thorsen, P., Mortensen, P., Deleuran, B., Eaton, W.W. and Parner, E.T. (2009) Association of family history of autoimmune diseases and autism spectrum disorders. *Pediatrics* **124**(2), 687-694.

Auerbach, J.G., Berger, A., Atzaba-Poria, N., Arbelle, S., Cypin, N., Friedman, A. and Landau, R. (2008) Temperament at 7, 12 and 25 months in children at familiar risk for ADHD. *Infant and Child Development* **17**(4), 321-338.

Australian Centre for Posttraumatic Mental Health (2007) *Australian guidelines for the treatment of adults with acute stress disorder and posttraumatic stress disorder*. Melbourne: Author.

Aveyard, P., Massey, L., Parsons, A., Manaseki, S. and Griffin, C. (2009) The effect of transtheoretical model based interventions on smoking cessation. *Social Science and Medicine* **68**(3), 397-403.

Ayman-Nolley, S. and Taira, L.L. (2000) Obsession with the dark side of adolescence: A decade of psychological studies. *Journal of Youth Studies* **3**, 35-48.

Azrin, N., Ehle, C. and Beaumont, A. (2006) Physical exercise as a reinforcer to promote calmness of an ADHD child. *Behaviour Modification* **30**(5), 564-570.

Bahrick, H.P., Bahrick, P.O. and Wittinger, R.P. (1975) Fifty years of memory for names and faces: A cross-sectional approach. *Journal of Experimental Psychology* **104**, 54-75.

Bailey, A., Phillips, W. and Rutter, M. (1996) Autism: towards an integration of clinical, genetic, neuropsychological, and neurobiological perspectives. *Journal of Child Psychology and Psychiatry, and Allied Disciplines* **37**(1), 89-126.

Ballantyne, A., Trenwith, L., Zubrinich, S. and Corlis, M. (2010) 'I feel less lonely': What older people say about participating in a social networking website. *Quality in Ageing and Older Adults* **11**(3), 25-35.

Bandura, A. (1965) Influences of models' reinforcement contingencies on the acquisition of initiative responses. *Journal of Personality and Social Psychology* **1**, 589-593.

Bandura, A. (1977a) *Social Learning Theory*. Englewood Cliffs, NJ: Prentice Hall.

Bandura, A. (1977b) Self-efficacy: Toward a unifying theory of behavioral change. *Psychological Review* **84**(2), 191-215.

Bandura, A. (2000) Health promotion from the perspective of social cognitive theory. In P. Norman, C. Abraham and M. Connor (eds) *Understanding and Changing Health Behaviour: From Health Beliefs to Self-Regulation*. Switzerland: Harwood Academic, pp. 229-242.

Bandura, A., Ross, D. and Ross, S.A. (1961) Transmission of aggression through imitation of aggressive models. *Journal of Abnormal and Social Psychology* **63**, 575-582.

Banja, J.D. (2007) My what? *American Journal of Bioethics* **7**(11), 13-15.

Barbarich, N.C., McConaha, C.W., Halmi, K.A., Gendall, K., Sunday, S.R., Gaskill, J., La Via, M. and Kaye, W.H. (2004) Use of nutritional supplements to increase the efficacy of fluoxetine in the treatment of anorexia nervosa. *International Journal of Eating Disorders* **35**, 10-15.

Barber, C. (2011) Understanding learning disabilities: An introduction. *British Journal of Healthcare Assistance* **5**(4), 168-169.

Barber, J. (1998) The mysterious persistence of hypnotic analgesia. *International Journal of Clinical and Experimental Hypnosis* **46**(1), 28-43.

Barch, D.M. (2005) The cognitive neuroscience of schizophrenia. *Annual Review of Clinical Psychology* **1**, 321-353.

Barlow, J., Wright, C., Sheasby, J., Turner, A. and Hainsworth, J. (2002) Self-management approaches for people with chronic conditions: A review. *Patient Education and Counseling* **48**(2), 177-187.

Baroletti, S. (2010) Medication adherence in cardiovascular disease. *Circulation: Journal of the American Heart Association* **121**, 1455-1458.

Baron, R.A. (2001) *Psychology* (5th edn). Boston, MA: Allyn and Bacon.

Bartlett, D. (1998) *Stress: Perspectives and Processes*. Buckingham: Open University Press.

Bartrop, R.W., Lazarus, L., Luckhurst, E., Kiloh, L.G. and Penny, R. (1977) Depressed lymphocyte function after bereavement. *The Lancet* **309**(8016), 834-836.

Batelaan, N.M., De Graaf, R. and Van Balkom, A.J. (2006) Epidemiology of panic. *Tijdschrift voor Psychiatrie* **48**, 195-205.

Bates, T., Luciano, M., Castles, A., Coltheart, M., Wright, M. and Martin, N. (2007) Replication of reported linkages for dyslexia and spelling and suggestive evidence for novel regions on chromosomes 4 and 17. *European Journal of Human Genetics* **15**(2), 194-203.

Bazillier, C., Verlhiac, J.F., Mallet, P. and Rouesse, J. (2011) Predictors of intentions to eat healthily in 8-9 year old children. *Journal of Cancer Education* **26**(3), 572-576.

Beach, R. and Proops, R. (2009) Respecting autonomy in young people. *Postgraduate Medical Journal* **85**, 181-185.

Bebbington, P. and Delemos, I. (1996). Pain in the family. *Journal of Psychosomatic Research* **40**(5), 451-456.

Bebbington, P.E., Bowen, J., Hirsch, S.R. and Kuipers, E.A. (1995) Schizophrenia and psychosocial stresses. In S.R. Hirsch and D.R. Weinberger (eds.) *Schizophrenia*. Oxford, England: Blackwell Science, pp. 587-604.

Becker, M. (1974) *The Health Belief Model and Personal Health Behavior*. Thorofare, NJ: Slack.

Bee, H. (2006) *The Developing Child*. 11th edn. London: Addison Wesley.

Beecher, H.K. (1959) Generalisation from pain of various types and diverse origins. *Science* **130**, 267-268.

Beinhoff, U., Tumani, H. and Riepe, M.W. (2009) Applying new research criteria for a diagnosis of early Alzheimer's disease: sex and intelligence matter. *International Journal of Alzheimer's Disease, V;2009*. DOI: 10.4061/2009/638145.

Beltran, R.O., Scanlan, J.N., Hancock, N. and Luckett, T. (2007) The effect of first year mental health fieldwork on attitudes of occupational therapy students towards people with mental illness. *Australian Occupational Therapy Journal* **54**, 42-48.

Bendtsen, L. and Jensen, R. (2011) Treating tension-type headache - an expert opinion. *Expert Opinion on Pharmacotherapy* **12**(7), 1099-1109.

Bennett, P. (2011) *Abnormal and Clinical Psychology: An introductory text.* (3rd edn.) New York: Open University Press.

Bennett, P., Williams, Y., Page, N., Hood, K., Woollard, M. and Vetter, N. (2005) Associations between organisational and incident factors and emotional distress in emergency ambulance personnel. *British Journal of Clinical Psychology* **44**(2), 215-226.

Berk, L., Hallam, K.T., Colom, F., Vieta, E., Hasty, M., Macneil, C. and Berk, M. (2010) Enhancing medication adherence in patients with bipolar disorder. *Human Psychopharmacology Clinical and Experimental* **25**(1), 1-16.

Berry, D. (2004) *Risk, Communication and Health Psychology*. Maidenhead: Open University Press/McGraw-Hil.

Bettelheim, B. (1967) *The Empty Fortress*. New York: Free Press.

Bettelheim, B. (1973) Bringing up children. *Ladies' Home Journal* **90**, 28.

Bibace, R. and Walsh, M.E. (1980) Development of children's concept of illness. *Paediatrics* **66**(6), 912-917.

Biederman, J. and Faraone, S.V. (2003) Current concepts on the neurobiology of attention-deficit/hyperactivity disorder. *Journal of Attention Disorder* **6**(1), 7-18.

Bigby, C. (2003) *Ageing with a Lifelong Disability. A Guide to Practice, Program and Policy Issues for Human Services and Professionals*. London: Jessica Kingsley Publishers.

Binderup, A., Arendt-Nielsen, L. and Madeleine, P. (2010) Cluster analysis of pressure pain threshold maps from the trapezius muscle. *Computer Methods in Miomechanics and Biomedical Engineering* **13**(6), 677-683.

Birch, S., Hesselink, J.K., Jonkman, F., Hekker, T. and Bos, A. (2004) Clinical research on acupuncture: Part 1. What have reviews of the efficacy and safety of acupuncture told us so far? *Journal of Alternative Complementary Medicine* **10**(3), 468-480.

Bishop, D.V.M. (2009) Genes, cognition, and communication. *Annals of the New York Academy of Sciences* **1156**, 1–18.

Bissell, K. and Hays, H. (2011) Understanding anti-fat bias in children: The role of media and appearance anxiety in third to sixth graders' implicit and explicit attitudes toward obesity. *Mass Communication and Society* **14**(1), 113–140.

Bisson, J. and Andrew, M. (2009) Psychological treatments of post-traumatic stress disorder (PTSD) (Review) The Cochrane Library, 2009 (2), http://www.thecochranelibrary.com.

Bodrova, E. and Leong, D.J. (2007) *Tools of the Mind: The Vygotskian Approach to Early Childhood Education* (2nd edn.) Upper Saddle River, NJ: Merrill/Prentice Hall.

Bogels, S.M. and Voncken, M. (2008) Social skills training versus cognitive therapy for social anxiety disorder characterized by fear of blushing, trembling, or sweating. *International Journal of Cognitive Therapy* **1**(2), 138–150.

Bohm, H. and Stewart, M.G. (2009) Brief report: on the concordance percentages for autistic spectrum disorder of twins. *Journal of Autism and Developmental Disorders* **39**(5), 806–808.

Bolivor, M. (2009) Treatment of complex regional pain syndrome. *Infome Medico* **11**(6), 347–353.

Bornstein, R. (2010) Gender schemas, gender roles, and expressive writing: Towards a process-focused model. *Sex Roles* **63**(3/4), 173–177.

Bosma, H., van Boxtel, M.P.J., Ponds, R.W.H.M., Haux, P.J.H. and Jolles, J. (2003) Education and age related cognitive decline: The contribution of mental workload. *Educational Gerontology* **29**(1), 165.

Bosmans, J., Geertzen, J., Post, W., van der Schans, C. and Dijkstra, P. (2010) Factors associated with phantom limb pain: a 31/2-year prospective study. *Clinical Rehabilitation* **24**(5), 444–453.

Bougarel, L., Guitter, J., Zimmer, L., Vaugeois, J. and Yacoubi, M. (2011) Behaviour of a genetic mouse model of depression in the learned helplessness paradigm. *Psychopharmacology* **215**(3), 595–605.

Bovbjerg, D.H., Redd, W.H., Jacobsen, P.B., Manne, S.L., Taylor, K.L., Surbone, A., Crown, J.P., Norton, L., Gilewski, T.A., Hudis, C.A., Reichman, B.S., Kaufman, R.J., Currie, V.E. and Hakes, T,B. (1992) An experimental analysis of classically conditioned nausea during cancer chemotherapy. *Psychosomatic Medicine* **54**(6), 623–637.

Bowlby, J. (1969) *Attachment and Loss.* New York: Basic Books.

Bowling, A. (1995) *Measuring Disease.* Buckingham: Open University Press.

Boyle, E. (2011) Management of pain in the neonatal unit: options, challenges and controversies. *Infant* **7**(3), 88–91.

Bradley, L. and Bryant, P.E. (1985) *Rhyme and Reason in Reading and Spelling.* Ann Arbor, MI: University of Michigan Press.

Bragard, I., Etienne, A., Merckaert, I., Libert, Y. and Razavi, D. (2010) Efficacy of a communication and stress management training on medical residents' self-efficacy, stress to communicate and burnout. *Journal of Health Psychology* **15**(7), 1075–1081.

Breggin, P. (1997) *Brain-disabling Treatment in Psychiatry.* New York: Springer.

Bridgeman, E.S. and Malinoski, A. (2009) The disclosure of unanticipated medical outcomes: Better communication, better care, better patient satisfaction. *Journal of Legal Nurse Consulting* **20**(1), 13-18.

British Crime Survey (2009) Retrieved 14 December 2011, from http://www.esds.ac.uk/findingData/snDescription.asp?sn=6627

Broadbent, D. (1958) *Perception and Communication.* London: Pergamon Press.

Brown, I. (2006) Nurses' attitudes towards adult patients who are obese: Literature review. *Journal of Advanced Nursing* **53**(2), 221-232.

Brown, I. and Brown, R.I. (2009) Choice as an aspect of quality of life for people with intellectual disabilities. *Journal of Policy and Practice in Intellectual Disabilities* **6**, 10-17.

Brown, J., Vanable, P., Carey, M. and Elin, L. (2010) The development of a computer administered cognitive-behavioural intervention to promote stress management among HIV+ women. *Journal of Cognitive Psychotherapy* **24**(4), 265-280.

Brown, L., Russell, J., Thornton, C. and Dunn, S. (1997) Experiences of physical and sexual abuse in Australian general practice attenders and eating disordered population. *Australian and New Zealand Journal of Psychiatry* **31**(3), 398-404.

Brown, R.I. and Shearer, J. (2004) Challenges for inclusion within a quality of life model for the 21st century. In D. Mitchell (ed.) *Special Educational Needs and Inclusive Education: Major Themes in Education* **2**, 139-156. London: Routledge Falmer.

Brown, S. and Locker, E. (2009) Defence responses to an emotive anti-alcohol message. *Psychology and Health* **24**(5), 517-512.

Brummett, B.H., Barefoot, J.C., Siegler, I.C., Clapp-Channing, N.E., Lytle, B.L.L., Bosworth, H.B., Williams, R.B. and Mark, D.B. (2001) Characteristics of socially isolated patients with coronary artery disease who are at elevated risk for mortality. *Psychosomatic Medicine* **63**(2), 267-272.

Bruner, J. (1983) Play, thought, and language. *Peabody Journal of Education* **60**(3), 60-69.

Bruster, S., Jarman, B., Bosanquet, N., Weston, D., Erens, R. and Delbanco, T.L. (1994) National survey of hospital patients. *British Medical Journal* **309**(6968), 1542-1546.

Bryans, A., Cornish, F. and McIntosh, J. (2009) The potential of ecological theory for building an integrated framework to develop the public health contribution of health visiting. *Health and Social Care in the Community* **17**(6), 564-572.

Budney, A.J., Radonovich, K.J., Higgins, S.T. and Wong, C.J (1998) Adults seeking treatment for marijuana dependence: A comparison with cocaine dependent treatment seekers. *Experimental and Clinical Psychopharmacology* **6**, 419-426.

Bugental, J. (1965) *The Search for Authenticity: An Existential-Analytic Approach to Psychotherapy.* London: Holt, Rinehart and Winston.

Buitelaar, A.J., van der Wees, M., Swaab-Barneveld, H. and van der Gaag, R. (1999) Theory of mind and emotion-recognition functioning in autistic spectrum disorders in psychiatric control and normal children. *Development and Psychopathology* **11**, 39-58.

Bulik, C.M., Sullivan, P.F., Tozzi, F., Furberg, H., Lichtenstein, P. and Pedersen, N.L. (2006) Prevalence, heritability, and prospective risk factors for anorexia nervosa. *Archives of General Psychiatry* **63**, 305-312.

Bunker, S.J., Colquhoun, D.M., Esler, M.D., Hickie, I.B., Hunt, D., Jelinek, V.M., Oldenburg, B.F., Peach, H.G., Ruth, D., Tennant, C.C. and Tonkin, A.M. (2003) Stress and coronary heart disease: Psychosocial risk factors. National Heart Foundation of Australia Position Statement Update. *Medical Journal of Australia* **178**(6), 272-276.

Burgess, L., Page, S. and Hardman, P. (2006) Changing attitudes in dementia care and the role of nurses. *Nursing Times* **99**(18), 18-19.

Burish, T.G., Shartner, C.D. and Lyles, J.N. (1981) Effectiveness of multiple muscle-site EMG biofeedback and relaxation training in reducing the aversiveness of cancer chemotherapy. *Biofeedback and Self-Regulation* **6**(4), 523-535.

Burke, B.L., Arkowitz, H. and Menchola, M. (2003) The efficacy of motivational interviewing: A meta-analysis of controlled clinical trials. *Journal of Consulting and Clinical Psychology* **71**, 843-861.

Burns, A. and Hope, T. (1997) Clinical aspects of the dementias of old age. In R. Jacoby and C. Oppenheimer (eds) *Psychiatry in the Elderly* (5th edn). Oxford: Oxford University Press, pp. 456-493.

Burns, V.E., Carroll, D. Ring, C., Harrison, L.K. and Drayson, M. (2002) Stress, coping, and hepatitis B antibody status. *Psychosomatic Medicine* **64**(2), 287-293.

Bush, T. (2003) Communicating with patients who have dementia. *Nursing Times* **99**(42), 42-45.

Buss, A.H., Plomin, R. and Willerman, L. (1973) The inheritance of personality traits. *Journal of Personality* **41**, 513-524.

Byrne, M.K., Deane, F.P. and Coombs, T. (2005) Nurse's beliefs and knowledge about medications are associated with their difficulties using patient treatment adherence strategies. *Journal of Mental Health* **14**(5), 513-521.

Cabaniss, R. (2011) Educating nurses to impact change in nursing's image. *Teaching and Learning in Nursing* **6**(3), 112-118.

Cacioppo, J.T. and Petty, R.E. (1979) Effects of message repetition and position on cognitive response, recall and persuasion. *Journal of Personality and Social Psychology* **37**, 97-109.

Campbell, M., Adams, P., Perry, R., Spencer, E.K. and Overall, J.E. (1988) Tardive and withdrawal dyskinesias in autistic children: A prospective study. *Psychopharmacology Bulletin* **24**, 251-255.

Cannon, W.B. (1932) *The Wisdom of the Body.* New York: Norton.

Cappell, H. and Greeley J. (1987) Alcohol and tension reduction: An update on research and theory. In H.T. Blane and K.E. Leonard (eds) *Psychological Theories of Drinking and Alcoholism.* New York: Guilford Press, pp. 15-54.

Cardozo, B.L., Kaiser, R., Gotway, C.A. and Agani, F. (2003) Mental health, social functioning, and feelings of hatred and revenge in Kosovar Albanians one year after the war in Kosovo. *Journal of Traumatic Stress* **16**, 351-360.

Carey, P. (1985) Manner and meaning in West Sumatra: The social-context of consciousness. *The Times Literary Supplement* **4305**, 112.

Cargin, J.W., Maruff, P., Collie, A. and Masters, C. (2006) Mild memory impairment in healthy older adults is distinct from normal aging. *Brain and Cognition* **60**, 146-155.

Caris-Verhallen, M., Kerkstra, A. and Bensing, J.M. (2001) Non-verbal behaviour in nurse-elderly patient communication. *Journal of Advanced Nursing* **29**(1), 808-818.

Carlson, N.R. and Buskist, W. (1997) *Psychology: The Science of Behaviour* (5th edn). Needham Heights, MA: Allyn and Bacon.

Caroll, D., Moore, R.A., McQuay, H.J., Fairman, F., Gramer, M. and Leijon, G. (2006) Transcutaneous electrical nerve stimulation (TENS) for chronic pain. *The Cochrane Database of Systematic Reviews,* Issue 4. Chichester: Wiley.

Carpenter, C.J. (2010) A meta-analysis of the effectiveness of health belief model variables in predicting behaviour. *Health Communication* **25**(8), 661-669.

Carr, A. (2010) Thematic review of family therapy journals 2009. *Journal of Family Therapy* **32**(4), 409-427.

Carter, J.C., McFarlane, T.L., Bewell, C., Olmsted, M.P., Woodside, D.B., Kaplan, A.S. and Crosby, R.D. (2009) Maintenance treatment for anorexia nervosa: A comparison of cognitive behavior therapy and treatment as usual. *International Journal of Eating Disorders* **42**(3), 202-207.

Carter, L.E., McNeil, D.W., Vowles, K.E., Sorrell, J.T., Turk, C.L., Ries, B.J. and Hopko, D.R. (2002) Effects of emotion on pain reports, tolerance and physiology. *Pain Research and Management* **7**(1), 21-30.

Carter, M.A. (2009) Trust, power, and vulnerability: A discourse on helping in nursing. *Nursing of North America* **44**(4), 393-405.

Cartwright, M., Wardle, J., Steggles, N., Simon, A.E., Croker, H. and Jarvis, M.J. (2003) Stress and dietary practices in adolescents. *Health Psychology* **22**(4), 362-369.

Carver, C.S., Scheier, M.F. and Segerstrom, S.C. (2010) Optimism. *Clinical Psychology Review* **30**(7), 879-889.

Casey, B., Jones, R.M., Levita, L., Libby, V., Pattwell, S.S., Ruberry, E.J., Soliman, F. and Somerville, L.H. (2010) The storm and stress of adolescence: Insights from human imaging and mouse genetics. *Developmental Psychobiology* **52**, 225-235.

Casey, A. and Wallis, A. (2011) Effective communication: Principle of Nursing Practice E. *Nursing Standard* **25**(32), 35-37.

Castellanos, (2002) Brain size linked to ADHD. *Brown University Psychopharmacology Update* **13**(11), 4.

Castro, L. and Wasserman, E. (2010) Animal learning. *Wiley Interdisciplinary Reviews: Cognitive Science* **1**(1), 89-98.

Chakraborti, S. (2011) Thyroid functions and bipolar affective disorder. *Journal of Thyroid Research,* 1-13.

Chakraborty, A., Selby, D., Gardiner, K., Myers, J., Moravon, V. and Wright, T. (2011) Malignant bowel obstruction: Natural history of a heterogeneous patient population followed prospectively over two years. *Journal of Pain and Symptom Management* **41**(2), 412-420.

Chan, C., Richardson, A. and Richardson, J. (2011) Managing symptoms in patients with advanced lung cancer during radiotherapy: Results of a psychoeducational randomized controlled trial. *Journal of Pain and Symptom Management* **41**(2), 347-357.

Chandola, T., Britton, A., Brunner, E., Hermingway, H., Kumari, M., Badrick, E., Kivimaki, M. and Marmot, M. (2008) Work stress and coronary heart disease: What are the mechanisms? *European Heart Journal* **29**(5), 640-648.

Chapman, S. (2011) Chronic pain syndrome in cancer survivors. *Nursing Standard* **25**(2), 35–41.

Charles, E. and Rivera, S. (2009) Object permanence and method of disappearance: Looking measures further contradict reaching measures. *Developmental Science* **12**(6), 991–1006.

Charney, D.S., Nagy, L.M., Bremner, J.D., Goddard, A.W., Yehuda, R. and Southwick, S.M. (2000) Neurobiological mechanisms of human anxiety. In B.S. Fogal (ed.) *Synopsis of Neuropsychiatry*. Philadelphia: Lippincott Williams and Wilkins, pp. 273–288.

Chen, C. and Farruggia, S. (2002) Culture and adolescent development. In W.J. Lonner, D.L. Dinnel, S.A. Hayes and D.N. Sattler (eds) *Online Readings in Psychology and Culture* (Unit 11, Chapter 2) Bellingham, Washington: Western Washington University, Center for Cross-Cultural Research. http://www.wwu.edu/~culture

Chen, Y., Lai, Y., Shun, S., Chi, N., Tsai, P. and Liao, Y. (2011) The Chinese behaviour pain scale for critically ill patients: Translation and psychometric testing. *International Journal of Nursing Studies* **48**(4), 438–448.

Cheng, J.O., Lo, R.S., Chan, F.M., Kwan, B.H. and Woo, J. (2010) An exploration of anticipatory grief in advanced cancer patients. *Psycho-oncology* **19**(7), 693–700.

Cherry, C. (1966) *On Human Communication: A Review, a Survey, and a Criticism*. (2nd edn). Cambridge, MA: MIT Press.

Chiang, E.S., Byrd, S.P. and Molin, A.J. (2011) Children's perceived cost for exercise: Application of an expectancy-value paradigm. *Health Education and Behaviour* **38**(2), 143–149.

Chronis, A.M., Chacko, A., Fabiano, G.A., Wymbs, B.T. and Pelham, W.E. (2004) Enhancements to the behavioural parent training paradigm for families of children with ADHD: A review and future directions. *Clinical Child and Family Psychology Review* **7**, 1–27.

Chugani, D.C., Muzik, O., Behen, M., Rothermel, R., Janisse, J.J., Lee, J. and Chugani, H.T. (1999) Developmental changes in brain serotonin synthesis capacity in autistic and nonautistic children. *Annals of Neurology* **45**(3), 287–295.

Clark, A. (2003) 'It's like an explosion in your life . . .': Lay perspectives on stress and myocardial infarction. *Journal of Clinical Nursing* **12**, 544–553.

Cleland, J.A., Palmer, J.A. and Venzke, W.J. (2005) Ethnic differences in pain perception. *Physical Therapy Reviews* **10**, 113–122.

Closs, S.J., Barr, B., Briggs, M., Cash, K. and Seers, K. (2004) A comparison of five pain assessment scales for nursing home residents with varying degrees of cognitive impairment. *Journal of Pain and Symptom Management* **27**(3), 196–205.

Coelho, C.M. and Purkis, H.M. (2009) The origins of specific phobias: Influential theories and current perspectives. *Review of General Psychology* **13**(4), 335–348.

Cohen, D., Taieb, O., Flament, M., Benoit, N., Chevret, S., Corcos, M., Fossati, P. and Basquin M. (2000) Absence of cognitive impairment at long-term follow-up in adolescents treated with ECT for severe mood disorder. *American Journal of Psychiatry* **157**(3), 460–462.

Cohen, L., Savary, C. and de Moor, C. (2000) Stress and social support affect immune function in cancer patients receiving vaccine treatment. *Psychosomatic Medicine* **62**(1), 1137.

Cohen, S. (2005) The Pittsburgh Common Cold Studies: Psychosocial predictors of susceptibility to respiratory infectious illness. *International Journal of Behavioural Medicine* **12**(3), 123-131.

Cohen, S., Frank, E., Doyle, W.J., Skoner, D.P., Rabin, B.S. and Gwaltney Jr, J.M. (1998) Types of stressors that increase susceptibility to the common cold in healthy adults. *Health Psychology* **17**(3), 214-223.

Cohen, S., Kessler, R.C. and Gordon, L.U. (1997) Stategies for measuring stress in studies of psychiatric and physical disorders. In S. Cohen, R.C. Kessler and L.U. Gordon (eds) *Measuring Stress: A Guide for Health and Social Scientists*. New York: Oxford University Press.

Cohn, N.J. and Squire, L.R. (1980) Preserved learning and retention of pattern-analyzing skill in amnesia: Dissociation of knowing how and knowing that. *Science* **210**(4466), 207-210.

Coleman, I. and Ataullahjan, A. (2010) Life course perspectives on the epidemiology of depression. *Canadian Journal of Psychiatry* **55**(10), 622-632.

Coleman, M.A. (2009) *Oxford Dictionary of Psychology*. London: Oxford University Press.

Coll, A.M., Jamal, A. and Mead, D. (2004) Postoperative pain assessment tools in day surgery: Literature review. *Journal of Advanced Nursing* **46**(2), 124-133.

Colver, A. (2006) Study protocol: SPARCLE - a multi-centre European study of the relationship of environment to participation and quality of life in children with cerebral palsy. *BMC Public Health* **6**, 105-110.

Combes, C. and Feral, F. (2010) Drug compliance and health locus of control in schizophrenia. *L'encéphale* **37**(1), 11-18.

Conklin, H.M. and Iacono, W.G. (2002) Schizophrenia: A neurodevelopmental perspective. *Current Diagnosis in Psychological Science* **11**, 33-37.

Conner, M. and Norman, P. (1996) *Predicting Health Behavior. Search and Practice with Social Cognition Models*. Ballmore, Buckingham: Open University Press.

Conway, K.P., Compton, W., Stinson, F.S. and Grant, B.F. (2006) Lifetime comorbidity of DSM-IV mood and anxiety disorders and specific drug use disorder: Result from the national epidemiologic survey of alcohol and related conditions. *Journal of Clinical Psychiatry* **67**(2), 247-257.

Cook, D., Levinson, A., Garside, S., Dupras, D., Erwin, P. and Montori, V. (2010) Instructional design variations in internet-based learning for health professions education: A systematic review and meta-analysis. *Academic Medicine* **85**(5), 909-922.

Cooper, J. (2007) *Cognitive Dissonance: 50 years of a Classic Theory*. London: Sage.

Coudin, G. and Alexopoulos, T. (2010) 'Help me! I'm old!' How negative aging stereotypes create dependency among older adults. *Aging and Mental Health* **14**(5), 516-523.

Cox, A., Rutter, M., Newman, S. and Bartak, L. (1975) A comparative study of infantile autism and specific developmental language disorders. 2: Parental characteristics. *British Journal of Psychiatry* **126**, 146-159.

Cox, F. (2010) Basic principles of pain management: Assessment and intervention. *Nursing Standard* **25**(1), 36-39.

Coyne, I. (2006) Consultation with children in hospital: Children, patients' and nurses' perspectives. *Journal of Clinical Nursing* **15**, 61-71.

Craik, F.I.M. and Lockhart, R.S. (1972) Levels of processing: A framework for memory research. *Journal of Verbal Learning and Verbal Behavior* **11**, 671-684.

Crain, W. (2005) *Theories of Development* (5th edn). Upper Saddle River, NJ: Prentice Hall.

Cramer, J.A. and Rosenheck, R. (1998) Compliance with medication regimens for mental and physical disorders. *Psychiatry Service* **49**, 196-201.

Craske, M.G. and Barlow, D.H. (2007) Panic disorder and agoraphobia. In D. Barlow (ed.) *Clinical Handbook of Psychological Disorders* (4th edn). New York: Guilford Press, pp. 1-64.

Craske, M.G. and Waters, A.M. (2005) Panic disorder, phobias, and generalized anxiety disorder. *Annual Review of Clinical Psychology* **1**, 197-226.

Crockenberg, S. and Leerkes, E. (2003) Infant negative emotionality, caregiving, and family relationships. In A.C. Crouter and A. Booth (eds) *Children's Influence on Family Dynamics*. Mahwah, NJ: Erlbaum, pp. 57-78.

Crowe, M., Whitehead, L., Gagon, M., Baxtor, G., Pankhurst, A. and Valledar, V. (2010) Listening to the body and talking to myself – the impact of chronic lower back pain: a qualitative study. *International Journal of Nursing Studies* **47**(5), 586-592.

Cuetos, F., Herrera, E. and Ellis, A.W. (2010) Impaired word recognition in Alzheimer's disease: The role of age of acquisition. *Neuropsychologia* **48**(11), 3329-3334.

Cumming, E. and Henry, W.E. (1961) *Growing Old: The Process of Disengagement*. New York: Basic Books.

Curran, J., Machin, C. and Gournay, K. (2006) Cognitive behavioural therapy for patients with anxiety and depression. *Nursing Standard* **21**(7), 44-52.

Curtis, K., Tzarnes, A. and Rudge, T. (2011) How to talk to doctors: A guide for effective communication. *Nursing Standard* **58**(1), 13-20.

daCosta, M.D., Gupta, S., Mcdonald, M. and Sadosky, A. (2011) Evaluating the health and economic impact of osteoarthritis pain in the workforce: Results from the National Health and Wellness Survey. *BMC Musculoskeletal Disorders* **12**(1), 83-91.

Dahlgren, G. and Whitehead, M. (1991) *Policies and Strategies to Promote Social Equity in Health*. Stockholm: Institute of Futures Studies.

Dandana, A., Gammoudi, I., Ferchichi, S., Chahed, H., Limam, H., Addad, F. and Abdelhedi, M. (2011) Correlation of oxidative stress parameters and inflammatory markers in Tunisian coronary artery disease patients. *International Journal of Biomedical Science* **7**(1), 6-13.

Dare, C. and Eisler, I. (1997) Family therapy for anorexia nervosa. In D. Garner and P.E. Garfinkel (eds) *Handbook of Treatment for Eating Disorders* (2nd edn). Chichester, UK: Wiley, pp. 333-349.

Dave, J.M., An, L.C., Jeffery, R.W. and Ahluwalia, J.S. (2009) Relationships of attitudes toward fast food and frequency of fast-food intake in adults. *Obesity* **17**(6), 1164-1170.

Davey, G. (2008) *Psychopathology: Research, Assessment and Treatment in Clinical Psychology*. BPS Blackwell.

Davey, G.C.L. (2007) Psychopathology and treatment of specific phobias. *Psychiatry* **6**(6), 247-253.

David, A.S. (2009) Basic concepts in neuropsychiatry. In A.S. David, S. Fleminger, M.D. Kopelman, S. Lovestone, and J.D.C. Mellers (eds) *Lishman's Organic Psychiatry: A Textbook of Neuropsychiatry.* (4th edn). Oxford: Wiley-Blackwell, pp. 3–28.

Davidhizar, R. (1983) Critique of the health-belief model. *Journal of Advanced Nursing* **8**(6), 467–472.

Davidson, P.W., Prasher, V.P. and Janicki, M.P. (2003) *Mental Health, Intellectual Disabilities and the Aging Process.* Oxford: Blackwell.

Dean, C. and Surtees, P.G. (1989) Do psychological factors predict survival in breast cancer? *Journal of Psychosomatic Research* **33**(5), 561–569.

Deardorff, W. (2003) The gate control theory of chronic pain. Retrieved 13 December 2011 from http://www.spine-health.com

Dehghani, M., Sharpe, L. and Nicholas, M. (2003) Selective attention to pain-related information in chronic musculoskeletal patients. *Pain* **105**(1–2), 37–46.

Denney, C.B. (2001) Stimulant effects in attention-deficit/hyperactivity disorder. *Journal of Clinical Child Psychology* **30**, 98–109.

Derenne, A. and Breitstein, M. (2010) Gradient shifts with naturally occurring human face stimuli. *The Psychological Record* **56**(3), 3.

Deschamps, M., Band, P.R. and Coldman, A.J. (1988) Assessment of adult cancer pain: shortcomings of current methods. *Pain* **32**(2), 133–139.

Devi, P.S. (2011) A timely referral to palliative care team improves quality of life. *Indian Journal of Palliative Care (suppl)* S14–16.

Devonshire, V., Lapierre, Y., Macdonell, R., Romo-Tello., Patti, F, Fontarura, R. and Kieseier, B.C. (2011) The global adherence progect (GAP): A multicentre observational study on adherence to disease-modifying therapies in patients with relapsing-remitting multiple sclerosis. *European Journal of Neurology* **18**(1), 69–77.

Dimond, E.G., Kittle, C.F. and Crockett, J.E. (1960) Comparison of internal mammary artery ligation and sham operation for angina pectoris. *American Journal of Cardiology* **5**, 483–486.

Dillworth, T. and Jensen, M.P. (2010) The role of suggestions in hypnosis for chronic pain: A review of the literature. *Open Pain Journal* **3**(1), 39–51.

Dobson, K.S., Hollon, S.D., Dimidjian, S., Schmaling, K.B., Kohlenberg, R.J., Gallop, R.J., Rizvi, S.L. and Jacobson, N.S. (2008) Randomized trial of behavioral activation, cognitive therapy, and antidepressant medication in the prevention of relapse and recurrence in major depression. *Journal of Consulting and Clinical Psychology* **76**, 468–477.

Docherty, N.M., St-Hilaire, A., Aakre, J.M. and Seghers, J.P. (2009) Life events and high-trait reactivity together predict psychotic symptom increases in schizophrenia. *Schizophrenia Bulletin* **35**(3), 638–645.

DoH (2001) *Valuing People: A New Strategy for Learning Disability for the 21st Century.* London: Department of Health.

DoH (2005) *Creating a Patient-led NHS: Delivering the NHS Improvement Plan.* London: Department of Health.

DoH and Care Service Improvement Partnership (2005) Integrated mental health services for older adults: a service development guide. Retrieved 12 October 2011, from http://www.nmhdv.org.uk/silo/files/factsheetserviceusersandcarers.pdf

Dolbier, C.L., Cocke, R.R., Leiferman, J.A., Steinhardt, M.A., Schapiro, S.J., Nehete, P.N., Perlman, J.E. and Sastry, J. (2001) Differences in functional immune responses of high versus low hardy healthy individuals. *Journal of Behavioural Medicine* **24**(3), 219–229.

Donaldson, M. (1978) *Children's Minds*. London: Fontana.

Donfrancesco, R., Iozzino, R., Caruso, B., Ferrante, L., Mugnaini, D., Talamo, A., and Masi, G. (2010) Is season of birth related to developmental dyslexia? *Annals of Dyslexia* **60**(2), 175–182.

Donnelly, E. and Hinterlong, J. (2010) Changes in social participation and volunteer activity among recently widowed older adults. *Gerontologist* **50**(2), 158–169.

Donovan, J.L. and Blake, D.R. (1992) Patient compliance: Deviance or reasoned decision making? *Social Science and Medicine* **34**, 507–513.

Drew, D. (2006) Growing, living and learning at end of life. *International Journal of Palliative Nursing* **12**(11), 504.

Duncan, G.E., Sheitman, B.B. and Leberman, J.A. (1999) An integrated view of pathophysiological models of schizophrenia. *Brain Research Reviews* **29**, 250–264.

Dunn, C., Deroo, L. and Rivara, F.P. (2001) The use of brief interventions adapted from motivational interviewing across behavioral domains: A systematic review. *Addiction* **96**, 1725–1742.

Durkin, K. (1995) *Developmental Social Psychology: From Infancy to Old Age*. Oxford: Wiley Blackwell.

Durston, S., Hulshoff Pol, H.E., Schnack, H.G., Buitelaar, J.K., Buitelaar, J.K., Steenhuis, M.P., Minderaa, R.B., Kahn, R.S. and van England, H. (2004) Magnetic resonance imaging of boys with attention-deficit/hyperactivity disorder and their unaffected siblings. *Journal of American Academy of Child and Adolescent Psychiatry* **43**, 332–340.

Dysvik, E., Sommerseth, R. and Jacobson, F. (2011) Living a meaningful life with chronic pain from a nursing perspective: Narrative approach to a case story. *International Journal of Nursing Practice* **12**(1), 36–42.

Eamon, M.K. and Mulder, C. (2005) Predicting antisocial behaviour among Latino young adolescents: An ecological sytem analysis. *American Journal of Orthopsychiatry* **75**(1), 117–127.

Edvardsson, K., Edvardsson, D. and Hornsten, A. (2009) Raising issues about children's overweight maternal and child health nurses' experiences. *Journal of Advanced Nursing* **65**(12), 2542–2551.

Egan, G. (2002) *The Skilled Helper: A Problem-management and Opportunity-development Approach to Helping* (7th edn). Pacific Grove, CA: Brooks/Cole.

Eisenberg, M.E., Neumark-Sztainer, D., Story, M. and Perry, C. (2005) The role of social norm and friends' influences on unhealthy weight-control behaviours among adolescent girls. *Social Science and Medicine* **60**(6), 1165–1173.

Eiser, C. (1997) Children's quality of life measures. *Archives of Disease in Childhood* **77**, 350–354.

Eiser, C. (1989) Children's understanding of illness: A critique of the 'stage' approach. *Psychology and Health* **3**, 93-101.

Eisler, I. (2011) Family-based treatment increases full emission at 1-year follow-up compared with adolescent-focused individual therapy in adolescents with anorexia nervosa. *Evidence Based Mental Health* **14**(1), 27.

Eisler, I., Simic, M., Russell, G.M.F. and Dare, C. (2007) A randomised controlled treatment trial of two forms of family therapy in adolescent anorexia nervosa: A five-year follow-up. *Journal of Child Psychology and Psychiatry* **48**, 552-560.

Ekman, I., Schaufelberger, M., Kjellgren, K.I., Swedberg, K. and Granger, B. (2007) Standard medication information is not enough: Poor concordance of patient and nurse perceptions. *Journal of Advanced Nursing* **60**(2), 181-186.

Elbert, A., Lovett, M., Cate-Carter, T., Pitch, A., Kerr, E. and Barr, C. (2011) Genetic variation in the KIAA0319 5' region as a possible contributor to dyslexia. *Behaviour Genetics* **41**(1), 77-89.

Elfant, E., Burns, J.W. and Zeichner, A. (2008) Repressive coping style and suppression of pain-related thoughts: Effects on responses to acute pain induction. *Cognition and Emotion* **22**(4), 671-696.

Elia, J. and Vetter, V. (2010) Cardiovascular effects of medications for the treatment of attention-deficit hyperactivity disorder. *Pediatric Drugs* **12**(3), 165-175.

Elliott, A.M., Smith, B.H., Penny, K.I., Smith, W.C. and Chambers, W.A. (1999) The epidemiology of chronic pain in the community. *Lancet* **354**(9186), 1248-1252.

Ellis, A. (1962) *Reason and Emotion in Psychotherapy*. Secaucus, NJ: Prentice-Hall.

Emerson, E. (1998) Working with people with challenging behaviour. In E. Emerson, C. Haton, J. Bromley and A. Caine (eds) *Clinical Psychology and People with Intellectual Disabilities*. Chichester: Wiley.

Emerson E., Hatton, C., Robertson, J., Roberts, H., Baines, S. and Glover, G. (2010) *People with Learning Disabilities in England*. Learning Disabilities Observatory, University of Lancaster. http://tinyurl.com/learndis-england-2010 (Accessed 20 July 2011)

Emmelkamp, P.M.G. (1982) *Phobic and Obsessive-compulsive Disorders: Theory, Research, and Practice*. New York: Plenum Press.

Emmelkamp, P.M.G., Bowman, T.K.O. and Scholing, A. (1995) *Anxiety Disorders. A Practitioner's Guide*. Chichester, UK: John Wiley.

Engel, G.L. (1980) The clinical application of the biopsychosocial model. *American Journal of Psychiatry* **137**(5), 535-544.

Erickson, C., Stigler, K., Wink, L., Mullett, J., Kohn, A., Posey, D. and McDougle, C. (2011) A prospective open-label study of aripiprazole in fragile X syndrome. *Psychopharmacology* **216**(1), 85-90.

Evans, D.L., Leserman, J., Perkins, D.O., Stern, R.A., Murphy, C., Zheng, B., Gettes, D., Longmate, J.A., Silva, S.G., van der Horst, C.M., Hall, C.D., Folds, J.D., Golden, R.N. and Petitto, J.M. (1997) Severe life stress as a predictor of early disease progression in HIV infection. *American Journal of Psychiatry* **154**(5), 630-634.

Everson-Rose, S.A. and Lewis, T.T. (2005) Psychosocial factors and cardiovascular diseases. *Annual Review of Public Health* **26**, 469-500.

Eysenck, M.W. and Flanagan, C. (2007) *Psychology for A2 Level*. East Sussex: Psychology Press.

Eysenck, W.M. and Keane, T.M. (2010) *Cognitive Psychology: A Student's Handbook*. (6th edn). New York: Psychological Press.

Ezzo, J., Berman, B., Hadhazy, V.A., Jadad, A.R., Lao, L. and Singh, B.B. (2000) Is acupuncture effective for the treatment of chronic pain? A systematic review. *Pain* **86**(3), 217-225.

Fairburn, C.G. (1997) Eating disorders. In D.M. Clark and C.G. Fairburn (eds) *Science and Practice of Cognitive Behaviour Therapy*. London: Oxford University Press, pp. 209-241.

Fairburn, C.G., Shafran, R. and Cooper, Z. (1999) A cognitive behavioural theory of anorexia nervosa. *Behaviour Research and Therapy* **37**, 1-13.

Fallon, P. (2008) Life events; their role in onset and relapse in psychosis, research utilizing semi-structured interview methods: a literature review. *Journal of Psychiatric and Mental Health Nursing* **15**(5), 386-392.

Faraone, S.V. and Khan, S.A. (2006) Candidate gene studies of attention-deficit/hyperactivity disorder. *Journal of Clinical Psychiatry* **67**, 13-21.

Farrar, J., Polomano, R., Berlin, J. and Strom, B. (2010) A comparison of change in the 0-10 numeric rating scale to a pain relief scale and global medication performance scale in short-term clinical trial of breakthrough pain intensity. *Anaesthesiology* **112**(6), 1464-1472.

Fazel, S. and Danesh, J. (2002) Serious mental disorder in 23 000 prisoners: A systematic review of 62 surveys. *Lancet* **359**(9306), 545-550.

Feeney, T. (2010) There's always something that works: Principles and practices of positive support for individuals with traumatic brain injury and problem behaviours. *Seminars in Speech and Language* **31**(1), 145-161.

Feil, N. (1996) Validation: Techniques for communicating with confused old-old persons and improving their quality of life. *Topics in Geriatric Rehabilitation* **11**(4), 34-42.

Feiler, A. and Watson, D. (2010) Involving children with learning and communication difficulties: The perspectives of teachers, speech and language therapists and teaching assistants. *British Journal of Learning Disabilities* **39**(2), 113-120.

Feingold, B.F. (1979) *The Feingold Cookbook for Hyperactive Children*. New York: Random House.

Feldt, K.S. (2000) The Checklist of Nonverbal Pain Indicators (CNPI) *Pain Management Nursing* **1**(1), 13-21.

Fernandez, E. and Towery, S.A. (1996) Parsimonious set of verbal descriptors of pain sensation derived from the McGill Pain Questionnaire. *Pain* **66**(1), 31-37.

Ferns, T. (2007) Factors that influence aggressive behaviour in acute care settings. *Nursing Standard* **21**(33), 41-45.

Ferri, C.P., Prince, M., Brayne, C., Brodaty, H., Fratiglioni, L., Ganguli, M., Hall, K., Hasegawa, K., Hendrie, H., Huang, Y., Jorm, A., Mathers, C., Menezes, P.R., Rimmer, E., Scazufca, M. and Alzheimer's Disease International (2005) Global prevalence of dementia: a Delphi consensus study. *Lancet* **366**(9503), 2112-2117.

Festinger, L. (1957) *A Theory of Cognitive Dissonance*. Stanford, CA: Stanford, University Press.

Fieldsen, D. and Wood, D. (2011) Dealing with phantom limb pain after amputation. *Nursing Times* **107**(1), 21–23.

Filges, I., Rothlisberger, B., Blattner, A., Boesch, N., Demaugin, P., Wenzel, F. and Miny, P. (2011) Deletion in Xp22.11: PTCHD1 is a candidate gene for X-linked intellectual disability with or without autism. *Clinical Genetics* **79**(1), 79–85.

Fillingham, A. (2010) Stress and coping. In A. Berman and S. Snyder (eds) *Kozier and Erb's. Fundamentals of Nursing*. Frenchs Forest, NSW, Australia: Pearson.

Figueroa-Moseley, C., Jean-Pierre, P., Roscoe, J.A., Ryan, J.L., Kohli, S., Palesh, O.G., Ryan, E.P. and Morrow, G.R. (2007) Behavioral interventions in treating anticipatory nausea and vomiting. *Journal of the National Comprehensive Care* **5**(1), 44–50.

Findley, J. (2004) The gate control theory of pain: Applying theory to practice. *Journal of Neonatal Nursing* **10**(2), 38–40.

First, M. and Pincus, H. (1999) ICD-10 v. DSM-IV. A response. *British Journal of Psychiatry* **175**, 205–209.

Fischer, B., Oviedo-Joekes, E., Blanken, P., Haasen, C., Rehm, J., Schechter, M.T., Strang, J. and van den Brink, W. (2007) Heroin-assisted treatment (HAT) a decade later: A brief update on science and politics. *Journal of Urban Health* **84**, 552–562.

Fishbein, M. (1967) Attitude and the prediction of behavior. In M. Fishbein (ed.) *Readings in Attitude Theory and Measurement*. New York: Wiley, pp. 477–492.

Fishbein, M. and Ajzen, I. (1975) *Belief, Attitude, Intention, and Behavior: An Introduction to Theory and Research*. Ontario: Addison-Wesley.

Fiske, S.T. and Taylor, S.E. (1991) *Social Cognition* (2nd edn) New York: McGraw-Hill.

Flaskerud, J. (2010) DSM proposed changes, Part 1: Criticisms and influences on changes. *Issues in Mental Health Nursing* **31**(10).

Foa, E.B. (2010) Cognitive behavioural therapy of obsessive-compulsive disorder. *Dialogues in Clinical Neuroscience* **12**(2), 199–207.

Foa, E.B., Franklin, M.E. and Kozak, M.J. (1998) Psychosocial treatments for obsessive compulsive disorder: A literature review. In R.P. Swinson, M.M. Antony, S. Rachman and M.A. Richter (eds) *Obsessive-compulsive Disorder: Theory, Research and Treatment*. New York: Guildford Press, pp. 258–276.

Folkman, S. and Lazarus, R.S. (1988) Coping as a mediator of emotion. *Journal of Personality and Social Psychology* **54**(3), 466–475.

Folstein, S.E. and Rosen-Sheidley, B. (2001) Genetics of autism: Complex aetiology for a heterogeneous disorder. *Nature Reviews Genetics* **2**(12), 943–955.

Fordyce, W.E., Lansky, D., Calsyn, D.A., Shelton, J.I., Stolov, W.C. and Roch, D.I. (1984) Pain measurement and pain behaviour. *Pain* **18**(1), 53–69.

Forgas, J. and George, J.M. (2001) Affective influences on judgements and behaviour in organisations: An information processing perspective. *Organisational Behaviour & Human Decision Processes* **86**(1), 3–34.

Fox, J. and Bailenson, J. (2009) Virtual self-modelling: The effects of vicarious reinforcement and identification on excessive behaviours. *Media Psychology* **12**(1), 1–25.

Francati, V., Vermetten, E. and Bremner, J.D. (2007) Functional neuroimaging studies in posttraumatic stress disorder: Review of current methods and findings: *Depression and Anxiety* **24**, 202-218.

Francis, J.J., Stockton, C., Eccles, M.P. Johnston, M., Cuthbertson, B.H., Grimshaw, J.M., Hyde, C. and Tinmouth, A. (2010) Evidence-based selection of theories for designing behaviour change interventions: Using methods based on theoretical constructions domains to understand clinicians' blood transfusion behaviour. *British Journal of Health Psychology* **14**(4), 625-646.

Frank, A.J.M., Moll, J.M.H. and Hort, J.F. (1982) A comparison of three ways of measuring pain. *Rheumatology* **21**, 211-217.

Frasure-Smith, N., Lesperance, F., Gravel, G., Masson, A., Juneau, M., Talajic, M. and Bourassa, M.G. (2000) Social support, depression, and mortality during the first year after myocardial infarction. *Circulation* **101**(16), 1919-1924.

French, S.E., Lenton, R., Walter, V. and Eyles, J. (2000) An empirical evaluation of an expanded nursing stress scale. *Journal of Nursing Measurement* **8**, 161-178.

Friedman, M. and Rosenman, R.H. (1974) *Type A Behavior and Your Heart*. New York: Knopf.

Fuller, B., Simmering, M.J., Marler, L.E., Cox, S.S., Bennett, R.J. and Cheramie, R.A. (2011) Exploring touch as a positive workplace behaviour. *Human Relations* **64**(2), 231-256.

Furlan, A.D., van Tulder, M., Cherkin, D., Tsukayama, H., Lao, L., Koes, B. and Berman, B. (2005) Acupuncture and dry-needling for low back pain: An updated systematic review within the framework of the Cochrane Collaboration. *Spine* **30**(8), 944-963.

Galaburda, A.M. (1993) *Dyslexia and Development: Neurobiological Aspects of Extraordinary Brains*. Cambridge, MA: Harvard University Press.

Gamus, D., Meshulam-Atzmon, V., Pintov, S. and Jacoby, R. (2008) The effect of acupuncture therapy on pain perception and coping strategies: A preliminary report, *Journal of Acupuncture and Meridian Studies* **1**(1), 51-53.

Garrison, M.M., Christakis, D.A., Ebal, B.E., Wiehe, S.E. and Rivara, F.P. (2003) A systematic review of smoking cessation interventions for adolescents. *Paediatric Research* **53**(4), 3206.

Garsson, B. (2004) Psychological factors and cancer development: Evidence after 30 years of research. *Clinical Psychology Review* **24**(3), 315-338.

Gatchel, R.J., Bo Peng, Y., Peters, M.L., Fuchs, P.H. and Turk, D.C. (2007) The biopsychosocial approach to chronic pain: Scientific advances and future directions. *Psychological Bulletin* **133**, 581-624.

Gates, B. (2007) *Learning Disabilities: Toward Inclusion*. (5th edn). Burlington, MA: Elsevier Churchill Livingstone.

Gates, B. (2010) When a workforce strategy won't work: Critique on current policy direction in England UK. *Journal of Intellectual Disability* **14**(4), 251-258.

Geurts, H.M., Broeders, M. and Nieuwland, M.S. (2010) Thinking outside the executive functions box: Theory of mind and pragmatic abilities in attention deficit/hyperactivity disorder. *European Journal of Developmental Psychology* **7**(1), 135-151.

Ghali, N. and Josifova, D. (2009) Genetic investigations in children with learning difficulties. *Current Medical Literature: Pediatrics* **22**(1), 1-9.

Gibbons, C., Dempster, M. and Moutray, M. (2011) Stress, coping and satisfaction in nursing students. *Journal of Advanced Nursing* **67**(3), 621–632.

Gilboa-Schechtman, E., Franklin, M.E. and Foa, E.B. (2000) Anticipated reactions to social events: Differences among individuals with generalized social phobia, obsessive compulsive disorder and non-anxious controls. *Cognitive Therapy and Research* **24**, 731–747.

Gladstone, G.L. (2004) Behavioural inhibition: Measurement and assessment of aetiology and outcome in adults. *Dissertation Abstracts International. Section B. Sciences and Engineering* **65**(6b), 3158.

Glanzer, M. and Cunitz, A.R. (1966) Two storage mechanisms in free recall. *Journal of Verbal Learning and Verbal Behaviour* **5**, 351–360.

Glasper, A. (2011) Every nurse needs to know about learning disabilities. *British Journal of Nursing* **30**(8), 514–515.

Gleeson, M. and Higgins, A. (2009) Touching in mental health nursing: An exploratory study of nurses' views and perceptions. *Journal of Psychiatric and Mental Health Nursing* **16**(4), 382–389.

Glisky, E.L., Rubin, S.R. and Davidson, P.S. (2001) Source memory in older adults: An encoding or retrieval problem? *Journal of Experimental Psychology: Learning, Memory & Cognition* **27**, 1131–1146.

Gloaguen, V., Cottraux, J., Cucherat, M. and Blackburn, I.M. (1998) A meta-analysis of the effects of cognitive therapy in depressed patients. *Journal of Affective Disorder* **49**: 59–72.

Goh, Y., Sewang, S. and Oei, T.P.S. (2010) The revised transactional model (RTM) of occupational stress and coping: An improvement process approach. *Australian and New Zealand Journal of Organisational Psychology* **3**(1), 13–20.

Goldimond, I. (1974) Toward a constructional approach to social problems: Ethical and constitutional issues raised by applied behaviour analysis. *Behaviourism* **2**, 1–84.

Goldschneider, A. (1920) *Das Schmerz Problem*. Berlin: Springer.

Goll, P.S. (2004) Mnemonic strategies: Creating schemata for learning enhancement. *Education* **125**(2), 306–314.

Gonzales, E.A., Ledesma, R.J.A., McAllister, D.J., Perry, S.M., Dyer, C.A. and Maye, J.P. (2010) Effects of guided imagery on postoperative outcomes in patients undergoing same-day surgical procedures: A randomized, single-blind study. *American Association of Nurse Anesthetists* **73**(3), 181–188.

Gotestam, K.G. and Agras, W.S. (1995) General population-based epidomological study of eating disorders in Norway. *International Journal of Eating Disorders* **18**(2), 119–126.

Gottesman, I.I. (1991) *Schizophrenia Genesis: The Origins of Madness*. New York: W.H. Freeman.

Gottesman, I.I. and Reilly, J.L. (2003) Strengthening the evidence for genetic factors in schizophrenia (without abetting genetic discrimination) In M.F. Lenzenweger and J.M. Hooley (eds) *Principles of Experimental Psychopathology: Essays in Honor of Brendan A. Maher*. Washington, DC: American Psychological Association, pp. 31–44.

Gough, B., Fry, G., Grogan, S. and Conner, M. (2009) Why do young adult smokers continue to smoke despite the health risks? A focus group study. *Psychology and Health* **24**(2), 203–220.

Gould, R.A., Otto, M.W. and Pollack, M.H. (1995) A meta-analysis of treatment outcome for panic disorder. *Clinical Psychology Review* **15**, 819-844.

Goyette, G.H., Connors, C.K., Petti., T.A. and Curtis, L.E. (1978) Effects of artificial colors on hyperkinetic children: A double-blind challenge study. *Psychopharmacology Bulletin* **14**, 39-40.

Graf, P. and Schacter, D.L. (1985) Implicit and explicit memory for new associations in normal and amnesic subjects. *Journal of Experimental Psychology: Learning, Memory, and Cognition* **11**, 501-518.

Graham, C., Bond, S., Gerkovich, M. and Cook, M. (1980) Use of the McGill Pain Questionnaire in the assessment of cancer pain: Replicability and consistency. *Pain* **8**(3), 377-387.

Gray, J.E. (1983) A theory of anxiety: The role of the limbic system, *Encephale* **9** (Suppl 2), 161B-166B.

Gray, J.R. and Kagan, J. (2000) The challenge of determining which children with attention deficit hyperactivity disorder will respond positively to methylphenidate. *Journal of Applied Developmental Psychology* **21**, 471-489.

Gray-Toft, P. and Anderson, J.G. (1981) The nursing stress scale: Development of an instrument. *Journal of Behavioural Assessment* **3**(1), 11-23.

Greenberger, E., Chen, C., Tally, S. and Dong, Q. (2000) Family, peer, and individual correlates of depressive symptomatology in U.S. and Chinese adolescents. *Journal of Consulting and Clinical Psychology* **68**, 202-219.

Greenfield, P.M. (2004) *Weaving Generations Together: Evolving Creativity in the Maya of Chippas.* Santa Fe, NM: School of American Research.

Greer, S., Morris, T. and Pettingale, K.W. (1979) Psychological response to breast cancer: Effect on outcome. *Lancet* **2**(8146), 785-787.

Greer, S., Morris, T., Pettingale, K.W. and Haybittle, J.L. (1990) Psychological responses to breast cancer and 15 year outcome. *Lancet* **335**(8680), 49-50.

Greener, M. (2009) Tackling the burden of pain. *Nurse Prescribing* **7**(9), 398-402.

Gregson, R.A.M. and Stacey, B.G. (1981) Components of some New Zealand attitudes to alcohol and drinking in 1978-79: A preliminary report. *New Zealand Psychologist* **9**, 29-33.

Gremigni, P., Bacchi, F., Turrini, C., Cappelli, G., Albertazzi, A., Enrico, P. and Bitti, R. (2007) Psychological factors associated with medication adherence following renal transplantation. *Clinical Transplantation* **21**(6), 710-715.

Gross, R. (2010) *Psychology: The Science of Mind and Behaviour.* (6th edn). London: Hodder Education.

Gross, R. and Kinnison, N. (2007) *Psychology for Nurses and Allied Health Professionals.* London: Hodder Arnold.

Grossman, P., Tiefenthaler-Gilmer, U., Raysz, A. and Kesper, U. (2007) Mindfulness training as an intervention for fibromyalgia: evidence of postintervention and 3-year follow-up benefits in well-being. *Psychotherapy and Psychosomatics* **76**(4), 226-233.

Gude, D. (2011) Battling chemotherapy induced nausea and vomiting in cancer palliative care. *Indian Journal of Palliative Care* **17**(1), 78-79.

Gullaspie, M. (2010) Better pain management after total joint replacement surgery: A quality improvement approach. *Orthopaedic Nursing* **29**(1), 20-26.

Gumpel, T. (2007) Are social competence difficulties caused by performance or acquisition deficits? The importance of self-regulatory mechanisms. *Psychology in the Schools* **44**(4), 351-372.

Guo, Y., Le, W.D., Jankovic, J., Yang, H.-R., Xu, H.B., Xie, W.J., Song, Z. and Deng, H. (2011) Systematic genetic analysis of the PITX3 gene in patients with Parkinson disease. *Movement Disorder* **26**(9), 1729-1732.

Gupta, M.A. and Johnson, A.M. (2000) Non-weight-related body image concerns among female eating-disordered patients and nonclinical controls: Some preliminary observations. *International Journal of Eating Disorders* **27**, 304-309.

Gwaltney, C., Metrik, J., Kahler, C. and Shiffman, S. (2009) Self-efficacy and smoking cessation: A meta-analysis. *Psychology of Addictive Behaviours* **23**(1), 56-66.

Hagger, S. (2009) Personality, individual differences, stress and health. *Journal of the International Society for the Investigation of Stress* **25**(5), 381-386.

Hajek, P., Taylor, T. and McRobbie, H. (2010) The effect of stopping smoking on perceived stress levels. *Addiction* **105**(8), 1466-1471.

Hall, G.R. (1988) *Evaluating a Low Stimulus Nursing Home Unit for Residents with Chronic Dementing Illnesses*. Master's thesis. Iowe City, Iowa: The University of Iowa College of Nursing.

Halperin, J.M. and Healey, D.M. (2011) The influences of environmental enrichment, cognitive enhancement, and physical exercise on brain development: Can we alter the developmental trajectory of ADHD? *Neuroscience & Biobehavioural Reviews* **35**(3), 621-634.

Halterman, J.S., Borrelli, B., Conn, K.M., Tremblay, P. and Blaakman, S. (2010) Motivation to quit smoking among parents of unborn children with asthma. *Patient Education and Counselling* **79**(2), 152-155.

Hana, Y., Sue, K., Hea-Kung, H. and Hee-soon, K. (2011) The effects of an animation distraction intervention on pain response of preschool children during venipuncture. *Applied Nursing Research* **24**(2), 94-100.

Hand, M.W. (2002) Quality queries: Seven key questions to evaluate temporary nursing personnel agencies. *Nursing Spectrum (West)* **3**(1), 18.

Hanley, J.R. and Thomas, A. (1984) Maintenance rehearsal and the articulatory loop. *British Journal of Psychology* **75**(4), 521-527.

Harlow, H.F. (1959) Love in infant monkeys. *Scientific American* **200**(6), 64-74.

Harrison, E., Shankar, J., Theriaque, D., Burns, S. and Sherrill, L. (2006) The gluten-free, casein-free diet in autism: Results of a preliminary double blind clinical trial. *Journal of Autism & Developmental Disorders* **36**(3), 413-420.

Haskard, K.B., DiMetteo, M., Robin, M. and Heritage, J. (2009) Affective and instrumental communication in primary care interactions: Predicting the satisfaction of nursing staff and patients. *Health Communication* **24**(1), 21-32.

Hatch, J.P., Prihoda, T.J., Moore, P.J., Cyr-Provost, M., Borcherding, S., Boutros, N.N. and Seleshi, E. (1991) A naturalistic study of the relationships among electromyographic activity, psychological stress, and pain in ambulatory tension-type headache patients and headache-free controls. *Psychosomatic Medicine* **53**(5), 576-584.

Haynes, R.B., Taylor, D.W. and Sackett, D.L. (1979) *Compliance in Healthcare*. Baltimore, MD: Johns Hopkins University Press.

Healey, D.M., Flory, J.D., Miller, C. and Halperin, J.M. (2011) Maternal positive parenting style is associated with better functioning in hyperactive/inattentive preschool children. *Infant and Child Development* **20**(2), 148-161.

Health and Age (2006) The importance of empathy when nursing patients. *Health and Age*, 27 November.

Heffer, K.L., Kiecolt-Glaser, J.K., Loving, T.J., Glaser, R. and Malarkey, W.B. (2004) Spousal support satisfaction as a modifier of physiological responses to marital conflict in younger and older couples. *Journal of Behavioural Medicine* **27**(3), 233-254.

Helgeson, V.S. (2002) Social support and quality of life. *Quality of Life Research: An International Journal of Quality of Life Aspects of Treatment, Care and Rehabilitation* **12**(Suppl 1), 25-31.

Hellzen, O., Kristiansen, L. and Norbergh, K.G. (2003) Nurses' attitudes towards older residents with long-term schizophrenia. *Journal of Advanced Nursing Practice* **43**(6), 616-622.

Hennessy, M.B., Deak, T. and Schiml-Webb, P.A. (2009) Early attachment-figure separation and increased risk for later depression: Potential mediation by proinflammatory processes. *Neuroscience and Biobehavioural Reviews* **34**(6), 782-790.

Henrich, C., Brookmeyer, K., Shrier, L. and Shahar, G. (2011) Supportive relationships and sexual risk behaviour in adolescence: An ecological-transactional approach. *Journal of Pediatric Psychology* **31**(3), 286-297.

Henriques, G. (2011) The problem of psychology. *Behavioural Science* **1**, 29-42.

Herzog, D.B., Nussbaum, K.M. and Marmor, A.K. (1996) Comorbidity and outcome in eating disorders. *Psychiatric Clinics of North America* **19**(4), 843-859.

Heslop, P., Smith, G.D., Carroll, D., Macleod, J., Hyland, F. and Hart, C. (2001) Perceived stress and coronary heart disease risk factors: The contribution of socio-economic position. *British Journal of Health Psychology* **6**(2), 167-178.

Hibbard, J.H. and Pope, C.R. (1993) The quality of social roles as predictors of morbidity and mortality. *Social Science and Medicine* **36**(3), 217-225.

Hill, J. (2003) Early identification of individuals at risk for antisocial personality disorder. *British Journal of Psychiatry* **182**, 11-14.

Hirschfeld, R.M. and Goodwin, F.K. (1988) Mood disorders. In J.A. Talbott, R.E. Hales and S.C. Yudosfsky (eds) *The American Psychiatric Press Textbook of Psychiatry,* Vol. 7. Washington, DC: American Psychiatric Press.

Hjermstad, M., Fayers, P., Haugen, D., Caraceni, A., Hanks, G., Loge, J., Fainsinger, R., Aass, N., Kaasa, S. and European Palliative Care Research Collaborative (EPCRC) (2011) Studies comparing numerical rating scales, verbal rating scales and visual analogue scales for assessment of pain intensity in adults: A systematic review. *Journal of Pain and Symptom Management* **41**(6).

Hoffman, L. (2009) The use of psychoanalytic knowledge during the implementation of penal measures. *International Forum of Psychoanalysis* **18**, 3-10.

Hoffman, L. (2010) One hundred years after Sigmund Freud's lectures in America: Towards an integration of psychoanalytic theories and techniques within psychiatry. *History of Psychiatry* **21**(4), 455-470.

REFERENCES

Hoffman, S., Sawyer, A., Witt, A. and Oh, D. (2010) The effect of mindfulness-based therapy on anxiety and depression: A meta-analytic review. *Journal of Counselling and Clinical Psychology* **78**(2), 169-183.

Hogart, A., Wu, D., Lasalle, J. and Schanen, N. (2010) The comorbidity of autism with genomic disorders of chromosome 12q11.2-q13. *Neurobiology of Disease* **38**(2), 181-191.

Hogg, M.A. and Vaughan, G.M. (2005) *Social Psychology* (4th edn) Harlow: Pearson Education.

Hogg, M.A. and Vaughan, G.M. (2008) *Social Psychology* (5th edn) Harlow: Pearson Education.

Hollins, M. and Bull, P. (2008) Obedience and conformity in clinical practice. *British Journal of Midwifery* **16**(8), 506-509.

Holmes, T.H. and Rahe, R.H. (1967) The social readjustment rating scale. *Journal of Psychosomatic Research* **11**, 213-218.

Holt-Lunstad, J., Smith, T.B. and Layton, B. (2010) Social relationships and mortality risk: A meta-analytic review. *PLoS Medicine* **7**(7): e1000316.

Hommel, K.A., Odell, S., Sander, E., Baldassano, R.N. and Barg, F.K. (2011) Treatment adherence in paediatric inflammatory bowel disease: Perceptions from adolescent patients and their families. *Health and Social Care in the Community* **16**(1), 80-88.

Horne, R. and Weinmann, J. (1999) Patients' beliefs about prescribed medicines and their role in adherence to treatment in chronic physical illness. *Journal of Psychosomatic Research* **47**, 555-567.

Horwitz, A.V., Widom, C.S., McLaughlin, J. and White, H.R. (2001) The impact of childhood abuse and neglect on adult mental health: A prospective study. *Journal of Health and Social Behavior* **42**(2), 184-201.

Hougaard, E. (2010) Placebo and antidepressant treatment for major depression: Is there a lesson to be learned for psychotherapy? *Nordic Psychology* **62**(2), 7-26.

Hough, M. (2002) *A Practical Approach to Counselling.* Harlow: Pearson Education.

Houldin, A.D. (2000) *Patients with Cancer: Understanding Psychological Pain.* Philadelphia: Lippincott, Williams and Wilkins.

Houts, P.S., Doak, C.C., Doak, L.G. and Loscalzoc, M.G. (2006) The role of pictures in improving health communication: A review of research on attention, comprehension, recall, and adherence. *Patient Education and Counseling* **61**(2), 173-190.

Hovland, C.I., Janis, I.L. and Kelley, H.H. (1953) *Communication and Persuasion.* New Haven, CT: Yale University Press.

HSE (2005) Psychosocial working conditions in Great Britain in 2005. Health and Safety Executive. Retrieved 18 November 2008, from http://www.hse.gov.uk/statistics/causdis/pwc2005.pdf

HSE (2011) Stress and mental health and work. Health and Safety Executive. http://www.hse.gov.uk/stress/furtheradvice/stressandmentalhealth.htm

Hubble, M.A., Duncan, B.L. and Miller, S.D. (1999) *The Heart and Soul of Change.* Washington DC: American Psychological Association.

Hudson, J.I., Hiripi, E., Pope, H.G. and Kessler, R.C. (2007) The prevalence and correlates of eating disorders in the National Comorbidity Survey Replication. *Biological Psychiatry* **61**, 348-358.

Huguet, A., Stinson, J. and McGrath, P. (2010) Measurement of self-reported pain intensity in children and adolescents. *Journal of Psychosomatic Research* **68**(4), 329-336.

Hunot, V., Churchill, R., Silva de Lima, M. and Teixeira, V. (2007) Psychological therapies for generalised anxiety disorder. *Cochrane Database of Systematic Reviews* **24**(1), CD001848.

Hunt, P. and Pearson, D. (2001) Motivating change. *Nursing Standard* **16**(2), 45-52.

Huque, M.F. (1988) Experiences with meta-analysis in NDA submissions. *Proceedings of the Biopharmaceutical Section of the American Statistical Association* **2**, 28-33.

Hurley, A., Tomasulo, D.J. and Pfadt, A.G. (1998) Individual and group psychotherapy approaches for persons with intellectual disabilities and developmental disabilities. *Journal of Developmental and Physical Disabilities* **10**, 365-386.

Husson, O., Mols, F. and Poll-Franse, L.V. van de (2011) The relation between information disclosure and health-related quality of life and psychological distress among cancer survivors: A systematic review. *Annals of Oncology* **22**, 761-772.

Hutson, M. (2008) Know your audience. *Psychology Today* **41**(4), 27.

IASP (1992) *Classification of Chronic Pain* (2nd edn). Seattle: International Association for the Study of Pain, IASP.

Ibrahim, N.K., Attia, S., Sallam, S., Fetohy, E. and El-Seovi, F. (2010) Physicians' therapeutic practice and compliance of diabetic patients attending rural primary health care units in Alexandria. *Journal of Family and Community Medicine* **17**(3), 121-128.

Iigen, M., Schulenberg, J., Kloska, D., Czyz, E., Johnston, L. and O'Malley, P. (2011) Addictive behaviours (Article in press).

Ilott, N., Saudino, K.J, Wood, A. and Asherson, P. (2010) A genetic study of ADHD and activity level in infancy. *Genes, Brain and Behavior* **9**(3), 296-304.

Iliffe, S. and Drennan, V. (2001) *Primary Care and Dementia*. London: Jessica Kingsley.

Inman, A. (2010) The cancer journey. *Biofeedback* **38**(1), 24-27.

Ishikawa, H., Hashimoto, H., Kinoshita, M. and Yano, E. (2010) Can nonverbal communication skills be taught? *Medical Teacher* **32**(10), 860-863.

Iwata, B.A., Pace, G.M., Dorsey, M.F., Zarcone, J.R., Vollmer, T.R., Smith, R.G., Rodgers, T.A., Lerman, D.C., Shore, B.A., Mazalesk, J.L., Goh, H., Cowdery, E.G., Kalsher, M.J., McCosh, K.C. and Willis, K.D. (1994) The functions of self-injurious behaviour: An experimental-epidemiological study. *Journal of Applied Behaviour Analysis* **23**, 99-110.

Jacobson, E. (1938) *Progressive Relaxation*. Chicago: University of Chicago Press.

Jacobson, R., Moldrup, C. and Christrup, L. (2010) Psychological and behavioural predictors of pain management outcomes in patients with cancer. *Scandinavian Journal of Caring Sciences* **12**(4), 781-790.

Janis, I.L. (1967) Effect of fear arousal on attitude change: Recent developments in theory and experimental research. In L. Berkowitz (ed.) *Advances in Experimental Social Psychology*. New York: Academic Press, pp. 167-224.

Jensen, M.P. (2011) Psychosocial approaches to pain management: An organizational framework. *Pain* **152**(4), 717-725.

Jensen, M.P., Ehde, D.M., Gertz, K.J., Stoelb, B.L., Dillworth, T.M., Hirsh, A.T., Molton, I.R. and Kraft, G.H. (2011) Effects of self-hypnosis training and cognitive restructuring on daily pain intensity and catastrophizing in individuals with multiple sclerosis and chronic pain. *International Journal of Clinical and Experimental Hypnosis* **59**(1), 45-63.

Jensen, M. and Patterson, D.R. (2006) Hypnotic treatment of chronic pain. *Journal of Behavioural Medicine* **29**(1), 95-124.

Johnson, S., Batey, M. and Holdsworth, J. (2009) Personality and health: The mediating role of trait emotional intelligence and work locus of control. *Personality and Individual Differences* **47**(5), 470-475.

Johnston, C. and Mash, E.J. (2001) Families of children with attention-deficit/hyperactivity disorder: Review and recommendations for future research. *Clinical Child and Family Psychology Review* **4**(3), 183-207.

Jones, A., Spindler, H., Jorgensen, M.M. and Zachariae, R. (2002) The effect of situation-evoked anxiety and gender on pain report using the cold pressor test. *Scandinavian Journal of Psychology* **43**(4), 307-313.

Jones, H. (1993) Altered images. *Nursing Times* **89**(5), 58-60.

Jones, J.R., Huxtable, C.S. and Hodgson, J.T. (2006) *Self-Reported Work-Related Illness in 2004/05: Results from The Labour Force Survey.* Caerphilly: Health and Safety Executive.

Jones, S.E. and Yarbrough, A.E. (1985) A naturalistic study of the meanings of touch. *Communication Monographs* **52**, 19-56.

Jones, S.H. (2006) Cognitive therapy and bipolar disorder. *Expert Review of Neurotheraputics* **2**(4), 573-581.

Jootun, D. and McGhee, G. (2011) Effective communication with people who have dementia. *Nursing Standard* **25**(25), 40-46.

Joubert, J., Reid, C., Borton, D., Cumming, T., McLean, A., Joubert, L., Barlow, J., Ames, D. and Davis, S. (2009) Integrated care improves risk-factor modification after stroke: Initial results of the integrated care for the reduction of secondary stroke model. *Journal of Neurology, Neurosurgery and Psychiatry* **80**, 279-284.

Joyce, D. (2006) Basic science of pain. *Journal of Bone and Joint Surgery* **88**(2), 58-62.

Kang, Y., Moyle, W. and Venturato, L. (2011) Korean nurses' attitudes towards older people with dementia in acute care settings. *International Journal of Older People Nursing* **6**(2), 143-152.

Kanner, A.D., Coyne, J.C., Schafer, C. and Lazarus, R.S. (1981) Comparison of two modes of stress measurement: Daily hassles and uplifts versus major life events. *Behavioral Medicine* **4**(4), 1-39.

Kaptchuk, T.J., Friedlander, E., Kelley, J.M., Sanchez, M.N., Kokkotou, E., Singer, J.P., Kowalczykowski, M., Miller, F.G., Kirsch, I. and Lembo, A.J. (2010) Placebos without deception: A randomized controlled trial in irritable bowel syndrome. *Plus One* **5**(12), 1-7.

Karling, M., Renstrom, M. and Ljungman, G. (2002) Acute and postoperative pain in children. *Acta Paediatric* **91**(6), 660-666.

Kastenbaum, R. (1979) *Growing Old - Years of Fulfilment.* London: Harper and Row.

Kater, K.J., Rohwer, J. and Levine, M.P. (2000) An elementary school project for developing healthy body image and reducing the risk factors for unhealthy and disordered eating. *Eating Disorders*, 3-15.

Katic, B.J., Krause, S.J., Tepper, S.J., Hu, H.X. and Bigal, M.J. (2009) Adherance to acute migraine medication: What does it mean, why does it matter? *Headache: The Journal of Head and Face Pain* **50**(1), 117-129.

Katon, W.J. (2006) Panic disorder. *New England Journal of Medicine* **35**, 2360-2367.

Kaye, W.H., Nagata, T., Weltzin, T.E, Hsu, L.K., Sokol, M.S., McConaha, C., Plotnicov, K.H. and Deep, D. (2001) Double-blind placebo-controlled administration of fluoxetine in restricting – and restricting purging-type anorexia nervosa. *Biological Psychiatry* **49**, 644-652.

Kazdin, A.E. and Bass, D. (1989) Power to detect differences between alternative treatments in comparative psychotherapy outcome research. *Journal of Consulting and Clinical Psychology* **57**, 138-147.

Kean, S. (2010) Children and young people visiting an adult intensive care unit. *Journal of Advanced Nursing* **66**(4), 868-877.

Keck, P.E. Jr, McIntyre, R.S. and Shelton, R.C. (2007) Bipolar depression: Best practices for the outpatient. *CNS Spectrums* **12**(20), 1-14.

Keel, P.K., Heatherton, T.F., Dorer, D.J., Joiner, T.E. and Zalta, A.K. (2006) Point prevalence of bulimia nervosa in 1982, 1992, and 2002. *Psychological Medicine* **36**, 119-127.

Keenan, T. (2002) *An Introduction to Child Development*. London: Sage.

Kerr, R., McHugh, M. and McCrory, M. (2009) HSE Management standards and stress-related work outcomes. *Occupational Medicine* **59**(8), 574-579.

Keller, P.A. and Block, L.G. (1995) Increasing the persuasiveness of fear appeals: The effect of arousal and elaboration. *Journal of Consumer Research* **22**, 448-459.

Kelly, J. (1995) Making sense of drug compliance. *Nursing Times* **91**(40), 40-41.

Kelsoe, J.R. (2003) Arguments for the genetic basis of the bipolar spectrum. *Journal of Affective Disorders* **73**, 183-197.

Kemeny, M.E. (2003) The psychology of stress. *Current Directions in Psychological Science* **12**(4), 124-129.

Kendler, K. and Schaffner, K. (2011) The dopamine hypothesis of schizophrenia: An historical and philosophical analysis. *Philosophy, Psychiatry and Psychology* **18**(1), 41-63.

Kessels, R.P.C. (2003) Patients' memory for medical information. *Journal of Royal Society Medicine* **96**, 219-222.

Kessler, R.C., Berglund, P.A., Bruce, M.L., Koch, J.R., Laska, E.M., Leaf, P.J., Manderscheid, R.W. and Wang, P.S. (2001) The prevalence and correlates of untreated serious mental illness. *Health Services Research* **36**, 987-1007.

Kessler, R.C., Berglund, P., Demler, O., Jin, R., Merikangas, M.R. and Walters, E.E. (2005a) Lifetime prevalence and age-of-onset distributions of *DSM-IV* disorders in the National Comorbidity Survey Replication. *Archives of General Psychiatry* **62**, 593-602.

Kessler, R.C., Burglund, P., Demler, O., Jin, R., Koretz, D., Merikangas, K.R., Rush, A.J. and Wang, P.S. (2003) The epidemiology of major depressive disorder: Results from the National Comorbidity Survey Replication (NCR-R) *Journal of the American Medical Association* **289**, 3095-3105.

Kessler, R.C., Demler, O., Frank, R.G., Olfson, M., Pincus, H.A., Walters, E.E. and Wang, P. (2005b) Prevalence and treatment of mental disorders, 1990-2003. *The New England Journal of Medicine* **352**(24), 2515-2523.

Kessler, R.C., Gruber, M., Hettema, J.M., Hwang, I., Sampson, N. and Yonkers, K.A. (2008) Comorbid major depression and generalized anxiety disorders in the National Comorbidity Survey follow-up. *Psychological Medicine* **38**(3), 365-374.

Keys, T.R., Morant, K.M. and Stroman, C.R. (2009) Black youth's personal involvement in the HIV/AIDS issue: Does the public service announcement still work? *Journal of Health Communication* **14**(2), 189–202.

Khadilkar, A., Odebiyi, D.O., Brosseau, L. and Wells, G.A. (2008) Transcutaneous Electrical Nerve Stimulation (TENS) versus placebo for chronic low-back pain. *Physical Therapy Reviews* **13**(5), 355–365.

Khanna, M.S. and Kendall, P.C. (2010) Computer-assisted cognitive behavioral therapy for child anxiety: Results of a randomized clinical trial. *Journal of Consulting and Clinical Psychology* **78**(5), 737–745.

Kiecolt-Glaser, J.K., Fisher, L.D., Ogrocki, P., Stout, J.C., Speicher, C.E. and Glaser, R. (1987) Marital quality, marital disruption, and immune function. *Psychosomatic Medicine* **49**(1), 13–34.

Kiecolt-Glaser, J.K. and Glaser, R. (1992) Psychoneuroimmunology: Can psychological interventions modulate immunity? *Journal of Consulting and Clinical Psychology* **60**(4), 569–575.

Kiecolt-Glaser, J.K., Loving, T.J., Stowell, J.R., Malarkey, W.B., Lemeshow, S., Dickinson, S.L. and Glaser, R. (2005) Hostile marital interactions, proflammatory cyrokine production, and wound healing. *Archives of General Psychiatry* **62**, 1377–1384.

Kiernan, C., Reeves, D., Hatton, C., Alborz, A., Emerson, E., Mason, H., Swarbrick, R., and Mason, L. (1997) *The HARC Challenging Behaviour Project. Report 1: The Persistence of Challenging Behaviour*. Hester Adrian Research Centre: Manchester.

Kim, P., Sorcar, P., Um, S., Chung, H. and Lee, Y.S. (2009) Effects of episodic variations in web-based avian influenza education: Influence of fear and humor on perception, comprehension, retention and behaviour. *Health Education Research* **24**(3), 369–380.

Kindermann, T.A. (2011) Commentary: The invisible hand of the teacher. *Journal of Applied Psychology* (in press). DOI: 10.1016/j.appdev.2011.04.005.

King, D.W., King, L.A., Foy, D.W., Keane, T.M. and Fairbank, F.A. (1999) Posttraumatic stress disorder in a national sample of female and male Vietnam veterans: Risk factors, war-zone stressors, and resilience-recovery variables. *Journal of Abnormal Psychology* **108**, 164–170.

King, K.A., Vidourek, R. and Schwiebert, M. (2009). Disordered eating and job stress among nurses. *Journal of Nursing* **17**(7), 861–869.

King-Sears, M.E., Mercer, C.D. and Sindelar, P.T. (1992) Toward independence with keyword mnemonics: A strategy for science vocabulary instruction. *Remedial and Special Education* **13**(5), 22–33.

Kitwood, T. (1997) *Dementia Reconsidered: The Person Comes First*. Buckingham: Open University Press.

Klages, U., Kianifard, S., Ulusoy, Ö. and Wehrbein, H. (2006) Anxiety sensitivity as predictor of pain in patients undergoing restorative dental procedures. *Community Dentistry and Oral Epidemiology* **34**: 139–145. doi: 10.1111/j.1600-0528.2006.00265.x

Kliem, S., Kroger, C. and Kosfelder, J. (2010) Dialectical behavior therapy for borderline Personality Disorder: A meta-analysis using mixed-effects modeling. *Journal of Consulting and Clinical Psychology* **78**(6), 936–951.

Knivsberg, A.M., Reichelt, K.L., Hoien, T. and Nodland, M. (1998) Parents' observations after one year of dietary intervention for children with autistic syndromes. *Psychobiology of Autism: Current Research and Practice*, 13-24.

Ko, D.M. and Kim, H.S. (2010) Message framing and defensive processing. A cultural examination. *Health Communication* **25**(1), 61-68.

Kobasa, S.C. (1979) Stressful life events, personality, and health: Inquiry into hardiness. *Journal of Personality and Social Psychology* **37**(1), 1-11.

Koegel, R.L., Koegel, L.K and McNerney, E.K. (2001) Pivotal areas in intervention for autism. *Journal of Clinical Child Psychology* **30**, 19-32.

Kofler, M.J., Rapport, M.D., Bolden, J., Sarver, D.E., Raiker, J.S. and Alderson, M.R. (2011) Working memory deficits and social problems in children with ADHD. *Journal of Abnormal Child Psychology* **39**(6), 805-817.

Koolhaas, J.M., de Boer, S.F., Coppens, C.M. and Buwalda, B. (2010) Neuroendocrinology of coping styles: Towards understanding the biology of individual variation. *Frontiers in Neuroendocrinology* **31**(3), 307-321.

Koons, C.R., Robins, C.J., Tweed, J.L., Lynch, T.R., Gonzalez, A.M., Morse, J.Q. and Bastian, L.A. (2001) Efficacy of dialectical behaviour therapy in women veterans with borderline personality disorder. *Behavior Therapy* **32**(2), 371-390.

Korinek, L. (1991) Self management for the mentally retarded. In R.A. Gable (ed.) *Advances in Mental Retardation and Developmental Disabilities* (Vol. 4). London: Jessica Kingsley.

Kozulin, A. (ed.) (2003) *Vygotsky's Educational Theory in Cultural Context*. Cambridge, UK: Cambridge University Press.

Koszycki, D., Talijaird, M., Segal., Z. and Bradwejn, J. (2011) A randomized trial of sertraline, self-administered cognitive behavior therapy, and their combination for panic disorder. *Psychological Medicine* **41**(2), 373-383.

Kramer, U. (2010) Coping and defence mechanisms: What's the difference? - Second act. *Psychology and Psychotherapy: Theory, Research and Practice* **83**(2), 207-221.

Kraus, G. and Reynolds, D.J. (2001) The "ABC's" of the Cluster B's: Identifying, understanding, and treating Cluster B personality disorders. *Clinical Psychology Review* **21**, 345-373.

Kreitler, S. (1999) Denial in cancer patients. *Cancer Investigation* **17**, 514-534.

Kremer, E., Atkinson, J.H. and Ignelzi, R.J. (1981) Measurement of pain: Patient preference does not compound pain measurement. *Pain* **10**(2), 241-248.

Kreuter, M.W., Chheda, S.G. and Bull, F.C. (2000) How does physician advice influence patient behaviour? *Archives of Family Medicine* **9**, 426-433.

Kroenke, C.H., Hankinson, S.E., Schernhammer, E.S., Coditz, G.A., Kawachi, I. and Holmes, M.D. (2004) Caregiving stress, endogenous sex steroid hormone levels, and breast cancer incidence. *American Journal of Epidemiology* **159**(11), 1019-1027.

Krueger, P.M. and Chang, V.W. (2008) Being poor and coping with stress: Health behaviors and the risk of death. *American Journal of Public Health* **98**(5), 889-896.

Krueger, R.F., Watson, D. and Barlow, D.H. (2005) Introduction to the special section: Toward a dimensionally based taxonomy of psychopathology. *Journal of Abnormal Psychology* **114**, 491-493.

Kübler-Ross, E. (1969) *On Death and Dying*. New York: Macmillan.

Kuhn, S., Cooke, K., Collins, M., Jones, J.M. and Mucklow, J.C. (1990) Perceptions of pain after surgery. *British Medical Journal* **300**, 1687-1690.

Lachlan, K.A., Burke, J., Spence, P.R. and Griffin, D. (2009) Risk perceptions, race, and Hurricane Katrina. *Howard Journal of Communication* **20**(3), 295-309.

Lai, H.F. and Chang, P. (2009) What makes nurses perceive differently on the usability of same system? *Studies in Health Technology and Informatics* **149**, 743-744.

Lakatos, P.L. (2009) Prevalence predictors and clinical consequences of medical adherence in IBD: How to improve it? *World Journal of Gastroenterology* **15**(34), 4234-4239.

Lakhan, S.E. and Viera, K.F. (2009) Schizophrenia pathophysiology: Are we any closer to a complete model? *Annals of General Psychiatry* **8**, 1-8.

Lam, D. and Gale, J. (2000) Cognitive behaviour therapy: Teaching a client the ABC model - the first steps towards the process of change. *Journal of Advanced Nursing* **31**(2), 444-451.

Lam, K.S.L., Aman, M.G. and Arnold, L.E. (2006) Neurochemical correlates of autistic disorder: A review of the literature. *Research in Developmental Disabilities* **27**, 254-289.

Landolt, A.S. and Milling, L. (2011) The efficacy of hypnosis as an intervention for labour and delivery pain: A comprehensive methodological review. *Clinical Psychology Review* **31**(6), 1022-1031.

Langley, P., Fonseca, J. and Iphofen, R. (2006) Psychoimmunology and health from a nursing perspective. *British Journal of Nursing* **15**(20), 1126-1129.

Latif, S. and McNicoll, L. (2009) Medication and non-adherence in the older adult. *Medicine and Health/Rhode Island* **92**(12), 418-419.

Latter, S. (2010) Promoting concordance in prescribing interactions. In M. Courtney, M. Griffiths and J. Crown, *Independent and Supplementary Prescribing: An Essential Guide.* (2nd edn). Cambridge: Cambridge University Press.

Launder, W., Davidson, G., Anderson, I. and Barclay, A. (2005) Self-neglect: The role of judgments and applied ethics. *Nursing Standard* **19**(18), 45-51.

Lavie, N. (2010) Attention, distraction, and cognitive control under load. *Current Directions in Psychological Science* **19**(3), 143-148.

Lavoie, A. (2008) Pain hurts more if the person hurting you means it. Retrieved 20 January 2009, from http://www.medicalnewstoday.com/articles/133127.php

Lavretsky, H. (2008) History of schizophrenia as a psychiatric disorder. In K.T. Mueser and D.V. Jeste (eds) *Clinical Handbook of Schizophrenia.* New York: Guilford Press, pp. 3-13.

Lawrie, S.M., McIntosh, A.M., Hall, J., Owens, D.G.C. and Johnstone, E.C. (2008) Brain structure and function changes during the development of schizophrenia: The evidence from studies of subjects as increased genetic risk. *Schizophrenia Bulletin* **34**, 330-340.

Lazarus, R.S. and Folkman, S. (1984) *Stress, Appraisal, and Coping.* New York: Springer.

Lazarus, R.S. and Folkman, S. (1987) Transactional theory and research on emotions and coping. *European Journal of Personality* **1**, 141-170.

Lazarus, R.S. and Launier, R. (1978) Stress related transactions between person and environment. In L.A. Pervin and M. Lewis (eds) *Perspectives in International Psychology.* New York: Plenum, pp. 287-327.

Leaver, R. (2001) Urology. The empowerment of patients with chronic urinary tract infection. *Professional Nurse* 17(4), 238-241.

Leaviss, J. (2010) The role of usability usefulness and frame in persuasive health communication. PhD thesis. University of Nottingham.

Lee, H., Schmidt, K. and Ernst, E. (2005) Acupuncture for the relief of cancer-related pain: A systematic review. *European Journal of Pain* 9(4), 437-444.

Lee, M. and Rotheram-Borus, M.J. (2001) Challenges associated with increased survival among parents living with HIV. *American Journal of Public Health* 91(8), 1303-1309.

Leider, H., Dhaliwal, J., Davis, E., Kulakadlu, M. and Buikema, A. (2011) Healthcare costs and nonadherence among chronic opioid users. *American Journal of Managed Care* 17(1), 32-40.

Lennmarken, C. and Sydsjo, G. (2007) Psychological consequences of awareness and their treatment. *Best Practice and Research. Clinical Anaesthesiology* 21(3), 357-367.

Lerner, R.M., Villarruel, F.A. and Castellino, D.R. (1999) *Adolescence: Developmental Issues in the Clinical Treatment of Children*. Boston, MA: Allyn and Bacon, pp. 125-136.

Leserman, J. (2003) HIV disease progression: Depression, stress and possible mechanisms. *Biological Psychiatry* 54(3), 295-306.

Leventhal, H., Prochaska, T.R. and Hirschman, R.S. (1985) Preventive health behaviour across the lifespan. In J.C. Rosen and L.J. Solomon (eds) *Prevention in Health Psychology*. Hanover, NH: University Press of New England.

Levett-Jones, T. and Lathlean, J. (2009) 'Don't rock the boat': Nursing students' experiences of conformity and compliance. *Nursing Education Today* 29(3), 342-349.

Levy-Storms, L. (2008) Therapeutic communication training in long-term care institutions: Recommendations for future research. *Patient Education and Counseling* 73(1), 8-21.

Lewin, K. (1946) Action research and minority problems. In E. Hart and M. Bond (eds) *Action Research for Health and Social Care: A Guide to Practice*. Buckingham: Open University Press.

Lewinsohn, P.M., Youngren, M.A. and Grosscup, S.J. (1979) Reinforcement and depression. In R.A. Dupue (ed.) *The Psychobiology of Depressive Disorders: Implications for the Effects of Stress*. New York: Academic Press, pp. 291-316.

Ley, P. (1979) Memory for medical information. *British Journal of Social Clinical Psychology* 18, 245-255.

Ley, P. (1981) Professional non-compliance: A neglected problem. *British Journal of Clinical Psychology* 20, 151-154.

Ley, P. (1989) Improving patients' understanding, recall, satisfaction and compliance. In A. Boome (ed.) *Health Psychology*. London: Chapman and Hall.

Ley, R. (1987) Panic disorder and agoraphobia: Fear of fear or fear of the symptoms produced by hyperventilation? *Journal of Behavioural Therapy and Experimental Psychiatry* 18(4), 305-316.

Liddell, C., Rae, G., Brown, T.R., Johnston, D., Coates, V. and Mallet, J. (2004) Giving patients an audiotape of their GP consultation: A randomized control trial. *British Journal of General Practice* 54(506), 667-672.

Liddle, H. and Hogue, A. (2000) A family-based, developmental-ecological preventative intervention for high-risk adolescents. *Journal of Marital and Family Therapy* 26(3), 265-279.

Lieb, R., Wittchen, H-U., Hofler, M., Fuetsch, M., Stein, M.B. and Merikangas, K.R. (2000) Parental psychopathology, parenting styles, and the risk of social phobia in offspring: A prospective/longitudinal community study. *Archives of General Psychiatry* **57**, 859-866.

Lieberman, J.A., Kinon, B.J. and Loebel, A.D. (1990) Dopaminergenic mechanisms in idiopathic and drug-induced psychoses. *Schizophrenia Bulletin* **16**, 97-109.

Lillberg, K., Verkasalo, P.K., Kapiro, J., Teppo, L., Helenius, H. and Koskenvuo, M. (2003) Stressful life events and risk of breast cancer in 10,808 women: A cohort study. *American Journal of Epidemiology* **157**, 415-423.

Lin Bing, Yu Xu-yan and Lin Yu (2007) Insight of schema theory into interpretation practice. *US-China Foreign Language* **5**(10), 13-17.

Lin, M.F., Chiou, J.H., Chou, M.H. and Hsu, M.C. (2006) Significant experience of token therapy from the perspective of psychotic patients. *Journal of Nursing Research* **14**(4), 315-323.

Linebarger, J.S., Sahler, O.J.Z. and Egan, K.A. (2009) Coping with death. *Pediatrics in Review* **30**(9), 350-356.

Lingam, R. and Scott, J. (2003) Treatment non-adherence in affective disorders. *Acta Psychiatrica Scandinavica* **105**(3), 164-172.

Li-Rong and Nian Yue (2010) Application of schema theory in teaching college English reading. *Canadian Social Science* **6**(1), 59-65.

Liston, C., Cohen, M., Teslovich, T., Levenson, D. and Casey, B. (2011) Atypical prefrontal connectivity in attention-deficit/hyperactivity disorder: Pathway to disease or pathological end point? *Biological Psychiatry* **69**(12), 1168-1177.

Livsey, K. (2009) Structural empowerment and professional nursing practice behaviours of baccalaureate nursing students in clinical learning environments. *International Journal of Nursing Education Scholarship* **6**(1).

Lock, J., and Le Grange, D. (2005) Family-based treatment of eating disorders. *International Journal of Eating Disorders* **37**, 64-67.

Loeber, R., Green, S.M. and Lahey, B.B. (2003) Risk factors for adult antisocial personality. In D.P. Farrington and J.W. Coid (eds) *Early Prevention of Adult Antisocial Behaviour.* Cambridge, England: Cambridge University Press, pp. 79-108.

Lolak, S., Connors, G.L., Sheridan, M.J. and Wise, T.N. (2008) Effects of progressive muscle relaxation training on anxiety and depression in patients enrolled in an outpatient pulmonary rehabilitation programme. *Psychotherapy and Psychosomatics* **77**(2), 119-125.

Lovaas, O.I. (1987) Behavioural treatment and normal educational and intellectual functioning in young autistic children. *Journal of Consulting and Clinical Psychology* **55**, 3-9.

Lovell, B. and Wetherell, M.A. (2011) The caregiver control model of chronic stress: Endocrine and immune implications in elderly and non-elderly caregivers. *Neuroscience & Biobehavioural Reviews* **35**(6), 1342-1352.

Lowe, G. (1995) Alcohol and drug addiction. In A.A. Lazarus and A.M. Coleman (eds) *Abnormal Psychology.* London: Longman.

Lowe, J., Maclean, P.C., Shaffer, M.L. and Watterberg, K. (2009) Early working memory in children born with extremely low birth weight: Assessed by object permanence. *Journal of Child Neurology* **24**(4), 410-415.

Lueboonthavathchi, P. (2009) Role of stress areas, stress severity and stressful life events on the onset of depressive disorder: A case-control study. *Journal of the Medical Association of Thailand* **92**(2), 1240–1249.

Luengo-Fernandez, R., Leal, J. and Gray, A. (2010) *Dementia 2010. The Prevalence, Economic Cost and Research Funding of Dementia Compared with Other Major Diseases.* www.alzheimers-research.org.uk/assets/docs/2010020 1103600Dementia2010Exec.pdf. retrieved online (19/12/2010)

Lumsdaine, A.A. and Janis, I.L. (1953) Resistance to 'counterpropaganda' produced by one-sided and two-sided 'propaganda' presentations. *Public Opinion Quarterly* **17**, 311–318.

Luo, L., and Craik, F. (2009) Age differences in recollection: Specificity effects at retrieval. *Journal of Memory and Language* **60**(4), 421–436.

Lundberg, U. (2006) Stress, subjective and objective health. *International Journal of Social Welfare* **15**(1) (suppl.), s41–s48.

Luszczynska, A., Benight, C. and Cieslak, R. (2009) Self-efficacy and health-related outcomes of collective trauma: A systematic review. *European Psychologist* **14**(1), 51–62.

Lysaker, P.H. and Davis, L.W. (2004) Social function in schizophrenia and schizoaffective disorder: Associations with personality, symptoms and neurocognition. *Health & Quality of Life Outcomes* **2**, 15.

Lyons, G. (2005) The Life Satisfaction Matrix: an instrument and procedure for assessing the subjective quality of life of individuals with profound multiple disabilities. *Journal of Intellectual Disability Research* **49**(10), 766–769.

Ma, S.H. and Teasdale, J.D. (2004) Mindfulness-based cognitive therapy for depression: Replication and exploration of differential relapse prevention effects. *Journal of Consulting and Clinical Psychology* **72**(1), 31–40.

Madden, A. and Parkes, J. (2010) Impact of learning disability on the health, participation and quality of life of children with cerebral palsy. *Learning Disability Practice* **13**(10), 28–33.

Mahalik, J.R. and Burns, S.M. (2011) Predicting health behaviours in young men that put them at risk for heart disease. *Psychology of Men and Masculinity* **12**(1), 1–12.

Mancini, J. and Huebner, A. (2004) Adolescent risk behavior patterns: Effects of structured time-use, interpersonal connections, self-system characteristics, and socio-demographic influences. *Child and Adolescent Social Work Journal* **21**(6), 647–668.

Markovitz, P.J. (2004) Recent trends in the pharmacotherapy of personality disorders. *Journal of Personality Disorder* **18**(1), 90–101.

Marks, D.F. (2005) *Health Psychology: Theory, Research and Practice*. London: Sage.

Maslow, A. (1954) *Motivation and Personality*. New York: Harper and Row.

Maslow, A. (1970) *Motivation and Personality*. (2nd edn). New York: Harper and Row.

Massé, R. (2000) Qualitative and quantitative analyses of psychological distress: Methodological complementarity and ontological incommensurability. *Qualitative Health Research* **10**(3), 411–423.

Matarazzo, J.D. (1982) Behavioural health's challenge to academic, scientific and professional psychology. *American Psychologist* **37**, 1–14.

Matjasko, J., Needham, B., Grunden, L. and Farb, A. (2010) Violent victimisation and perpetration during adolescence: Developmental stage dependent ecological models. *Journal of Youth and Adolescence* **39**(9), 1053–1066.

Matthews, G. and Campbell, S.E. (2009) Sustained performance under overload: Personality and individual differences in stress and coping. *Theoretical Issues in Ergonomics* **10**(5), 417–442.

Matthys, J., Elwyn, G., Van Nuland, M., Van Maele, G., De Sutter, A., De Meyere, M. and Deveugele, M. (2009) Patients' ideas, concerns, and expectations (ICE) in general practice: Impact on prescribing. *British Journal of General Practice* **59**(558), 29–36.

Matziou, V., Galanis, P., Tsoumakas, C., Gymnopoulou, E., Perdikaris, P. and Brokalaski, H. (2009) Attitudes of nurse professionals and nurse students towards children with disabilities. Do nurses really overcome children's physical and mental handicaps? *International Nursing Reviews* **56**, 456–460.

Maynard, T. and Thomas, N. (2009) *An Introduction to Early Childhood Studies*. (2nd edn). London: Sage.

McAllister-Williams, R.H., Foran, K., Forrest, S., Ingram, G., McMahon, L., Taylor, M., Rajwal, M. and Cornwall, L. (2006) NICE guidelines on antidepressants. *British Journal of General Practice* **56**(531), 798–800.

McCabe, C. and Timmins, F. (2006) *Communication Skills for Nursing Practice.* Basingstoke: Palgrave Macmillan.

McDonald, H.P., Garg, A.X. and Haynes, R.B. (2002) Interventions to enhance patient adherence to medication prescriptions: Scientific review. *Journal of the American Medical Association* **288**, 2868–2879.

McGregor, B.A., Antoni, M.H., Boyers, A., Alferi, S.M., Blomberg, B.B. and Carver, C.S. (2004) Cognitive-behavioural stress management increases benefit finding and immune function among women with early-stage cancer. *Journal of Psychosomatic Research* **56**(1), 1–8.

McGue, M. and Iacono, W.G. (2005) The association of early adolescents' problem behaviour with adult psychopathology. *American Journal of Psychiatry* **162**, 1118–1124.

McGuire, W.J. (1969) The nature of attitude and attitude change. In G. Lindzey and E. Aronson (eds) *Handbook of Social Psychology* (2nd edn), vol. 3. Reading, MA: Addison-Wesley.

McGuire, W.J. (1986) The vicissitudes of attitudes and similar representational constructs in twentieth century psychology. *European Journal of Social Psychology* **16**, 89–130.

McHorney, C.A. and Gadkari, A.S. (2010) Individual patients hold different beliefs to prescription medications to which they persist vs nonpersist and persist vs nonfulfill. *Patient Preference and Adherence* **21**(4), 187–195.

McLean, S.A. and Clauw, D.J. (2005) Biomedical models of fibromyalgia. *Disability and Rehabilitation* **27**(12), 659–665.

McLeod, J. (2001) *Qualitative Research in Counselling and Psychotherapy*. London: Sage.

McMain, S.F., Links, P.S., Gnam, W.H., Guimond, T., Cardish, R.J., Korman, L. and Streiner, D.L. (2009) A randomized trial of dialectical behavior therapy versus general psychiatric management for borderline personality disorder. *American Journal of Psychiatry* **166**(12), 1365-1374.

McQuillan, A., Nicastro, R., Guenot, F., Girard, M., Lissner, C. and Ferrero, F. (2005) Intensive dialectical behavior therapy for outpatients with borderline personality disorder who are in crisis. *Psychiatric Services* **56**(2), 193-197.

McVilly, K. and Rawlinson, R. (1998) Quality of life: Issues in the development and evaluation of services for people with intellectual disability. *Journal of Intellectual and Developmental Disability* **23**, 199-218.

Mearns, J. (2008) *The Social Learning Theory of Julian B. Rotter.* Retrieved 12 January 2009 from http://psych.fullerton.edu/jmearns/rotter.htm

Meeus, J., Nijs, J., Oosterwijck, J., Alsenay, V. and Traujen, S. (2010) Pain physiology education improves pain beliefs in patients with chronic fatigue syndrome compared with pacing and self-enhancement education: A double blind randomised controlled trial. *Archives of Physical Medicine and Rehabilitation* **91**(8), 1153-1159.

Mehr, D.R., Binder, E.F., Kruse, R.L., Zweig, S.C., Madsen, R., Popejoy, L. and D'Agostino, R.B. (2001) Mortality in nursing home residents with lower respiratory tract infection. *Journal of the American Medical Association* **286**(19), 2427-2436.

Meichenbaum, D.M. and Cameron, R. (1983) Stress inoculation training: Toward a general paradigm for training coping skills. In D. Meichenbaum and M.E. Jaremko (eds) *Stress Reduction and Prevention.* New York: Plenum.

Melamed, B.G., Hawes, R.R., Heiby, E. and Gluck, J. (1975) Use of filmed modelling to reduce uncooperative behaviour of children during dental treatment. *Journal of Dental Research* **54**(4), 797-801.

Melin-Johansson, C., Axelsson, B., Gaston-Johansson, F. and Danielson, E. (2010) Significant improvement in quality of life of patients with incurable cancer after designation to a palliative homecare team. *European Journal of Cancer Care* **19**: 243-250.

Melzack, R. (1975) The McGill Pain Questionnaire: Major properties and scoring methods. *Pain* **1**, 277-299.

Melzack, R. (1993) Pain, past present and future. *Canadian Journal of Experimental Psychology* **47**(1), 149-170.

Melzack, R. and Katz, J. (2001) The McGill Pain Questionnaire: Appraisal and current status. In D. Turk and R. Melzack (eds) *Handbook of Pain Assessment* (2nd edn). New York: Guilford Press, 35-52.

Melzack, R. and Wall, P.D. (1965) Pain mechanisms: A new theory. *Science* **150**, 971-979.

Melzack, R. and Wall, P.D. (1973) *The Challenge of Pain.* New York: Basic Books.

Metcalf, C., Smith, G.D., Wadsworth, E., Sterne, J.A., Heslop, P., Macleod, J. and Smith, A. (2003) A contemporary validation of the Reeder Stress Inventory. *British Journal of Health Psychology* **8**, 83-94.

Michael, Y.L., Carlson, N.E., Chlebowski, R.T., Aickin, M., Weihs, K.L., Ockene, J.K., Bowen, D.J. and Ritenbaugh, C. (2009) Influence of stressors on breast cancer incidence in the Women's Health Initiative. *Health Psychology* **28**(2), 137-146.

Michelotti, A., Farella, M., Tedesco, A., Cimino, R. and Martina, R. (2000) Changes in pressure-pain thresholds of the jaw muscles during a natural stressful condition in a group of symptom-free subjects. *Journal of Orofacial Pain* **14**, 279-285.

Milgram. S (1963) Behavioural study of obedience. *Journal of Abnormal and Social Psychology* **67**, 371-378.

Miller, B., Bemson, B. and Gailbraith, K. (2001) Family relationships and adolescent pregnancy risk: A research synthesis. *Developmental Review* **21**, 1-38.

Miller, E. and Morris, R. (1993) *The Psychology of Dementia*. Chichester: Wiley.

Miller, G. (2005) Genes that guide brain development linked to dyslexia. *Science* **310**(5749), 759.

Miller, G.A. (1956) The magical number seven, plus or minus two: Some limits on our capacity for processing information. *Psychological Review* **63**, 81-97.

Miller, W.R. and Rollnick, S. (2002) *Motivational Interviewing: Preparing People for Change*. New York: Guilford Press.

Milling, L.S. (2008) Recent developments in the study of hypnotic pain reduction: A new golden era of research? *Contemporary Hypnosis* **25**, 165-177.

Millward, C., Ferriter, M., Calver, S. and Connell-Jones, G. (2004) Gluten- and casein-free diets for autistic spectrum disorder, *Cochrane Database of Systematic Reviews*, Issue 2.

Minuchin, S., Baker, L., Rosman, B.L., Liebman, R., Milman, L. and Todd, T.C. (1975) Conceptual model of psychosomatic illness in children: Family organisation and family therapy. *Archives of General Psychiatry* **32**(8), 1031-1038.

Minuchin, S., Rosman, B.L. and Baker, L. (1978) *Psychosomatic Families: Anorexia Nervosa in Context*. Cambridge, MA: Harvard University Press.

Moffitt, T.E., Caspi, A., Rutter, M. and Silva, P.A. (2001) *Sex Difference in Antisocial Behaviour: Conduct Disorder, Delinquency, and Violence in the Dunedin Longitudinal Study*. Cambridge, England: Cambridge University Press.

Möller, J., Hallqvist, J., Diderichsen, F., Theorell, T., Reuterwall, C. and Ahlbom, A. (1990) Do episodes of anger trigger myocardial infarction? A case-crossover analysis in the Stockholm heart epidemiology program (SHEEP) *Psychosomatic Medicine* **61**, 842-849.

Montgomery, G.H. and Bovbjerg, D.H. (1997) The development of anticipatory nausea in patients receiving adjuvant chemotherapy for breast cancer. *Physiology and Behaviour* **61**(5), 737-741.

Moorey, S. (2010) Unplanned hospital admission: Supporting children, young people and their families. *Paediatric Nursing* **22**, 10.

Mori, K. and Arai, M. (2010) No need to fake it: Reproduction of the Asch experiment without confederates. *International Journal of Psychology* **45**(5), 390-397.

Morris, T., Moore, M. and Morris, F. (2011) Stress and chronic illness: The case of diabetes. *Journal of Adult Development* **18**(2), 70-80.

Morrison, A., Bentall, R., French, P., Walford, L., Kilcommons, A. and Lewis, S.W. (2002) A randomised controlled trial of early detection and cognitive therapy in individuals at risk of psychosis. *British Journal of Psychotherapy* **181**(43), 91-97.

Morrow, D., Weiner, M., Young, J., Steinley, D., Deer, M. and Murray, M. (2005) Improving medication knowledge among older adults with heart failure: A patient-centred approach to instruction design. *Gerontologist* **45**(4), 545-552.

Morrow, G.R. and Dobkin, P.L. (1988) Anticipatory nausea and vomiting in cancer patients undergoing chemotherapy treatment: Prevalence, aetiology and behavioural interventions. *Clinical Psychology Review* 8, 517-556.

Morrow, G.R. and Morrell, C. (1982) Behavioural treatment for the anticipatory nausea and vomiting induced by cancer chemotherapy. *New England Journal of Medicine* 307(24), 1476-1480.

Morrow, G.R. and Rosenthal, S.N. (1996) Models, mechanisms and management of anticipatory nausea and emesis. *Oncology* 53(Suppl 1), 4-7.

Morrow, G.R., Roscoe, J.A., Kirshner, J.J., Hynes, H.E. and Rosenbluth, R.J. (1998) Anticipatory nausea and vomiting in the era of 5-HT3 antiemetics. *Support Care Cancer* 6(3), 244-247.

Morton, I. (1997) Beyond validation. In I.N. Norman and S.J. Redfern (eds) *Mental Health Care for Elderly People*. Edinburgh: Churchill Livingstone.

Morton, I. (1999) *Person-Centred Approaches to Dementia Care*. Bicester: Winslow.

Moss, S., Emerson, E., Kiernan, C., Turner, S., Hatton, C. and Alborz, A. (2000) Psychiatric symptoms in adults with learning disability and challenging behaviour. *The British Journal of Psychiatry* 177, 452-456.

Muller, J., Karl, A., Denke, C., Mathier, F., Dittmann, J., Rohleder, N. and Knaevelsrud, C. (2009) Biofeedback for pain management in traumatised refugees. *Cognitive Behavioural Therapy* 38(3), 184-190.

Muller-Oerlinghausen, B., Berghofer, A. and Bauer, M. (2002) Bipolar disorder. *Lancet* 359, 241-247.

Munson, M.R., Floersch, J.E. and Townsend, L. (2010) Are health beliefs related to adherence among adolescents with mood disorders? *Administration and Policy in Mental Health & Mental Health Services Research* 37(5), 408-416.

Murray, C.J. and Main, A. (2005) Role modelling as a teaching method for student mentors. *Nursing Times* 101(26), 30-33.

Muuss, R.E. (2006) *Theories of Adolescence* (6th edn). New York: McGraw-Hill.

Myant, K.A. and Williams, J.M. (2005) Children's concept of health and illness: Understanding of contagious illnesses, non-contagious illnesses and injuries. *Journal of Health Psychology* 10(6), 805-819.

Nacasch, N., Foa, E.B., Huppert, J.D., Tzur, D., Fostick, L., Dinstein, Y., Polliack, M. and Zohar, J. (2010) Prolonged exposure therapy for combat- and terror-related posttraumatic stress disorder: A randomized control comparison with treatment as usual. *Journal of Clinical Psychiatry*. (Epub ahead of print)

National Institute for Health and Clinical Excellence (2004) Eating disorders: Core interventions in the treatment and management of anorexia nervosa, bulimia nervosa and related eating disorders. www.nice.org.uk/CG009

Navakatikyan, M. and Davison, M. (2010) The dynamics of the law of effects: A comparison of models. *Journal of Experimental Analysis of Behaviour* 93(1), 91-127.

Neal, J.A. and Edelmann, R.J. (2003) The etiology of social phobia: Towards a developmental profile. *Clinical Psychology Review* 23, 761-786.

Neale, B.M., Medland, S., Ripke, P., Anney, R.J.L., Asherson, P., Buitelaar, J. and Biederman, J. (2010) Case-control genome-wide association study of attention-deficit/hyperactivity disorder. *Journal of the American Academy of Child and Adolescent Psychiatry* 49, 906-920.

Neisser, U. (1967) *Cognitive Psychology*. Englewood Cliffs, NJ: Prentice-Hall.

Nelson, S.D. (2011) The posttraumatic growth path: An emerging model for prevention and treatment of trauma-related behavioral health conditions. *Journal of Psychotherapy Integration* 21(1), 1–42.

Nemeroff, C.B., Bremner, J.D., Foa, E.B., Mayberg, H.S. North, C.S. and Stein, M.B. (2006) Post traumatic stress disorder: A state of the science review. *Journal of Psychiatric Research* 40, 1-2.

Neva, M., Hakkinen, A., Isomaki, P. and Sokka, T. (2011) Chronic back pain in patients with rheumatoid arthritis and in a control population: Prevalence and disability – a 5-year follow up. *Rheumatology* 50(9), 1639.

NICE (2005a) Obsessive-compulsive disorder: core interventions in the treatment of obsessive-compulsive disorder and body dysmorphic disorder. National Institute for Health and Clinical Excellence www.nice.org.uk/CG31

NICE (2005b) Post-traumatic stress disorder. The management of PTSD in adults and children in primary and secondary care. National Institute for Health and Clinical Excellence www.nice.org.uk/Guidance/CG26

NICE (2006) Bipolar disorder: The management of bipolar disorder in adults, children and adolescents, in primary and secondary care. National Institute for Health and Clinical Excellence www.nice.org.uk/CG038

NICE (2009a) Borderline personality disorder: treatment and management. National Institute for Health and Clinical Excellence www.nice.org.uk/CG78

NICE (2009b) Antisocial personality disorder: Treatment, management and prevention. National Institute for Health and Clinical Excellence http://guidance.nice.org.uk/CG77

NICE (2009c) Schizophrenia: Core interventions in the treatment and management of schizophrenia in adults in primary and secondary care (update). National Institute for Health and Clinical Excellence http://guidance.nice.org.uk/CG82

NICE (2009d) Depression. The treatment and management of depression in adults. National Institute for Health and Clinical Excellence www.nice.org.uk/CG90.

Nielsen, N.R. and Brønbæk, M. (2006) Stress and breast cancer: A systematic update on the current knowledge. *Nature Clinical Practice Oncology* 3, 612–620.

Nielsen, N.R., Zhang Z.-F., Kristensen, T.S., Netterstrom, B., Schnohr, P. and Grownbaek, M. (2005) Self reported stress and risk of breast cancer: Prospective cohort study. *British Medical Journal* 331, 548–552.

Nikolas, M., Friderici, K., Waldman, I., Jernigan, K. and Nigg, J. (2010) Gene x environment interactions for ADHD: synergistic effect of 5HTTLPR genotype and youth appraisals of interparental conflict. *Behavioural and Brain Functions* 6, 23–37.

Nishizawa, Y., Saito, M., Ogura, N., Kudo, S., Saito, K. and Hanaya, M. (2006) The non-verbal communication skills of nursing students: Analysis of interpersonal behavior using videotaped recordings in a 5-minute interaction with a simulated patient. *Japan Journal of Nursing Science* 3, 15–22.

Nixon, T. and Aruguete, M. (2010) Healthcare attitudes, knowledge and decision making. *North American Journal of Psychology* 12(2), 355–364.

NMC (2008) *The Code: Standards of Conduct, Performance and Ethics for Nurses and Midwives. Standards 04.08*. Nursing and Midwifery Council

Nolen-Hoeksema, S. (2011) *Abnormal Psychology* (4th edn). New York: McGraw-Hill.

Norman, P. and Bennett, P. (1995) Health locus of control. In M. Conner and P. Norman (eds) *Predicting Health Behaviour*. Buckingham: Open University Press, pp. 62-94.

Novy, D., Nelson, D., Francis, D. and Turk, D. (1995) Perspectives of chronic pain: An evaluative comparison of restrictive and comprehensive models. *Psychological Bulletin* **118**(2), 238-247.

Novick, D., Haro, J.M., Suarez, D., Vieta, E. and Naber, D. (2009) Recovery in the outpatient setting: 36-month results from the Schizophrenia Outpatients Health Outcomes (SOHO) study. *Schizophrenia Research* **108**, 223-230.

O'Cathail, S.M., O'Connell, O.J., Long, N., Morgan, M., Eustace, J.A., Plant, B.J. and Haurihane, J.B. (2011) Association of cigarette smoking with drug use and risk taking behaviour in Irish teenagers. *Addictive Behaviours* **36**(5), 547-550.

Odell, J. and Holbrook, J. (2006) Improving the hospital experience for older people. *Nursing Times* **102**(23), 23-24.

Office for National Statistics (2011) Population Trends. Retrieved 12 October 2011 from http://www.ons.gov.uk/ons/rel/population-trends-rd/population-trends/no-145-autumn-2011/index.html

Ogden, J. (2007) *Health Psychology: A Textbook* (4th edn). Oxford: Open University Press.

Old, S.R. and Naveh-Benjamine, M. (2008) Differential effects of age on item and associative measures of memory: A meta-analysis. *Psychology and Aging* **23**(1), 104-118.

Oldham, A. (2007) Changing behaviour: Cognitive behavioural therapy: Linking thoughts and actions. *Journal of Primary Care Nursing* **4**(1), 26-29.

Oliver, S. and Ryan, S. (2004) Effective pain management for patients with arthritis. *Nursing Standard* **18**(50), 43-52.

Olsen, J. (1997) Nurse-expressed empathy, patient outcomes and development of a middle-range theory. *Journal of Nursing Scholarship* **29**(1), 71-76.

O'Neil, R.E., Horner, R.H., Albin, R.W., Storey, K. and Sprague, J.R. (1990) *Functional Analysis of Problem Behaviour: A Practical Assessment Guide*. Sycamore Publishing: Sycamore.

Ost, L.G. and Hugdahl, K. (1985) Acquisition of blood and dental phobia and anxiety response patterns in clinical patients. *Behaviour Research and Therapy* **23**(1), 27-34.

Oudshoorn, A., Ward-Griffin, C. and McWilliams, C. (2007) Client-nurse relationship in home-based palliative care: A critical analysis of power relations. *Journal of Clinical Nursing* **16**(8), 1435-1443.

Palviainen, P., Hietala, M., Routasalo, P., Suominen, T. and Hupli, M. (2003) Do nurses exercise power in basic care situations? *Nursing Ethics* **10**(3).

Papakostas, G.I. and Fava, M. (2010) *Pharmacotherapy for Depression and Treatment-Resistant Depression* (1st edn). Singapore: World Scientific Publishing.

Park, D.C., Morrell, R.W., Frieske, D. and Kincaid, D. (1992) Medication adherence behaviors in older adults: Effects of external cognitive supports. *Psychology and Aging* **7**, 252-256.

Park, S.G., Kim, H.C., Min, J.Y., Hwang, S.H., Park, Y.S. and Min, K.B. (2011) A prospective study of work stressors and the common cold. *Occupational Medicine* **61**(1), 53-56.

Parker, I. (2010) Psychoanalysis: the 'talking cure'. In M. Barker, A. Vossler and D. Longdridge (eds). *Understanding Psychotherapy*. London: Sage.

Parkes, C.M. (1972) *Bereavement, Studies of Grief in Adult Life*. Harmondsworth: Penguin.

Parkes, C.M. (1986) *Bereavement, Studies of Grief in Adult Life*. (2nd edn). London: Tavistock.

Patterson, D.R. and Jensen, M.P. (2003) Hypnosis and clinical pain. *Psychological Bulletin* **129**(4), 495-521.

Patterson, D.R., Wiechman, S.A., Jensen, M. and Sharar, S.R. (2006) Hypnosis delivered through virtual reality for burn pain: A clinical case series. *International Journal of Clinical and Experimental Hypnosis* **54**, 130-42.

Paul, G.L. and Lentz, R.J. (1977) *Psychosocial Treatment of Chronic Mental Patients: Milieu versus Social Learning Programs.* Cambridge, MA: Harvard University Press.

Pawlyn, J. and Carnaby, S. (2009) *Profound Intellectual and Multiple Disabilities: Nursing Complex Needs.* Wiley Blackwell.

Paykel, E.S., Brugha, T. and Fryers, T. (2005) Size and burden of depressive disorders in Europe. *European Neuropharmacology* **15**, 411-423.

Pearcey, P.A. and Elliot, B.E. (2004) Student impressions of clinical nursing. *Nurse Education Today* **24**(5), 382-387.

Pedersen, A., Zachariae, R. and Bovbjerg, D.H. (2010) Influence of psychological stress on upper respiratory infection: A meta-analysis of prospective studies. *Psychosomatic Medicine* **72**(8), 823-832.

Perivoliotis, D., Grant, P., Peters, E., Ison, R., Kuipers, E. and Beck, T. (2010) Cognitive insight predicts favourable outcome in cognitive behavioural therapy for psychosis. *Psychosis* **2**(1), 23-33.

Perner, J., Kain, W. and Barchfeld, P. (2002) Executive control and higher-order theory of mind in children at risk of ADHD. *Infant and Child Development* **11**, 141-158.

Perry, B. (2009) Role modelling excellence in clinical nursing practice. *Nursing Education in Practice* **9**(1), 36-44.

Persson, A.L., Veenhuizen, H., Zachrison, L. and Gard, G. (2008) Relaxation as treatment for chronic musculoskeletal pain: A systematic review of randomised controlled studies. *Physical Therapy Reviews* **13**(5), 355-365.

Peterson, C. and Seligman, M.E.P. (1984) Causal explanations as a risk factor for depression: Theory and evidence. *Psychological Review* **91**, 347-374.

Pettigrew, S. and Donovan, R. (2009) Older audiences' responses to mental health promotion messages. *International Journal of Mental Health Promotion* **11**(1), 23-31.

Petty, R.E. and Cacioppo, J.T. (1986) *Central and Peripheral Routes to Persuasion: The Role of Message Repetition.* New York: Springer.

Pharoah, F.M., Mari, J.J. and Streiner, D. (2000) Family intervention for schizophrenia. *Cochrane Library,* Issue 4. Oxford: Update software.

Phillips, L.J., Francey, S.M., Edwards, J. and McMurray, N. (2007) Stress and psychosis: towards the development of new models of investigation. *Clinical Psychology Review* **27**, 307-317.

Piaget, J. (1972) Intellectual evolution from adolescence to adulthood. *Human Development* **15**(1), 1-8.

Piaget, J. and Inhelder, B. (1956) *The Child's Conception of Space.* London: Routledge.

Piet, J. and Hougaard, E. (2011) Effect of mindfulness-based cognitive therapy for prevention of relapse in recurrent major depressive disorder: A systematic review and meta-analysis. *Clinical Psychology Review* **31**(6), 1032-1040.

Pike, K.M., Walsh, B.T., Vitousek, K., Wilson, G.T. and Bauer, J. (2003) Cognitive behaviour therapy in the post-hospitalization treatment of anorexia nervosa. *The American Journal of Psychiatry* **160**, 2046–2049.

Piton, A., Gautheir, J., Hamdon, F., Lafreniere, R., Yang, Y., Herion, E., Laurent, S., Noreau, A., Thibodeau, P., Karemera, L., Spiegelman, D., Kuku, F., Duguay, J., Destroismaisons, L., Jolivet, P., Côté, M., Lachapelle, K., Diallo, O., Raymond, A., Marineau, C., Champagne, N., Xiong, L., Gaspar, C., Rivière, J.B., Tarabeux, J., Cossette, P., Krebs, M.O., Rapoport, J.L., Addington, A., Delisi, L.E., Mottron, L., Joober, R., Fombonne, E., Drapeau, P. and Rouleau, G.A. (2011) Systematic resequencing of X-chromosome synaptic genes in autism spectrum disorder and schizophrenia. *Molecular Psychiatry* **16**(8), 867–880.

Piven, J. and Palmer, P. (1999) Psychiatric disorder and the broad autism phenotype: Evidence for a family study of multiple-incidence autism families. *American Journal of Psychiatry* **156**(4), 557–563.

Plant, A.E. and Sachs-Ericsson, N. (2004) Racial and ethical differences in depression: The roles of social support and meeting basic needs. *Journal of Consulting and Clinical Psychology* **72**(1), 41–52.

Planton, B.B., Adrell, P., Raner, C., Rudolph, M., Dvorestsky, A. and Mannheimer, C. (2010) High frequency, high intensity transcutaneous electrical nerve stimulation as treatment of pain after surgical abortion. *Pain* **148**(1), 114–119.

Plotnikoff, R.C., Lippke, S., Trinh, L., Courneya, K.S., Birkett, N. and Sigal, R.J. (2010) Protection motivation theory and the prediction of physical activity among adults with type 1 or type 2 diabetes in a large population sample. *British Journal of Health Psychology* **15**(3), 643–661.

Polemans, G., Buitelaar, J.K., Pauls, D.L. and Franke, B. (2011) A theoretical molecular network for dyslexia: Integrating available genetic findings. *Molecular Psychiatry* **16**(4), 365–382.

Porter, W.G. (2010) In their shoes: Helping patients and their families come to terms with terminal illness requires empathy and respect. *Medical Economics* **87**(22), 71–72.

Poulton, R. and Menzies, R.G. (2002) Non-associative fear acquisition: A review of the evidence from retrospective and longitudinal research. *Behaviour Research and Therapy* **40**(2), 127–149.

Powell, R. (2011) Research notes: Little Albert, lost or found: Further difficulties with the Douglas Merritte hypothesis. *History of Psychology* **14**(1), 106–107.

Powers, M.B., Halpern, J.M., Ferenschak, M.P., Gillihan, S.J. and Foa, E.B. (2010) A meta-analytic review of prolonged exposure for posttraumatic stress disorder. *Clinical Psychological Review* **30**, 635–641.

Powers, P.S., Santana, C.A. and Bannon, Y.S. (2002) Olanzapine in the treatment of anorexia nervosa: An open label trial. *International Journal of Eating Disorders* **32**, 146–154.

Prabhavalkar, K.S. and Chintamaneni, M. (2010) Diagnosis and treatment of mild cognitive impairment: A review. *Journal of Pharmacy Research* **3**(2), 338–392.

Pradel, F.G., Hartzema, A.G. and Bush, P.J. (2001) Asthma self-management: the perspective of children. *Patient Education and Counseling* **45**, 199–209.

Prasher, V. and Janicki, M.P. (2002) *Physical Health of Adults with Intellectual Disabilities*. Oxford: Blackwell.

Prati, G., Pietrontoni, L. and Cicognani, E. (2010) Self-efficacy moderates the relationship between stress appraisal and quality of life among rescue workers. *Anxiety, Stress and Coping* **23**(4), 463–470.

Premack, D. and Woodruff, G. (1978) Chimpanzee problem-solving: Test for comprehension. *Science* **202**, 532–535.

Preti, A., Girolamo, G., Vilagut, G., Alonso, J., Graaf, R., Bruffaerts, R., Demyttenaere, K., Pinto-Meza, A. and Morosini, P. (2009) The epidemiology of eating disorders in six European countries: Results of the ESEMeD-WMH project. *Journal of Psychiatric Research* **43**(14), 1125–1132.

Price, B. (2006) Exploring person-centred care. *Nursing Standards* **20**(50), 49–56.

Price, M., Mehta, N., Tone, E. and Anderson, P. (2011) Does engagement with exposure yield better outcomes? Components of presence as a predictor of treatmentresponse for virtual reality exposure therapy for social phobia. *Journal of Anxiety Disorders* **25**(6), 763–770.

Price, T., Cervero, F., Gold, M., Hammand, D. and Prescott, S. (2009) Chloride regulation in the pain pathway. *Brain Research Reviews* **60**(1), 149–170.

Prideaux, A. (2010) Male nurses and the protection of female dignity. *Nursing Standard* **25**(13), 42–49.

Prochaska, J.O. and DiClemente, C.C. (1982) Transtheoretical therapy: Toward a more integrative model of change. *Psychotherapy: Theory, Research and Practice* **19**, 276–288.

Prochaska, L., Teherani, A. and Hauer, K. (2007) Medical students' use of the stages of change model in tobacco cessation counselling. *Journal of General Internal Medicine* **22**(2), 223–227.

Quick, J.D., Nelson, D.L., Matuszek, P.A.C., Whittington, J.L. and Quick, J.C. (1996) Social support, secure attachments, and health. In Cary L.Cooper (ed.) *Handbook of Stress, Medicine, and Health*. Boca Raton, FL: CRC Press, pp. 267–287.

Quilty, L.C., Ameringen, M.V., Mancini, C., Oakman, J. and Farvolden, P. (2003) Quality of life and the anxiety disorders. *Journal of Anxiety Disorders* **17**, 405–426.

Quinn, C. (2009) Genetics research suggests links between common disorders. *Learning Disability Practice* **12**(9), 36–37.

Quintner, J., Cohen, M., Buchanan, D., Katz, J. and Williamson, O. (2008) Pain medicine and its models: Helping or hindering? *Pain Medicine* **9**(7), 824–834.

Radsma, J. and Bottorff, J.L. (2009) Counteracting ambivalence: Nurses who smoke and their health promotion role with patients who smoke. *Research in Nursing and Health* **32**(4), 443–452.

Ragland, J.D., Moelter, S.T., McGrath, C., Hill, S.K., Gur, R.E., Bilker, W.B., Siegel, S.J. and Gur, R.C. (2003) Levels of processes effect on word recognition in schizophrenia. *Biological Psychiatry* **54**(11), 1154.

Rahman, A., Reed, E., Underwood, M., Shipley, M.E. and Omar, R.Z. (2008) Factors affecting self-efficacy and pain intensity in patients with chronic musculoskeletal pain seen in a specialist rheumatology pain clinic. *Rheumatology* **47**(12), 1183–1192.

Raine, A. and Yang, Y. (2006) Neural foundations to moral reasoning and antisocial behaviour. *Social Cognitive and Affective Neuroscience* **1**(3), 203–213.

Rains, J.C., Penzien, D.B. and Lipchik, G.L. (2006) Behavioral facilitation of medical treatment of headache: Implications of non-compliance and strategies for improving adherence. *Headache* **46**(5), 5142–5143.

Rana, D. and Upton, D. (2009) *Psychology for Nurses*. Harlow, UK: Pearson Education.

Rampello, L., Nicoletti, F. and Nicoletti, F. (2000) Dopamine and depression: Therapeutic implications. *CNS Drugs* **13**, 35–45.

Raphaelson, M. (2004) Stimulants and attention-deficit/hyperactivity disorder. *Journal of the American Medical Association* **292**, 2214.

Rastam, M. (1992) Anorexia nervosa in 51 Swedish children and adolescents: Premorbid problems and comorbidity. *Journal of the American Academy of Child and Adolescent Psychiatry* **31**, 819-29.

Ratey, J. (2006, March 27) Commentary in L. Szabo, "ADHD treatment is getting a workout" *USA Today*, p. 6D.

Raudonis, B.M. and Acton, G.J. (1997) Theory-based nursing practice. *Journal of Advanced Nursing* **26**(1), 138-145.

Raven, B.H. (1965) Social influence and power. In I.D. Steiner and M. Fishbein (eds) *Current Studies in Social Psychology*. New York: Holt, Rinehart and Winston, pp. 371-382.

Reddy, K.S. (2005) Cytogenetic abnormalities and Fragile X syndrome in autism spectrum disorder. *BMC Medical Genetics* **6**, 3-16.

Reeves, G. and Schweitzer, J. (2004) Pharmacological management of attention deficit hyperactivity disorder. *Expert Opinions in Pharmacotherapy* **5**, 1313-1320.

Reiche, E.M., Nunes, S.O. and Morimoto, H.K. (2004) Stress, depression, the immune system, and cancer. *Lancet Oncology* **5**(10), 617-625.

Reichle, J., Johnson, L., Monn, E. and Harris, M. (2010) Task engagement and escape maintained challenging behaviour: Differential effects of general and explicit cues when implementing a signalled delay in delivery of reinforcement. *Journal of Autism & Developmental Disorders* **40**(6), 709-720.

Reid, S., Kauer, S., Dudgeon, P., Sanci, L., Shrier, L. and Patton, G. (2009) A mobile phone program to track young people's experiences of mood, stress and coping. *Social Psychiatry and Psychiatry Epidemiology* **44**(6), 501-507.

Reif, S., Mugavero, M., Raper, J., Thielman, N., Leserman, J., Whetten, K. and Pence, B.W. (2011) Highly stressed: stressful and traumatic experiences among individuals with HIV/AIDS in the Deep South. *AIDS Care* **23**(2), 152-162.

Reis, S.P., Wald, H.S., Monroe, A.D. and Brokan, J.M. (2010) Begin the Began (The Brown Educational Guide to the Analysis of Narrative): A framework for enhancing educational impact of faculty feedback to students' reflective writing. *Patient Education & Counselling* **8**(2), 253-259.

Reiss, A.L. and Freund, L. (1990) Fragile X syndrome, DSM-III-R, and autism. *Journal of the American Academy of Child and Adolescent Psychiatry* **29**(6), 885-891.

Reynolds, M. (2002) Reflecting on paediatric oncology nursing practice using Benner's helping role as a framework to examine aspects of caring. *European Journal of Oncology Nursing* **6**(1), 30-36.

Rhodes, N. and Wood, W. (1992) Self-esteem and intelligence affect influenceability: The mediating role of message reception. *Psychological Bulletin* **111**, 156-171.

Rice, K.G. and Van Arsdale, A.C. (2010) Perfectionism, perceived stress, drinking to cope, and alcohol-related problems among college students. *Journal of Counselling Psychology* **57**(4), 439-450.

REFERENCES

Rich, E.C., Loo, S.K., Yang, M., Dang, J. and Smalley, S.L. (2009) Social functioning in ADHD: Associations with PPD risk. *Clinical Child Psychology and Psychiatry* **14**(3), 329-344.

Rickles, N.M., Wertheimer, A.I. and Smith, M.C. (2010) *Social and Behavioural Aspects of Pharmaceutical Care.* (2nd edn) Sidbury, MA: Jones and Barlett.

Riddick-Grisham, S. and Deming, L.M. (2011) *Pediatric Life Care Planning and case management.* (2nd edn). Boca Raton, FL: CRC Press.

Robins, C.J. and Chapman, A.I. (2004) Dialectical behaviour therapy: Current status, recent developments, and future directions. *Journal of Personality Disorders* **18**(1), 73-89.

Robinson, T., Callister, M. and Jankoski, T. (2008) Portrayal of body weight on children's television sitcoms: A content analysis. *Body Image* **5**, 141-151.

Robles, D. (2011) The thin is in: Am I thin enough? Perfectionism and self-esteem in anorexia. *International Journal of Research & Review* **6**(1), 65-73.

Roeleveld, N., Zielhuis, G.A. and Gabeels, F. (1997) The prevalence of mental retardation: A critical review of recent literature. *Developmental Medicine & Child Neurology* **39**(2), 125-132.

Roelofs, J., Peters, M.L., De Jong, J.R. and Vlaeyen, J.W.S. (2002) Psychological treatment for chronic low back pain: Past, present and beyond. *Pain Reviews* **9**(1), 29-40.

Roemer, L., Orsillo, S.M. and Salters-Pedneault, K. (2008) Efficacy of an acceptance-based behaviour therapy for generalised anxiety disorder: evaluation in a randomised control trial. *Journal of Consulting and Clinical Psychology* **76**, 1083-1089.

Rogers, C. (1959) A theory of therapy, personality and interpersonal relationships as developed in the client-centered framework. In S. Koch (ed.) *Psychology: A Study of a Science. Vol. 3: Formulations of the Person and the Social Context.* New York: McGraw Hill.

Rogers, R.W. (1975) A protection motivation theory of fear appeals and attitude change. *Journal of Psychology* **91**, 93-114.

Rogers, R.W. (1983) Cognitive and physiological processes in fear appeals and attitude change: A revised theory of protection motivation. In J. Cacioppo and R. Petty (eds) *Social Psychophysiology.* New York: Guilford Press.

Rollins, A.L., Bond, G.R., Lysaker, P.H., McGrew, J.H. and Salyers, M.P. (2010) Coping with positive and negative symptoms of schizophrenia. *American Journal of Psychiatric Rehabilitation* **13**, 208-223.

Roper, N., Logan, W.W. and Tierney, A.J. (eds) (1983) *Using a Model for Nursing.* Edinburgh: Churchill Livingstone.

Roscoe, J.A., Morrow, G.R., Aapro, M.S., Molassiotis, A. and Olver, I. (2010) Anticipatory nausea and vomiting. Support Care Cancer. (Epub ahead of print.) dOI: 10.1007/s00520-010-0980-0

Rosenman, R.H., Friedman, M., Straus, R., Wurm, M., Kositchek, R., Haan, W. and Werthessen, N.T. (1964) A predictive study of coronary heart disease: The Western Collaborative Group Study. *Journal of the American Medical Association* **189**, 15.

Rosenstiel, A.K. and Keefe, F.J. (1983) The use of coping strategies in chronic low back pain patients: Relationship to patient characteristics and current adjustment. *Pain* **17**(1), 33-44.

Rosenstock, I. (1974) Historical origins of the Health Belief Model. *Health Education Monographs* **2**(4), 10.

Rosenthal, R. and Jacobson, L. (1968) *Pygmalion in the Classroom: Teachers' Expectations and Pupils' Intellectual Development*. New York: Holt.

Roskos-Ewoldsen, D.R. and Fazio, R.H. (1992) On the orienting value of attitudes: Attitude accessibility as a determinant of an object's attraction of visual attention. *Journal of Personality and Social Psychology* **63**, 198–211.

Roth, S. and Cohen, L.J. (1986) Approach, avoidance, and coping with stress. *American Psychologist* **41**, 813–819.

Rothman, A.J. and Salovey, P. (1997) Shaping perception to motivate healthy behaviour: The role of message framing. *Psychological Bulletin* **121**, 3–19.

Rotter, J.B. (1954) *Social Learning and Clinical Psychology*. New York: Prentice Hall.

Rotter, J.B. (1966) Generalized expectancies for internal versus external control of reinforcement. *Psychological Monographs* **80**(609).

Rovira, T., Edo, S. and Fernandez-Castro, J. (2010) How does cognitive appraisal lead to perceived stress in academic examinations? *Studying Psychology* **52**(3), 179–192.

Royal College of Physicians, British Geriatrics Society and British Pain Society (2007) *The Assessment of Pain in Older People: National Guidelines*. Concise guidance on good practice series, 8. London: RCP.

Ruef, M.B. and Turnbull, A.P. (2001) Stakeholder opinions on accessible informational products helpful in building positive, practical solutions to behavioral challenges of individuals with mental retardation and/or autism. *Education & Training in Mental Retardation & Developmental Disabilities* **36**(4), 441–456.

Ruppel, S.E., Jenkins, W.J., Griffin, J.L. and Kizer, J.B. (2010) Are they depressed or just old? A study of perceptions about the elderly suffering from depression. *North American Journal of Psychology* **12**(1), 31–42.

Ruscio, A.M., Brown, T.A., Chiu, W.T., Sareen, J., Stein, M.B. and Kessler, R.C. (2008) Social fears and social phobia in the USA: Results from the National Comorbidity Survey Replication. *Psychological Medicine* **38**, 15–28.

Russell, C., Crank, N., Herron, M., Knowels, N., Matteson, M., Peace, L. and Ponferrada, L. (2011) Motivational interviewing in dialysis adherence study (MIDAS) *Nephrology Nursing Journal* **38**(3), 229–236.

Russell, S., Daly, J., Hughes, E. and Hogg, C.O. (2003) Nurses and 'difficult' patients: Negotiating non-compliance. *Journal of Advanced Nursing* **43**(3), 281–287.

Rutter, D. and Quine, L. (2002) *Changing Health Behaviour: Intervention and Research with Social Cognition Models*. Milton Keynes: Open University Press.

Ryle, G. (1949) *The Concept of Mind*. London: Hutchinson.

Sagvolden, T., Johansen, E.B., Aase, H. and Russell, V.A. (2005) A dynamic developmental theory of attention-deficit/hyperactivity disorder (ADHD) predominantly hyperactive and combined subtypes. *Behavioural and Brain Sciences* **28**, 397–368.

Sahlsten, M.J., Larsson, I.E., Sjostrom, B. and Plos, K.A. (2009) Nurse strategies for optimising patient participation in nursing. *Scandinavian Journal of Caring Science* **23**(3), 490–497.

Salbach-Andrae, H., Lenz, K., Simmendinger, N., Klinkowski, N., Lehmkuhl, U. and Pfeiffer, E. (2008) Psychiatric comorbidities among female adolescents with anorexia nervosa. *Child Psychiatry and Human Development* **39**(3), 261–272.

Salehzadeh, M., Kalantari, M., Hoseien Molavi, H., Najafi, M.R. and Nouri, A. (2011) Effectiveness of cognitive-behavioral group therapy with focusing on dysfunctional attitudes in epilepsy on quality of life in intractable epileptic patients. *Behavioural Sciences* **4**(4), 255-260.

Salkovskis, P.M. (1985) Obsessive-compulsive problems: A cognitive-behavioural analysis. *Behaviour Research and Therapy* **23**, 571-583.

Sanson, A., Havighurst, S. and Zubrick, S. (2011) The science of prevention for children and youth. *Australian Review of Public Affairs* **10**(1), 79-93.

Santangelo, S.L. and Tsatsanis, K. (2005) What is known about autism: Genes, brain, and behavior. *American Journal of Pharmacogenomics* **5**, 71-92.

Sarafino, E.P. and Goehring, P. (2000) Age comparisons in acquiring biofeedback control and success in reducing headache pain. *Annals of Behavioral Medicine* **22**(1), 127-139.

Sarason, I.G., Levine, H.M., Basham, R.B. and Sarason, B.R. (1983) Assessing social support: The social support questionnaire. *Journal of Personality and Social Psychology* **44**(1), 127-139.

Sarlo, M., Buodo, G., Devigili, A., Munafo, M. and Palomba, D. (2011) Emotional sensitisation highlights the attentional bias in blood-injection-injury phobics: An ERP study. *Neuroscience Letters* **490**(1), 11-15.

Scanlan, J. (2009) Interventions to reduce the use of seclusion and restraint in inpatient psychiatric settings: What we know so far: a review of the literature. *International Journal of Social Psychiatry* **56**(4), 412-423.

Scerri, T.S. and Schult-Korne, G. (2010) Genetics of developmental dyslexia. *European Child and Adolescent Psychiatry* **19**(3), 179-197.

Schacter, D.L., Chiao, J.Y. and Mitchell, J.P. (2003) The seven sins of memory: Implications for self. *Annals of the New York Academy of Sciences* **1001**, 226-239.

Schafer, T., Wood, S. and Williams, P. (2011) A survey into student nurses' attitudes towards mental illness: Implications for nurse training. *Nurse Education Today* **31**(4), 328-332.

Schaie, K.W. and Willis, S.L. (2002) *Adult Development and Aging.* New York: Prentice Hall.

Schapiro, I.R., Ross-Petersen, L., Saelan, H., Garde, K., Olsen, J.H. and Johnsen, C. (2001) Extroversion and neuroticism and the associated risk of cancer: A Danish cohort study. *American Journal of Epidemiology* **153**(8), 757-763.

Scharfstein, L., Beidel, D., Finnell, L., Distler, A. and Carter, N. (2011) Do pharmacological and behavioural interventions differentially affect treatment outcome for children with social phobia? *Behavior Modification* **35**(5), 451-467.

Schechtman, E., Laufer, O. and Paz, R. (2010) Negative valence widens generalisation of learning. *Journal of Neuroscience* **30**(31), 10460-10464.

Scheff, T.J. (1975) *Labelling Madness.* Englewood Cliffs, NJ: Prentice-Hall.

Schernhammer, E. S., Hankinson, S. E., Rosner, B., Kroenke, C. H., Willett, W. C., Colditz, G. A. and Kawachi, I. (2004) Job stress and breast cancer risk. *American Journal of Epidemiology* **160**, 1079-1086.

Schildkraut, J.J., Green, A.I. and Mooney, J.J. (1985) Affective disorders: Biochemical aspects apects. In H.I. Kaplan and J. Sadock (eds) *Comprehensive Textbook of Psychiatry.* Baltimore, MD: Williams and Wilkins.

Schlotz, W., Hammerfald, K., Ehlert, U. and Gaab, J. (2011) Individual differences in the cortisol response to stress in young healthy men: Testing the roles of perceived stress reactivity and threat appraisal using multiphase latent growth curve modelling. *Biological Psychology* **87**(2), 257-264.

Schneiderman, N., Ironson, G. and Siegel, S, D. (2005) Stress and health: Psychological, behavioural and biological determinants. *Annual Review of Clinical Psychology* **1**, 607-628.

Schofield, P. (2010) It's your age: The assessment and management of pain in older adults. *Continuing Education in Anaesthesia, Critical Care & Pain* **10**(3), 93-98.

Schwarzer, R. (ed.) (1992) *Self Efficacy: Thought Control of Action.* Washington, DC: Hemisphere.

Scott, J., Harmsen, M., Prictor, M.J., Entwistle, V.A., Snowden, A.J. and Watt, I. (2006) Recordings or summaries of consultations for people with cancer (Cochrane Review). *Cochrane Library*, Issue 3. Oxford: Update Software/Chichester: John Wiley.

Scruggs, T.E., Mastropieri, M.A., Berkeley, S.L. and Marshak, L. (2010) Mnemonic strategies: Evidence based practice and practice based evidence. *Intervention in School and Clinic* **46**(2), 79-86.

Seligman, M.E.P. (1971) Phobias and preparedness. *Behaviour Therapy* **2**, 307-320.

Seligman, M.E.P. (1975) *Helplessness.* San Francisco, CA: Freeman.

Selye, H. (1956) What is stress? *Metabolism* **5**(5), 525-530.

Sengupta, J. and Johar, G.V. (2001) Contingent effects of anxiety on message elaboration and persuasion. *Personality and Social Psychology Bulletin* **27**, 139-150.

Shaddock, J. (2002) Appraising the quality of consumer health information leaflets. *Health Expectations* **5**(1), 84-87.

Shagam, J.Y. (2009) The many faces of dementia. *Radiologic Technology* **81**(2), 153-168.

Shahar, D.R., Henkin, Y., Rozen, G.S., Adler, D., Levy, O., Safra, C., Itzhak, B. and Shai, L. (2009) A controlled intervention study of changing health-providers' attitudes towards personal lifestyle habits and health promotion skills. *Nutrition* **25**(5), 532-539.

Shamaskin, A.M., Mikels, J.A. and Reed, A.E. (2010) Getting the message across: Age differences in the positive and negative framing of health care messages. *Psychology and Aging* **25**(3), 746-751.

Sharpe, L., Nicholson, P., Rogers, P., Dear, B.F., Nicholas, M.K. and Refshauge, K. (2010) A comparison of the effect of attention training and relaxation on respons to pain. *Pain* **150**(3), 347-357.

Shaughnessy P. and Cruse S. (2001) Health promotion with people who have a learning disability. Chapter 7. In J. Thomson and S. Pickering (eds) *Meeting the Health Needs of People Who Have a Learning Disability.* London: Harcourt.

Shaywitz, B.A., Shaywitz, S.E., Pugh, K.R. and Mencle, W.E (2002) Disruption of posterior brain systems for reading in children with developmental dyslexia. *Biological Psychiatry* **52**(2), 101-110.

Shaywitz, S.E. (2003) *Overcoming Dyslexia: A New and Complete Science-based Program for Reading Problems at Any Level.* New York: Alfred A. Knopf.

Shaywitz, S.E. and Shaywitz, B.A. (2005) Dyslexia (Specific Reading Disability). *Biological Psychiatry* **57**, 1301-1309.

Sheehan, J. (1985) Ethical considerations in nursing practice. *Journal of Advanced Nursing* **10**(4), 331-336.

Sherkow, S.P. (2011) The dyadic psychoanalytic treatment of a toddler with autism spectrum disorder. *Psychoanalytic Inquiry* **31**(3), 252-275.

Shih-Hsiang, L., Lian-Yu, L., Jing-Shiang, H., Yu-Yin, C., Chiau-Suang, L. and Jung-Der, W. (2010) Working the night shifts causes increased vascular stress and delayed recovery in young women. *Journal of Biological and Medical Rhythm Research* **27**(7), 1454-1468.

Shorney, R. (2004) A model of compliance: Understanding, satisfaction and recall in leg ulcer management. *Nurse 2 Nurse* **4**(7), 51-53.

Siegrist, J. and Marmot, M. (2004) Health inequalities and the psychosocial environment: Two scientific challenges. *Social Science and Medicine* **58**(8), 1463-1473.

SIGN (2007) *Risk Estimation and the Prevention of Cardiovascular Disease. A National Clinical Guideline*. Retrieved 18 November 2008, from http://www.sign.ac.uk/pdf/sign97.pdf

Simon, L., Greenberg, J. and Brehm, J. (1995) Trivialization: The forgotten mode of dissonance reduction. *Journal of Personality and Social Psychology* **68**, 247-260.

Simpson, H., Yuanjia, W., Maher, M., Yuanyuan, B., Foa, E. and Franklin, M. (2011) Patient adherence predicts outcome from cognitive behavioural therapy in obsessive-compulsive disorder. *Journal of Consulting & Clinical Psychology* **79**(2), 247-252.

Simpson, P.F. and Fothergill, A. (2004) Challenging gender stereotypes in the counselling of adult survivors of childhood sexual abuse. *Journal of Psychiatry and Mental Health Nursing* **11**(5), 589-594.

Slater, R. (1995) *The Psychology of Growing Old: Looking Forward. Rethinking Ageing.* Buckingham: Open University Press.

Smith, B.N. and Stasson, M.F. (2000) Social psychological predictors of AIDS-preventive behavioral intentions. *Journal of Applied Psychology* **30**, 443-463.

Smith, E.R., Broughton, M., Baker, R., Pachana, N.A., Angwin, J.A., Humphrys, M.S., Mitchell, L. and Chenery, H.J. (2010) Memory and communication support in dementia: Research based strategies for caregivers. *International Psychogeriatrics* **23**, 256-263.

Smith, L.A., Cornelius, V., Warnock, A., Bell, A. and Young, A.H. (2007) Effectiveness of mood stabilizers and antipsychotics in the maintenance phase of bipolar disorder: A systematic review of randomized controlled trials. *Bipolar Disorders* **9**(4), 394-412.

Snelgrove, S. (2006) Factors contributing to poor concordance in health care. *Nursing Times* **102**(2)

Snowden, A. (2008) Medication management in older adults: A critique of concordance. *British Journal of Nursing* **17**(2), 114-121.

Snowling, M.J., Duff, F., Petrou, A., Schiffeldrin, J. and Bailey, A.M. (2011) Identification of children at risk of dyslexia: The validity of teacher judgements using 'phonic phases'. *Journal of Research in Reading* **34**(2), 157-170.

Soderlund, A. (2009) Physical activity, diet and behaviour modification in the treatment of overweight and obese adults: A systematic review. *Perspectives in Public Health* **129**(3), 132-142.

Solowiej, K., Upton, D. and Mason, V. (2010) Psychological stress and pain in wound care, part 2: A review of pain and stress assessment tools. *Journal of Wound Care* **19**(3), 1109-1115.

Souze, L. and Frank, A. (2000) Subjective pain experience of people with chronic back pain. *Physiotherapy Research International* **5**(4), 207-219.

Spanos, N.P. and Katsanis, J. (1989) Effects of instructional set on attributions of nonvolition during hypnotic and nonhypnotic analgesia. *Journal of Personality and Social Psychology* **56**(2), 182-188.

Sparrenberger, F., Cichelero, F., Ascoli, A., Fonseca, P., Weiss, G., Berwanger, O., Fuchs, S.C., Morelia, L.B. and Fuchs, F.D. (2009) Does psychosocial stress cause hypertension? A systematic review of observational studies. *Journal of Human Hypertension* **23**(1), 12-19.

Speros, C.I. (2011) Promoting health literacy: A nursing imperative. *The Nursing Clinics of North America* **46**(3), 321-333.

Stallard, P., Richardson, T., Velleman, S. and Attwood, M. (2011) Computerized CBT (Think, Feel, Do) for depression and anxiety in children and adolescents: Outcomes and feedback from a pilot randomized controlled trial. *Behavioural and Cognitive Psychotherapy* **39**(3), 273-284.

Stayt, L. (2011) Clinical simulation: A *sine qua non* of nurse education or a white elephant? *Nurse Education Today*. (Article in press.)

Stayt, L.C. (2009) Death, empathy and self preservation: The emotional labour of caring for families of the critically ill in adult intensive care. *Journal of Clinical Nursing* **18**(9), 1267-1275.

Steiger, H., Léonard, S., Kin, N.Y., Ladouceur, C., Ramdoyal, D. and Young, S.N. (2000) Childhood abuse and platelet tritiated-paroxetine binding in bulimia nervosa: Implications of borderline personality disorder. *Journal of Clinical Psychiatry* **61**(6), 428-435.

Stein, M.B. and Kean, Y.M. (2000) Disability and quality of life in social phobia: Epidemiologic findings. *American Journal of Psychiatry* **157**, 1606-1613.

Steinberg, L. and Morris, S.A. (2001) Adolescent Development. *Annual Review in Psychology* **52**, 83-110.

Stephens, R.S., Roffman, R.A. and Curtin, L. (2000) Comparison of extended versus brief treatments for marijuana use. *Journal of Consulting and Clinical Psychology* **68**(5), 898-908.

Stevensen, J., Graham, P., Fredman, G. and McLoughlin, V. (1987) A twin study of genetic influences on reading and spelling ability and disability. *Journal of Child Psychology and Psychiatry and Allied Disciplines* **28**(2), 229-247.

Stice, E. (2002) Risk and maintenance factors for eating pathology: A meta-analytic review. *Psychological Bulletin* **128**, 825-848.

Stitzer, M.L., Iguchi, M.Y. and Felch, L.J. (1992) Contingent take-home incentive: Effects on drug use of methadone maintenance patients. *Journal of Consulting and Clinical Psychology* **60**, 927-934.

Stockhorst, U., Klosterhalfen, S. and Steingruber, H.J. (1998) Conditioned nausea and further side-effects in cancer chemotherapy: A review. *Journal of Psychophysiology* **12**(suppl. 1), 14-33.

Stone, J. and Cooper, J. (2001) A self-standards model of cognitive dissonance. *Journal of Experimental Social Psychology* **3**, 228-243.

Stranks, J.W. (2005) *Stress at Work: Management and Prevention*. Oxford: Elsevier Butterworth-Heinemann Press, p. 7.

Striegel-Moore, R.H. and Bulik, C.M. (2007) Risk factors for eating disorders. *American Psychologist* **62**, 181-198.

Stroebe, M.S. (1998) New directions in bereavement research: Exploration of gender differences. *Palliative Medicine* **12**, 5-12.

Stroebe, W. (2000) *Social Psychology and Health* (2nd edn) Buckingham, UK: Open University Press.

Stuart-Hamilton, I. (1997) Adjusting to later life. *Psychology Review* **4**(2), 20-23.

Stuart-Hamilton, I. (2007) *Dictionary of Psychological Testing, Assessment and Treatment*. London: Jessica Kingsley.

Sturmey, P. (2006) On some recent claims for the efficacy of cognitive therapy for people with intellectual disabilities. *Journal of Applied Research in Intellectual Disabilities* **19**, 109-118.

Suls, J.M. and Wallston, K.A. (2003) *Social Psychological Foundations of Health and Illness*. New York: Blackwell.

Suri, R. (2010) Working with the elderly: An existential-humanistic approach. *Journal of Humanistic Psychology* **50**(2), 175-186.

Sutton S. (2001) Back to the drawing board? A review of applications of the transtheoretical model to substance use. *Addiction* **96**, 175-186.

Swann, J. (2010) Helping patients manage pain and its symptoms. *British Journal of Healthcare Assistants* **4**(10), 494-497.

Swartz, M.S., Blazer, D., George, L. and Winfield, I. (1990) Estimating the prevalence of borderline personality disorder in the community. *Journal of Personality Disorders* **4**, 257-272.

Tai, S. and Turkington, D. (2009) The evolution of cognitive behaviour therapy for schizophrenia: Current practice and recent developments. *Schizophrenia Bulletin* **35**(5), 865-873.

Tait, T. and Genders, N. (2002) *Caring for People with Learning Disabilities*. London: Hodder Arnold.

Takano, Y. and Sogon, S. (2008) Are Japanese more collectivistic than Americans? Examining conformity in in-groups and the reference-group effect. *Journal of Cross-Cultural Psychology* **39**(3), 237-250.

Takkouche, B., Regueira C. and Gestal-Otero, J.J. (2001) A cohort study of stress and the common cold. *Epidemiology* **12**(3), 345-349.

Tancredi, L.R. (2009) Imaging and genetics: Future applications in the emergency room. *Primary Psychiatry* **16**(9), 54-59.

Taylor, E.S., Peplau, A.L. and Sears, O.D. (2003) *Social Psychology* (11th edn) Upper Saddle River, NJ: Prentice Hall.

Taylor, J., Novaco, R.W., Gillmere, B. and Thorne, I. (2002) Cognitive behavioural treatment of anger intensity among offenders with mental retardation. *Journal of Applied Research in Mental Retardation* **15**, 151-165.

Taylor, S. and Clark, D. (2009) Transdiagnostic cognitive-behavioural treatments for mood and anxiety disorders: Introduction to the special issue. *Journal of Cognitive Psychotherapy* **23**(1), 3-5.

Taylor, S.E. (2006) *Health Psychology* (4th edn) Boston: McGraw-Hill.

Tarrier, N. and Wykes, T. (2004) Is there evidence that cognitive behaviour therapy is an effective treatment for schizophrenia? A cautious or cautionary tale? *Behaviour Research and Therapy* **42**, 1377-1401.

Teachman, B.A., Clerkin, E.M. and Marker, C.D. (2010) Catastrophic misinterpretations as a predictor of symptom change during treatment for panic disorder. *Journal of Consulting and Clinical Psychology* **78**(6), 964-973.

Tebartz van Elst, L., Hesslinger, B., Thiel, T., Geiger, E., Haegele, K., Lemieux, L., Lieb, K. and Ebert, D. (2003) Frontolimbic brain abnormalities in patients with borderline personality disorder: A volumetric magnetic resonance imaging study. *Biological Psychiatry* **54**, 163-171.

Tennen, H., Affleck, G., Armeli, S. and Carney, M.A. (2000) A daily process approach to coping: Linking theory, research and practice. *American Psychologist* **55**, 626-636.

Thomas, R., Daly, M., Perryman, B. and Stockton, D. (2000) Forewarned is forearmed: Benefits of preparatory information on video cassette for patients receiving chemotherapy or radiotherapy – a randomised controlled trial. *European Journal of Cancer* **356**, 1536-1543.

Thomas, R.M. (2005) *Comparing Theories of Development* (5th edn) Belmont, CA: Wadsworth.

Thompson, D., Chair, S., Chan, S., Astin, F., Davidson, P. and Ski, C. (2011) Motivational interviewing: A useful approach to improving cardiovascular health? *Journal of Clinical Nursing* **20**(9/10), 1236-1244.

Thompson, G.O.B., Raab, G.M., Hepburn, W.S., Hunter, R., Fulton, M. and Laxen, D.P.H. (1989) Blood-lead levels and children's behaviour: Results from the Edinburgh lead study. *Journal of Child Psychology and Psychiatry* **30**, 515-528.

Thorn, B.E. and Kuhajda, M.C. (2006) Group cognitive therapy for chronic pain. *Journal of Clinical Psychology: In Session* **62**(11), 1355-1366.

Thorell, L.B. (2007) Do delay aversion and executive function deficits make distinct contributions to the functional impact of ADHD symptoms? A study of early academic skill deficits. *Journal of Child Psychology and Psychiatry* **48**(11), 1061-1070.

Tienari, P., Wynne, L.C., Laksy, K., Moring, J., Nieminen, P., Sorri, A., and Wahlberg, K.E. (2003) Genetic boundaries of the schizophrenia spectrum: Evidence from the Finnish adoptive family study of schizophrenia. *American Journal of Psychiatry* **160**(9), 1587-1594.

Tienari, P., Wynne, L.C., Moring, J., Laksy, K., Nieminen, P., Sorri, A. and Miettunen, J. (2000) Finnish adoptive family study: Sample selection and adoptee DSM-III-R diagnoses. *Acta Psychiatrica Scandinavica* **101**(6), 433-443.

Tillfors, M. (2004) Why do some individuals develop social phobia? A review with emphasis on the neurobiological influences. *Nordic Journal of Psychiatry* **58**(4), 267-276.

Timby, B.K. (2008) *Fundamental Nursing Skills and Concepts*. Philadelphia: Lippincott, Williams & Wilkins Press, p. 941.

Torgersen, S., Kringlen, E. and Cramer, V. (2001) The prevalence of personality disorders in a community sample. *Archives of General Psychiatry* **58**, 590-596.

Townsend, E., Dimigen, G. and Fung, D. (2000) A clinical study of child dental anxiety. *Behaviour Research and Therapy* **38**(1), 31-46.

Traeger, J. (2011) Patient information: Supporting your grieving child. *Journal of Palliative Medicine* **14**(1), 116-117.

Trani, M., Casini, M., Capuzzo, F., Gentile, S., Bianco, G., Menghini, D. and Vicari, S. (2011) Executive and intellectual functions in attention-deficit/hyperactivity disorder with and without comorbidity. *Brain & Development* **33**(6), 462-469.

Trossman, S. (2011) Overcoming stigma: Education and advocacy can make a difference in mental health care and services. *American Nurse* **43**(2), 1-9.

Troup, C. and Dewe, P. (2002) Exploring the nature of control and its role in the appraisal of workplace stress. *Work and Stress* **16**(4), 335-355.

Tubbs-Cooley, H.L., Santucci, G., Kang, T.I., Feinstein, J.A., Hexem, K.R. and Feudtner, C. (2011) Pediatric nurses' individual and group assessments of palliative, end-of-life, and bereavement care. *Journal of Palliative Care* **14**(5), 631-637.

Tulving, E. (1972) Episodic and semantic memory. In E. Tulving and W. Donaldson (eds) *Organization of Memory*. New York: Academic Press, pp. 381-403.

Tunnicliffe, P. and Oliver, C. (2011) Phenotype-environment interactions in genetic syndromes associated with severe or profound intellectual disability. *Research in Developmental Disabilities* **32**(2), 404-418.

Turk, C.L., Heimberg, R.G. and Hope, D.A. (2001) Social anxiety disorder. *Clinical Handbook of Psychological Disorder: A Step-by-step Treatment Manual*. (3rd edn) New York: Guilford Press, pp. 114-153.

Turk, Z. and Turk, E. (2009) Our experience with evaluation of communication among older patients and health workers. *HealthMED* **3**(3), 195-203.

Turnbull, C., Wilkie, F., McKenzie, K. and Powell, H. (2005) Health promotion: How to spread the word. *Learning Disability Practice* **8**(7), 16-19.

Turnbull, J. (1994) Facing up to the challenge: A view of the capacity of services to meet the needs of people with challenging behaviour. *Journal of Psychiatric and Mental Health Nursing* **1**(2), 67-75.

Twohig, M.P., Hayes, S.C. and Masuda, A. (2006) Increased willingness to experience obsessions: Acceptance and commitment Therapy as a treatment for obsessive-compulsive disorder, *Behavioural Therapy* **37**, 3-13.

Uchino, B.N. (2004) *Social Support and Physical Health: Understanding the Health Consequences of Relationships*. New Haven, CT: Yale University Press.

Unni, E.J. and Farris, K.B. (2011) Unintentional non-adherence and belief in medicines in older adults. *Patient Education and Counseling* **83**(2), 265-268.

Ustun, T.B., Rehm, J., Chatterji, S., Saxena, S., Trotter, R. Room, R., Bickenbach, J. and the WHO/NIH Joint Project CAR Study Group (1999) Multiple-informant ranking of the disabling effects of different health conditions in 14 countries. *Lancet* **354**(9173), 111-115.

Van den Bosch, L., Koeter, M., Stijnen, T., Verheul, R. and van den Brink, W. (2005) Sustained efficacy of dialectical behaviour therapy for borderline personality disorder. *Behaviour Research and Therapy* **43**(9), 1231-1241.

Van den Oord, E.J., Boomsma, D.I. and Verhulst, F.C. (1994) A study of problem behaviours in 10-15 year old biologically related and unrelated international adoptees. *Behaviour Genetics* **24**, 193-205.

Van Hecke, A., Gryponck, M. and Defloor, T. (2009) A review of why patients with leg ulcers do not adhere to treatment. *Journal of Clinical Nursing* **18**(3), 337-349.

Van Vlierberghe, L., Braet, C., Bosmans, G., Rosseel, Y. and Bogels, S. (2010) Maladaptive schemas and psychopathology in adolescence: On the utility of Young's schema theory in youth. *Cognitive Theory and Research* **34**(4), 316-332.

Varkula, L.C., Resler, R.M., Schulz, P.A. and McCue, K. (2010) Pre-school children's understanding of cancer: The impact of parental teaching and life experience. *Journal of Child Health Care* **14**(1), 24-34.

Vasudeva, S., Claggett, A.L., Tietjen, G.E. and McGrady, A.V. (2003) Biofeedback – assisted relaxation in migraine headache: Relationship to cerebral blood flow velocity in the middle cerebral artery. *Headache: The Journal of Head and Face* **43**(3), 245-250.

Verdugo, M.A. and Schalock, R.L. (2009) Quality of life: From concept to future applications in the field of intellectual disabilities. *Journal of Policy and Practice in Intellectual Disabilities* **6**, 62-64.

Videbeck, S.L. (2007) *Psychiatric Mental Health Nursing*. Philadelphia: Lippincott Williams and Wilkins Press, Chap. 13, p. 242.

Wade, C. and Tavris, C. (2003) *Psychology* (7th edn) Upper Saddle River, NJ: Pearson Education.

Wade, T.D., Bergin, J.L., Tiggemann, M., Bulik, C.M. and Fairburn, C.G. (2006) Prevalence and long term course of eating disorders in an adult Australian twin cohort. *Australian and New Zealand Journal of Psychiatry* **40**, 121-128.

Waldman, I.D. and Gizer, I.R. (2006) The genetics of attention deficit hyperactivity disorder. *Clinical Psychology Review*, **26**(4), 396-432.

Waldman, I.D. and Rhee, S.H. (2002) Behavioural and molecular genetic studies. In G. Davey (ed) *Psychopathology: Research, Assessment, and Treatment in Clinical Psychology.* Oxford: BPS Blackwell.

Walker, K. and Watts, R. (2009) Perceived early childhood family influence, perceived pain self-efficacy, and chronic pain disability: An exploratory study. *Adultspan: Theory Research and Practice* **8**(2), 102-113.

Wallbank, S. and Hatton, S. (2011) Reducing burnout and stress: The effectiveness of clinical supervision. *Community Practitioner* **84**(7), 31-35.

Wallston, K.A. and Wallston, B.S. (1982) Who is responsible for your health? The construct of health locus of control. In G. Sanders and J. Suls (eds) *Social Psychology of Health and Illness*. Hillsadle, NJ: Lawrence Erlbaum and Associates, pp. 65-98.

Walters, G. and Knight, R. (2010) Antisocial personality disorder with and without antecedent childhood conduct disorder: Does it make a difference? *Journal of Personality Disorders* **24**(1), 258-271.

Wampold, B.E., Minami, T., Baskin, T.W. and Callen, T.S. (2002) A meta-(re)analysis of the effects of cognitive therapy versus 'other therapies' for depression. *Journal of Affective Disorders* **68**, 159-165.

Wang, J.J., Hu, C.J. and Cheng, W.Y. (2011) Dementia patients: Effective communication strategies. *Journal of Nursing* **58**(1), 85-90.

Watson, J.B. (1913) Psychology as the behaviorist views it. *Psychological Review* **20**, 158-177.

Watson, P.W.B. and McKinstry, B. (2009) A systematic review of medical advice in healthcare consultations. *Journal of the Royal Society of Medicine* **102**(6), 235-243.

Webb, L. (2011) *Theory to Practice: Communicating Therapeutically*. Oxford: Oxford University Press.

Webster, S, Buckley, P. and Rose, I (2007) Psychosocial working conditions in Britain in 2007. Retrieved 15 December 2011 from http://www.hse-gov.UR/statistics/pdf/pwc2007.pdf

Weiss, G.L. and Larsen, D.L. (1990) Health value, health locus of control and the prediction of health protective behaviours. *Social Behaviour and Personality* **18**(1), 121-136.

Weiss, M. and Britten, N. (2003) What is concordance? *Pharmaceutical Journal* **271**(7270), 493.

Weissman, M.M., Bland, R.C., Canino, G.J., Faravelli, C., Greenwald, S., Hwu, H.G., Joyce, P.R. and Yeh, E.K. (1996) Cross-national epidemiology of major depression and bipolar disorder. *Journal of the American Medical Association* **276**(4), 293-299.

Wentzel, K.R. and Wigfield, A. (2009) *Handbook of Motivation at School*. New York: Routledge.

Wenzel, A., Sharp, I.R., Brown, G.K., Greenberg, R.L. and Beck, A.T. (2006) Dysfunctional beliefs in panic disorders: The panic belief inventory. *Behaviour Research and Therapy* **44**, 819-833.

Werner, S., Malaspina, D. and Rabinowitz, J. (2007) Socioeconomic status at birth is associated with the risk of schizophrenia: Population-based multilevel study. *Schizophrenia Bulletin* **33**(6), 1373-1378.

West, R. (2005) Time for a change: Putting the transtheoretical (stages of change) model to rest. *Addiction* **100**, 1036-1039.

Westen, D., Ludolph, P., Misle, B., Ruffins, S. and Block, J. (1990) Physical and sexual abuse in adolescent girls with borderline personality disorder. *American Journal of Orthopsychiatry* **60**, 55-66.

Wetherell, J.L., Afari, N., Ayers, C.R., Stoddard, J.A., Ruberg, J., Sorrell, J.T. and Patterson, T.L. (2011) Acceptance and Commitment Therapy for generalized anxiety disorder in older adults: A preliminary report. *Behavioural Therapy* **42**(1), 127-134.

Whitcher, S.J. and Fisher, J.D. (1979) Multidimensional reaction to therapeutic touch in a hospital setting. *Journal of Personality and Social Psychology* **37**, 87-96.

WHO (1946) Preamble to the Constitution of the World Health Organization as adopted by the International Health Conference, New York, 19-22 June. *Official Records of the World Health Organization*, 2, p. 100.

WHO (1992) *Tenth Revision of the International Classification of Diseases*. World Health Organization Geneva: WHO.

WHO (1996) *Diagnostic and Management Guidelines for Mental Disorders in Primary Care: ICD–10 Chapter V Primary Care Version*. World Health Organization Göttingen: Hogrefe & Huber.

WHO (1997) WHO QOL Measuring Quality of Life. World Health Organization Retrieved 14 December 2011 from http://www.who.int/mental_health/media/68.pdf

WHO (2007) Mental Health: Strengthening mental health promotion. Fact sheet No 220. World Health Organization Available at: http://www.who.int/mediacentre/factsheets/fs220/en/

Widiger, T.A. and Samuel, D.B. (2005) Diagnostic catogories or dimensions? A question for the Diagnostic and Statistical Manual of Mental Disorders: Fifth Edition. *Journal of Abnormal Psychology* **114**, 494-504.

Wieland, D. (2000) Abuse of older persons: An overview. *Holistic Nursing Practice* **14**(4), 40-50.

Wilkin, H. and Silvester, J. (2007) *Nurses Lacking Empathy Lower Patient Confidence*. Paper presented at the British Psychological Society's division of Occupational Psychology Annual Conference, Bristol.

Williams, R.B., Barefoot, J.C. and Schneiderman, N. (2003) Psychosocial risk factors for cardiovascular disease: More than one culprit at work. *Journal of the American Medical Association* **290**(16), 2190-2192.

Williamson, A. and Hoggart, B. (2005) Pain: A review of three commonly used pain rating scales. *Journal of Clinical Nursing* **14**(7), 798-804.

Wills, C.E. (2010) Sharing decisions with patients: Moving beyond patient-centred care. *Journal of Psychosocial Nursing and Mental Health Services* **48**(3), 4-5.

Wilson, E.J., MacLeod, C., Mathews, A. and Rutherford, E.M. (2006) The causal role of interpretative bias in anxiety reactivity. *Journal of Abnormal Psychology* **115**, 103-111.

Wilson, G.T. and Shafren, R. (2005) Eating disorder guidelines from NICE. *Lancet* **365**, 79-81.

Wilson, G.T., O'Leary, K.D., Nathan, P.E. and Clark, L.A. (1996). *Abnormal Psychology: Integrated Perspectives*. Needham Heights, MA: Allyn and Bacon.

Wilson, D., Williams, M. and Butler, D. (2009) Language and the pain experience. *Physiotherapy Research International* **14**(1), 56-65.

Winsler, A., Fernyhough, C. and Montero, I. (2009) *Private Speech, Executive Functioning, and the Development of Self-Regulation*. New York: Cambridge University Press.

Witte, K. and Allen, M. (2000) A meta-analysis of fear appeals: Implications for effective public health campaigns. *Health Education and Behaviour* **27**(5), 591-615.

Wolf, M., Bally, H. and Morris, R. (1996) Automaticity, retrieval processes, and reading: A longitudinal study in average and impaired readers. *Child Development* **57**, 988-1000.

Wolf, M.H., Putnam, S.M., James, S.A. and Stiles, W.B. (1978) The Medical Interview Satisfaction Scale: Development of a scale to measure patient perceptions of physician behavior. *Journal of Behavioral Medicine* **1**, 391-401.

Wood, C., Littleton, K. and Sheehy, K. (2006) (eds) *Developmental Psychology in Action*. Oxford: Blackwell.

Workman, E.A. and La Via, M.F. (1987) T-Lymphocyte polyclonal proliferation: Effects of stress and stress response style on medical students taking National Board examinations. *Clinical Immunology and Immunopathology* **43**(3), 308-313.

Yang, Y., Raine, A., Lencz, T., Bihre, S., LaCasse, L. and Colletti, P. (2005) Volume reduction in prefronfal gray matter in unsuccessful criminal psychopaths. *Biological Psychiatry* **57**(10), 1103-1108.

Yasuhara, D., Nakahara, T., Harada, T. and Inui, A. (2007) Olanzapine-induced hyperglycemia in anorexia nervosa. *American Journal of Psychiatry* **164**, 528-529.

Yehuda, R. and McEwen, B. (2004) Biobehavioral stress response: Protective and damaging effects - introduction. *Annals of the New York Academy of Sciences* **1032**, XI-XVI.

REFERENCES

Yoshida, K.A., Fennel, C.T., Swingley, D. and Werker, J.F. (2009) Fourteen-month-old infants learn similar sounding words. *Developmental Science* **12**(3), 412-418.

Young, J. (2010) Anorexia nervosa and estrogen: Current status of the hypothesis. *Neuroscience and Behavioural Reviews* **34**(8), 1195-1200.

Yousef, S., Adem, A., Zoubeidi, T., Kosanovic, M., Mabrouk, A.A. and Eapen, V. (2011) Attention deficit hyperactive disorder and environmental toxic mental exposure in the United Arab Emirates. *Journal of Tropical Pediatrics* [ahead of print] doi: 10.1093/tropej/fmq121

Zamanian, K. (2011) Attachment theory as defence: What happened to infantile sexuality? *Psychoanalytic Psychology* **28**, 33-47.

Zanarini, M.C., Williams, A.A., Lewis, R.E. and Reich, R.B. (1997) Reported pathological childhood experiences associated with the development of borderline personality disorder. *American Journal of Psychiatry* **154**, 1101-1106.

Zayas, V., Mischel, W., Shoda, Y. and Aber, J.L. (2011) Roots of adult attachment: Maternal caregiving at 18 months predicts adult peer and partner attachment. *Social Psycholgical and Personality* **2**(3), 289-297.

Zimmermann, G., Favrod, J., Trieu, V.H. and Pomini, V. (2005) The effect of cognitive behavioral treatment on the positive symptoms of schizophrenia spectrum disorders: A meta-analysis. *Schizophrenia Research* **1**(77), 1-9.

Zikmund-Fisher, B.J., Hofer, T.P., Klamerus, M.L. and Kerr, E.A. (2009) First things first: Difficulty with current medications is associated with patient willingness to add new ones. *Patient* **2**(4), 221-231.

Zolnierek, K.B.H. and DiMatteo, R.M. (2009) Physicians' communication and patient adherence to treatment: A meta-analysis. *Medical Care* **47**(8), 826-834.

Index

ABC (Antecedent-Behaviour-Consequence)
    chart 319
ABC model of cognitive behavioural therapy 59
action research 15-16, 316
acupuncture 243-4, 248
acute pain 222, 223, 239
    recurrent 224
ADHD *see* attention-deficit/hyperactivity disorder
    (ADHD)
adherence 135, 136, 137, 164-9
    causes of non-adherence 167-9
    and memory cues 163
    results of non-adherence 166-7
adolescence 22, 74, 75, 90-2
ageing population 92
Ainsworth, M. 84
alcohol abuse 205, 282, 283
Alcoholics Anonymous 286
Alzheimer's disease 98
ambivalent attachment 84
anal stage of development 37, 38
anorexia nervosa 278-9, 279-81
ANS (autonomic nervous system) 202
anticipatory nausea and vomiting (ANV) 42-4
antidepressant medication 268, 273, 274-5
    SSRIs (selective serotonin reuptake
      inhibitors) 273, 280-1
antipsychotic medication 264
antisocial personality disorder 275-7
ANV (anticipatory nausea and vomiting) 42-4
anxiety
    and CBT 58
    and defence mechanisms 35, 36
    and pain 230
    separation anxiety 77, 83
    and social learning theory 53
    stranger anxiety 84
    and stress 201, 213
    and systematic desensitisation 43
anxiety disorders 45, 265-71, 287
    diagnosis of 258, 259
    general anxiety disorder (GAD) 268-9
    obsessive compulsive disorder (OCD) 38, 58,
      269-70
    panic disorder 268
    and personality disorder 277

    phobias 265-8
    post-traumatic stress disorder (PTSD) 58, 260,
      270-1, 277
    and reinforcement 45
appraisal
    cognitive 107
    primary and secondary 194-5, 196, 210, 211
appraisal support 207
Archer, J. 104
Arnett, J.J. 90
Asch, S.E. 134-5
ASD *see* autism spectrum disorders (ASD)
Asperger's Syndrome 300, 307
Atkinson, R.C. 154
attachment 82-4
attention 156-60
attention-deficit/hyperactivity disorder
    (ADHD) 296, 300, 302-6
    behaviours associated with 303
    causes of 302-5
    treatment 306
attitudes 122-5, 127
autism 296, 306-12
    causes of 308-10
    diagnosis 308
    and echolalia 308
    treatment of 310-12
autism spectrum disorders (ASD) 287, 296, 306-12
    disorders associated with 307
autonomic nervous system (ANS) 202
autonomy 88-90
avoidant attachment 84

Bandura's theory of social learning 51-4, 55
Bartlett, D. 188
Beck, A. 58
Beecher, H.K. 227
behaviour, social norms of 18
behavioural approaches 6, 7-8, 9, 31, 40-7
    and autism 311
    and child development 76
    classical conditioning 40-4, 48, 51
    evaluation of 47
    and humanistic psychology 61
    operant conditioning 44-6, 48, 51
    pain and pain management 235-6, 245-6

behavioural approaches (*Continued*)
  and people with learning difficulties 318-21
  phobias 266
  and social learning theory 48, 55
  treatment based on 47
behavioural modification 47, 55
Berry, D. 318
Bettelheim, B. 310
between groups design 13
biofeedback 44, 242
biological factors
  in ADHD 304
  in autism 308-9
  in health and illness 17
  in pain 225
  in substance misuse 30
biological perspective 6
biopsychosocial model
  of autism 310
  of health and illness 17
  of mental health 288-9
  of pain 225-6
bipolar disorder (BD) 58, 272, 274-5, 287
Bobo doll experiment 52, 53
borderline personality disorder 277-8
Bovbjerg, D.H. 42
Bowlby, J. 83
brain abnormalities
  and ADHD 304-5
  and autism 309
  and dyslexia 301-2
  and schizophrenia 263
  see also neurotransmitters
breast cancer 199
Breuer, J. 31-2
Broadbent's filter theory of selective
    attention 156
Bronfenbrenner, U. 84-6, 91
buffer hypothesis
  of social support and stress 208
bulimia nervosa 58, 279-80, 281
burnout 213-14

cancer
  chemotherapy and ANV 42-4
  children and cancer care 107-8, 120
  pain associated with 224
  and stress 199
cannabis 283
Cannon's fight or flight model of stress 194, 202
Cartesian dualism 17
castration anxiety 37
catastrophising 243
categorical measures of pain 233
CBT *see* cognitive behavioural therapy (CBT)

central nervous system (CNS) 202
CET (cue exposure treatment) 285
challenging behaviour
  promoting behavioural change 318-19
CHD (coronary heart disease) 199
child development 22, 75-90
  attachment 82-4
  ecological systems theory 84-5
  Erikson's theory of personality
      development 88-90
  importance of studying 75
  Piaget's theory of cognitive development
      76-82, 92
  and understanding of death 101-4
  Vygotsky's sociocultural theory of 86-7
childhood disintegrative disorder 307
children
  and Bandura's theory of social learning 52-3
  and cancer care 107-8, 120
  childhood sexual abuse 277, 280
  conduct disorder in 276
  infantile sexuality and the Oedipus complex 37-8
  and pain
    assessment of 237-8
    management of 239, 244
  psychodynamic approach to childhood
      experiences 32
chromosomal disorders 309
chronic pain 222, 223-4
chunking information 157-8, 312
classical conditioning 40-4, 48, 51
  and anticipatory nausea and vomiting (ANV) 42
  conditioned response (CR) 41, 42
  conditioned stimulus (CS) 41, 42, 43
  Little Albert experiment 41
  stimulus generalisation 42
  systematic desensitisation 43
  unconditioned response (UCR) 41
  unconditioned stimulus (UCS) 41
CM (contingency management) 285
CNPI (checklist of nonverbal pain indicators) 236
CNS (central nervous system) 202
cocaine 283
coercive power 137
cognitive appraisal 107
cognitive behavioural therapy (CBT) 58-60, 67-8,
    273, 286
  and anxiety disorders 58, 267, 268, 269
  and bipolar disorder 275
  and eating disorders 281
  and pain management 244, 248
  and people with learning disabilities 319-21
  and schizophrenia 264-5
cognitive development
  Piaget's theory of 76-82

cognitive dissonance 124-5
cognitive impairment 95-6, 99, 313
cognitive models
  approaches to pain management 246-8
  of compliance 137
  and eating disorders 280
  of health behaviour 169-75
  phonological theory of dyslexia 302
cognitive psychology xiii, 6, 9, 21, 56-60
  assumptions of 56
  defining 147
  evaluation of 60
  information processing approach 28, 57
  schemas and scripts 57-8
cognitive science 21
colds 200
communication
  and memory 154
  and people with learning disabilities 313-14, 318
  persuasion 127-33
  see also information presentation; non-verbal
    communication (NVC)
community reinforcement approach (CRA) 285
comorbidities 260-1, 272
compliance 127, 134, 135-7, 139-40, 164-9
  cognitive hypothesis model of 167-8, 169
  see also adherence
concordance to treatment 164, 166
  see also adherence
conformity 134-5
congruence 65, 100
conscious mind 32, 33
context-dependent learning 55
contingency management (CM) 285, 286-7
coronary heart disease (CHD) 199, 213
counter-conditioning 43
CRA (community reinforcement approach) 285
Creating a patient-led NHS (government
    paper) xii
cues
  and behavioural approaches to autism 311
  cue exposure treatment (CET) 285
  in memory recall 162-3

Dahlgren, G. 19
DBT (dialectical behaviour therapy) 277-8
death and bereavement 22, 23, 101-6
  children's understanding of grief 101-4
  models of grief 104-6
declarative knowledge 160
defence mechanisms 35-7, 277
demand characteristics 55
dementia 98-101, 287
  carers and the immune system 204
  categories of 98, 99

communication with a patient with 100-1
  defining 98
  and non-verbal communication 117
denial 36
dental anxiety 53
depression
  and bipolar disorder 274
  and CT/CBT 58, 273
  and dementia 99
  major depression 272-3, 279, 287
  and personality disorder 277
  and reinforcement 45
  and stress 188, 201, 213
Descartes' explanation of pain 226
determinism
  and behaviourism 47
  and Freud's theories 39
developmental psychology 21
Dewey, J. 7
diagnosis and treatment 23
dialectical behaviour therapy (DBT) 277-8
diary studies 15
diet 20
  dietary control and autism 311
displacement 35
distraction 156, 248
Drew, D. 87
drug misuse 282-7
drug treatments see medication
dyscalculia 300
dysfunctional schemas 276
dysgraphia 300
dyslexia 296, 299-302, 312
dyspraxia 300

eating disorders 47, 277, 278-81, 287
eating and stress 205
echolalia 308
ecological model
  of learning disabilities and quality of
    life 315
ecological systems theory (Bronfenbrenner)
    84-5, 91
ecological validity 57
Ecstasy 283
ECT (electroconvulsive therapy) 273
the ego 33, 34, 39
  defence mechanisms 35-7, 39
elder abuse 35
Electra complex 38
electroconvulsive therapy (ECT) 273
electromyography (EMG) 234-5
EMDR (eye movement desensitization and
    reprocessing) 271
EMG (electromyography) 234-5

emotion-focused coping
  and pain 230
  and stress 196, 197
emotional arousal 55
emotional factors in health and illness 17-18
emotional support 207
emotional well-being
  and people with learning disabilities 317
empathy 64-5, 100, 117
empirical testing 11
endocrine system and stress 203
Engel, G.L. 188
environmental toxins
  and ADHD 304-5
episodic memory 159
Erikson's theory of personality development 88-90
esteem support 207
ethnicity 20
ethnocentrism 20
event schemas 161
exercise 20, 205, 306
existentialism 61
exosystem 84, 85
expectancies
  and social learning theory 48-9
expert power 138
explicit memory 159-60
exposure therapy 266-7
external health locus of control (HLoC) 50, 51
extinction 43
eye contact 117-19, 120-1
eye movement desensitization and reprocessing
      (EMDR) 271

facial expressions 117, 118, 121
family systems theory 280
family therapy 265, 281
fear-arousing messages 130, 131
Feil, N. 100
feminine Oedipus attitude 38
Ferns, T. 36
Festinger, L. 125
fixation 36
FLACC (Faces, Legs, Activity, Cry, Consolability)
      Scale 237-8
Fordyce, W.E. 245
Fragile X syndrome 309
Freud, S. 8, 31-2
  and anxiety disorders 266, 269, 270
  ego defence mechanisms 35-7
  evaluation of Freudian theory 38-9
  structural model of the mind 33-4
  theory of infantile sexuality 37-8
  topography of mind 32-3
functionalism 7

GAD (general anxiety disorder) 268-9
GAS (general adaptation syndrome) 193-4
gate control theory of pain 228-30
gender
  and Freud's theory of infantile sexuality 37-8
  and the psychosocial model of health and
      illness 20
  as a socio-cultural variable 20
  touching patients 120
general adaptation syndrome (GAS) 193-4
general anxiety disorder (GAD) 268-9
genetics 30
  and autism 309
  and dyslexia 301-2
  and learning disabilities 299
  and schizophrenia 263
genital phase of development 38
Gestalt theory 8, 9, 149-53
Glanzer, M. 155
goals
  and social learning theory 49-50
group interventions
  and pain management 248

hardy personalities 208-9
Harlow, H.F. 82
HBM (health belief model) 170-1
health behaviour
  cognitive models of 169-75
  social cognition models of 169, 173-5
health belief model (HBM) 170-1
health locus of control (HLoC) 50-1
health promotion
  and people with learning disabilities
      318, 321
  see also information presentation
hearing loss 313
heart attacks and stress 187, 188, 209
heart disease and stress 199, 209, 213
hepatitis 200
heroin 283
history of psychology xii, 6-9
HIV/AIDS and stress 199-200
holistic care 60
Holmes and Rahe SRRS scale 191, 201
homosexuality 38
hormonal system and stress 203
hospitals, family-centred care in 83
hostility and stress 209
Hough, M. 35
Houldin, A.D. 36
humanistic psychology 6, 8-9, 61-6
  evaluation of 65-6
  Maslow's hierarchy of needs 61-3, 66
  Rogers' person-centred approach 63-5, 66

Huque, M.F. 14
hypertension 213
hypnotism 31, 244
hypothesis testing 11
hypothetical constructs 12

IBS (irritable bowel syndrome) 240
iceberg analogy of the human mind 32-3
the id 33, 34, 37, 39
  and phobias 266
idiographic approach 39
immune system and stress 203-4, 213
implicit memory 159-60
infantile sexuality and the Oedipus complex 37-8
infectious diseases and stress 200
information presentation 160-9
  and attention 156-7
  cues in memory recall 162-3
  guidelines for improving information
    recall 168-9
  and learning disabilities 312
  levels of processing model of 162
  mnemonic aids 164, 165
  and perception 151
  persuasive communication of 127-33
  role of perceived importance in 163-4
  schema theory 161-2
  see also memory
information processing approach see cognitive
    psychology
information support 207
informational power 138
instrumental learning 44-5
instrumental support 207
intellectual disability 297
interaction model of stress 194-5, 210
internal health locus of control (HLoC) 50, 51
internet-based observational learning 52-3
interviews
  motivational interviewing (MI) 175, 178-80, 181
  and self-reported measures of pain 231-2
  structured 14
intractable-benign pain 224
introspection 7, 40, 56
irritable bowel syndrome (IBS) 240

James, W. 7
Jung, Carl 38

Kastenbaum, R. 93
Kessler, R.C. 267
Kiecolt-Glaser, J.K. 204
Klages, U. 247
Koegel, R.L. 310, 311
Kraepelin, E. 258

Kübler-Ross's five-stage bereavement model 105-6
Kuhn, T. 12

language of psychology 10
latency period of development 38
law of effect 44
learned helplessness 59, 272-3
learning disabilities xiii, 294-325
  causes of 299
  and communication 312-14, 318
  diagnostic criteria 297-8
  and emotional well-being 317
  and health promotion 318, 321
  and intellectual disability 297
  numbers of people with 296
  and the nurse workforce 296-7
  psychological approaches to 317-21
  and quality of life (QOL) 314-17
  specific learning disabilities (SpLDs) 299-312
  terminology used in relation to 297
legitimate power 138
Lewin, K. 16
Ley, P. 137
Liddell, C. 158-9
life stresses 191-3, 201
  and eating disorders 280
lifestyle factors 17, 20
linear-biomedical model of pain 226, 227
linguistics 21
locus of control (LoC) 50-1
long-term memory (LTM) 154-5, 159-60
longitudinal design 13, 14
Lovaas, I. 311
LSD 283
Lueboonthavatchi, P. 191

McGill pain questionnaire (MPQ) 233-4
macrosystems 84, 85
main effect hypothesis 208
maintenance rehearsal 158-9
male nurses
  and stereotyping 126
  and touch 120
Marks, D.F. 18
Maslow, A.
  hierarchy of needs 61-3, 66
Masse, R. 189-90
MBCT (mindfulness-based cognitive therapies) 273
medication
  for ADHD 306
  attitudes to 123-4
  for autism 310-11
  mnemonic aids to taking 165
  non-adherence to 166-7
  see also antidepressant medication

Melzack, R. 228, 233
memory 147, 153-60
  and attention 156-60
  deterioration 96
  encoding 153
  long-term memory (LTM) 154-5, 159-60
  mnemonic aids 164, 165
  primacy effect 155
  recency effect 155
  retrieval 153
  sensory 154-5, 156
  short-term memory (STM) 154-5, 157-9, 160
  stores 153, 154-5
  see also information presentation
menopause and stress 215-16
mental health xiii, 38, 254-93
  attitudes to 124
  biopsychosocial model of 288-9
  defining 257-8
  defining abnormal 257
  diagnostic classifications of 258-61
  and stress 201, 213
Mental Health Act 287-8
mesosystems 84, 85, 91
MET (motivational enhancement therapy) 286
meta-analysis 14
MI see motivational interviewing (MI)
microsystems 84, 91
Milgram, S. 138
mindfulness meditation training (MMT) 244
mindfulness-based cognitive therapies
        (MBCT) 273
MMT (mindfulness meditation training) 244
mnemonic aids 164
models 12
mood disorders 272-3
motivational enhancement therapy (MET) 286
motivational factors in health and illness 18
motivational interviewing (MI) 175, 178-80,
        181, 286
MPQ (McGill pain questionnaire) 233-4
Muller, J. 242
multidimensional measures of pain 233-4

narrative research 15
needs, Maslow's hierarchy of 61-3, 66
negative reinforcement 45
  of pain behaviours 245
negative schemas 58
Neisser, U. 147
nervous system
  and pain 224
  and stress 202-3
neuroleptics 310-11
neuropathic pain 224

neuroses 32, 38
neurotransmitters
  and ADHD 304
  and autism 309
  and eating disorders 280
  and schizophrenia 263-4
nicotine replacement therapy (NRT) 123
Nishizawa, Y. 116
nociceptive pain 224
nominal fallacy 66
non-nociceptive pain 224
non-verbal communication (NVC) 115-22
  eye contact 117-19, 120-1
  facial expressions 117, 118, 121
  and learning disabilities 312
  posture 118
  and SOLER 110
  sounds conveying understanding 118
  timing and pace 118
  tone of voice 118, 119
  touch 118, 119-20
non-verbal pain indicators 236
normative beliefs 174
numerical measures of pain 232-3
Nursing Stress Scale 214
NVC see non-verbal communication (NVC)

obedience 134, 138
object permanence 77
object relations theory 277
observational learning 52-3, 55, 122
observations 14
obsessive compulsive disorder (OCD) 38, 58,
        269-70
Oedipus complex 33, 37-8
older adults 22, 92-101
  activity theory of 97
  assessment of pain in 232-4, 237
  and cognitive impairments 95-6
  defining 92
  and dementia 98-101
  different age groups 92-3
  and memory 160
  negative stereotypes of 94-5
  and social disengagement theory (SDT) 96-7
O'Neill, R.E. 319, 320
operant conditioning 44-6, 48, 51
oral stage of development 37, 38

paedophilia 38
pain xiii, 21, 23, 219-53
  acute 222, 223, 239
    recurrent 224
  assessment of 231-8
    behavioural measures 235-6

categorical measures 233
  in children 237-8
  multidimensional measures 233-4
  numerical measures 232-3
  physiological measures 234-5
  self-report measures 231-2
  uni-dimensional measures 232
biopsychosocial model of 225-6
chronic 222, 223-4
concepts of 226-8
defining 223-4
gate control theory of 228-30
intractable-benign 224
linear-biomedical model of 226, 227
management of 239-50
  acupuncture 243-4, 248
  behavioural approaches to 245-6
  biofeedback 242
  cognitive approaches to 246-8
  drug treatments 239, 240
  hypnotism 244
  and medical intervention 239
  mindfulness meditation 244
  multi-modal methods of 239
  placebos 240, 244
  relaxation 242-3
  surgical methods 241
  transcutaneous electrical nerve stimulation
    (TENS) 241-2
nociceptive 224
non-nociceptive 224
pain behaviours (operants) 245-6
progressive 224
psychological factors influencing 230-1
recurrent acute 224
relevance to nursing practice 221-2
panic disorder 268
Parkes' model of grief 104-5
participatory action research 16, 316
patient management 55
pattern theory of pain 226
Paul, G.L. 46
Pavlov, I. 40-1
PCP/phencyclidine 283
PDD (pervasive developmental disorders) 306
peer mentoring 87
penis envy 38
perceived control 20, 175
perception 30, 147, 148-53
  closure principle 151
  continuity principle 151-2
  figure/ground grouping 150, 152
  proximity grouping 150, 152
  similarity grouping 151, 152
  top-down/bottom up processes of 148

performance accomplishments 54
person schemas 161
person-centred approach 63-5, 66
  and people with dementia 100
person-in-context approach to health
    improvement 86
personal agency 61
personality 30, 208-9
  Erikson's theory of personality
    development 88-90
personality disorders 275-8, 287
  clusters of 275, 278
  diagnosis of 258, 259, 275
persuasive communication 127-33
  audiences 131-2
  channels of 132-3
  content of the message 129-31
  factors involved in 127-9
pervasive developmental disorders (PDD) 306
phallic stage of development 37, 38
phantom limb pain 227
philosophy 21
phobias 53, 265-8
phonological theory of dyslexia 302
physiological measures of pain 234-5
physiological pathways
  and stress 201, 202-3
physiology 30
Piaget's theory of cognitive development 76-82
  application to practice 81-2
  concrete operational stage 79-80, 81
  formal operational stage 80-1, 92
  pre-operational stage 78-9, 81
  sensori-motor stage 77-8
placebos 13, 240, 244
PMR (progressive muscle relaxation) 44, 212,
    242-3
PMT (protection motivation theory) 171-2
PNI (psychoneuroimmunology) 204
positive reinforcement 45, 46
  and pain management 245, 248
post-traumatic stress disorder (PTSD) 58, 260,
    270-1, 277
power 137-9
pre-conscious mind 32, 33
pre-therapy 100
preparedness theory 266
primacy effect in memory 155
problem-focused coping
  and pain 230
  and stress 196, 197
procedural knowledge 160
progressive muscle relaxation (PMR) 44, 212,
    242-3
progressive pain 224

projection 36
protection motivation theory (PMT) 171-2
psychiatry 21
psychic determinism 32
psychoanalysis 33
psychoanalytic theory/psychodynamic
    approach 6, 8, 9, 28, 31-9
  and autism 310
  evaluation of 38-9
  and humanistic psychology 61
  language of 10
  see also Freud, S.
psychological approaches
  to learning disability nursing 317-21
psychological factors
  in ADHD 305-6
  in health and illness 3-4, 17, 18-20
  influencing pain 225, 230-1
psychology
  in health and nursing care 22-4
  researching 12-16
  role in nursing practice 4, 5
  as a science 10-12
  scope of 21
  WHO definition of 4
psychoneuroimmunology (PNI) 204
psychopathology 30
psychosis and CBT 58
psychosocial factors
  and schizophrenia 264
psychotherapy 21
PTSD (post-traumatic stress disorder) 58, 260,
    270-1

qualitative research 15
quality of life (QOL)
  and people with learning disabilities 314-17
questionnaires 14

randomised controlled trials (RCTs) 14-15, 240
Raudonis 66
Raven, B.H. 137
RCTs (randomised controlled trials) 14-15
reaction formation 36
recency effect in memory 155
recurrent acute pain 224
referent power 138
regression 36
rehearsing information 158-9, 162
reinforcement
  and autism 311
  and operant conditioning 45-6
  schedules 46
  value 49
  vicarious 52-3

reinforcers 45
relapse prevention (RP) 286
relaxation
  and pain management 242-3
repression 35
researching psychology 12-16
  action research 15-16
  between groups design 13
  cross-sectional studies 13
  longitudinal design 13, 14
  meta-analysis 14
  observations 14
  qualitative techniques 15
  questionnaires 14
  randomised controlled trials (RCTs) 14-15
  structured interviews 14
  surveys 14
  within participants design 13
Rett's disorder 308
reward power 137
risk behaviours
  in adolescence 90, 91-2
  strategies for changing 175-81
Roelofs, J. 246
Rogers' person-centred approach 61, 63-5, 66
role modelling 53, 54
role schemas 57, 161
Rosenstiel, A.K. 196
rote rehearsal 158-9, 162
Rotter's theory of social learning 48-50
RP (relapse prevention) 286

scaffolding 87
schema theory 161-2
schemas 57-8
  dysfunctional 276
schizophrenia 261-5, 287
  causes of 263-4
  and dementia 99
  diagnosis of 258, 259, 262
  non-adherence to medication 166
  symptoms 261, 262-3
  and token economies 46
  treatments for 264-6
science 10-12
  the induction-deduction method 11-12
scripts 57-8
SDT (social disengagement theory) 96-7
secure attachment 84
self-actualisation 61-2, 63
self-concept 63-4
self-efficacy 20, 54-5, 172
  and pain 230
  and people with learning difficulties 318
self-esteem 20

self-fulfilling prophecies 94, 126
self-report measures of pain 231-2
self-schemas 57, 161
Seligman, M.E.P. 266
semantic memory 159
semantic pragmatic disorder 300
sensory memory 154-5, 156
separation anxiety 77, 83
SES (socio-economic status) 20
sexuality, Freud's theory of infantile 37-8
Selye H. 189
short-term memory (STM) 154-5, 157-9, 160
SIT (stress-inoculation-training) 211
Skinner, B.F. 7, 44-5
SLT see social learning theory (SLT)
smoking 20
    and attitudes to 123, 127
    and stress 205
smoking cessation
    and motivational interviewing 179-81
    nicotine replacement therapy (NRT) 123
    stages of change model of 177-8
social anthropology 21
social cognition models
    of health behaviour 169, 173-5
social context of psychology xii
social disengagement theory (SDT) 96-7
social factors
    in health and illness 18-20
    in pain 225
    in substance misuse 30
social learning
    and communication 313
social learning theory (SLT) 28, 48-56
    assumptions of 48
    Bandura's theory of 51-4, 55
    and behaviourism 48, 55
    evaluation of 55-6
    locus of control (LoC) 50-1
    Rotter's theory of 48-50
    self-efficacy 54-5
social model
    of learning disabilities and quality of life 315
social norms of behaviour 18
social persuasion 54
social phobia 265, 267-8
social readjustment rating scale (SRRS) 191-2, 201
social support 21
    and pain management 248
    and stress 206-8
socio-economic status (SES) 20
sociology 21
somatic pain 224
specific learning disabilities (SpLDs) 299-312
    ADHD 296, 300, 302-6

autism spectrum disorders (ASD) 287, 296,
    306-12
dyslexia 296, 299-302, 312
and IQ tests 300
specificity theory of pain 226
speech disorders 313
SRRS (social readjustment rating scale) 191-2, 201
SSRIs (selective serotonin reuptake
    inhibitors) 273, 280-1
stages of change model 175-8
stereotypes 57, 125-6
    of nurses 161-2
    of older adults 94-5
stigma
    and mental health problems 260
STM (short-term memory) 154-5, 157-9, 160
stranger anxiety 84
stress xiii, 21, 185-218
    and CBT 58
    and changing behaviour 203
    coping with 195-8
        inappropriate coping mechanisms 204, 205
    defining 189-90
    and the general adaptation syndrome
        (GAS) 193-4
    and hardiness 208-9
    and health 198-206
        the hormonal system 203
        the immune system 203-4, 213
        physiology 201, 202-3
    interaction model of 194-5
    and life events 191-3, 201
    management techniques xiii, 188, 210-13
    and the menopause 215-16
    and nursing practice 213-14
    positive (eustress) 210
    primary and secondary appraisal 194-5, 196,
        210, 211
    psychological and physiological consequences
        of 198
    relevance of to nursing practice 188
    and social support 206-8
    and type A personality 209
stress-inoculation-training (SIT) 211
structural model of the mind 33-4
structuralism 6-7, 9
structured interviews 14
subjective norms 174-5
sublimation 35
substance misuse 30-1, 282-7
    diagnostic criteria for 282
    treatment for 285-7
suicide 277
the superego 33, 34, 37, 39
surgery and pain management 241

surveys 14
sympathetic pain 224
sympathy and empathy 65
systematic desensitisation 43

TABP (type A behaviour pattern) 209
tabula rasa view of mind 40, 47
talking cure 31
TENS (transcutaneous electrical nerve
    stimulation) 241-2
theory construction 11
theory of mind (TOM) deficits 305
theory of planned behaviour (TPB) 174-5
theory of reasoned action (TRA) 173-4
therapeutic touch 120
Thorndike, E. 44
token economy system 45-6
TOM (theory of mind) deficits 305
touching patients 118, 119-20
TPB (theory of planned behaviour) 174-5
TRA (theory of reasoned action) 173-4
transcutaneous electrical nerve stimulation
    (TENS) 241-2
transtheoretical model of change 175-8
tuberous sclerosis 309
twelve-step approaches 286
type A behaviour pattern (TABP) 209

unconditional positive regard 65, 100
unconscious mind 32, 33, 39
uni-dimensional measures of pain 232
urinary tract infections 200

validation therapy 100
variables 12
VAS (visual analogue scale) of pain 232-3, 234
vascular dementia 98
Vasudeva, S. 242
verbal persuasion 54
verbal rating scale (VRS) of pain 233
vicarious experience 54
vicarious reinforcement 52-3
virtual reality and hypnotism 244
visceral pain 224
visual analogue scale (VAS) of pain 232-3
visual imagery 212
    and pain management 248
VRD (verbal rating scale) of pain 233
Vygotsky's sociocultural theory of
    development 86-7

Wallston, K.A. and B.S. 50
Watson, John B. 7, 40
Whitehead, M. 19
Wilkin, H. 64
within participants design 13
Wong-Baker FACES Pain Rating Scale
    234, 235
work-related stress 198, 199
World Health Organisation (WHO)
    definition of health 4, 17
    definition of mental health 257-8
Wundt, W. 6-7

ZPD (zone of proximal development) 86